WHERE TO GET BREASTFEEDING SUPPORT

Details of where to go for breastfeeding support often appear at the end of a book like this. And that's where I originally put them. But then I realised that you might need support before even reading the book, or not get to the end for some reason and never find it. So I've put them here.

NATIONAL BREASTFEEDING HELPLINE

0300 100 0212

The National Breastfeeding Helpline is run by the Breastfeeding Network (BfN) and the Association of Breastfeeding Mothers (ABM). All the volunteers answering calls are women who have breastfed, and all have received extensive training in breastfeeding support. Calls are diverted to the next available ABM or BfN volunteer. Support is also available in Welsh.

THE BREASTFEEDING NETWORK

0300 100 0210

Phone lines are open 9.30am–9.30pm every single day of the year Live online support also available via webchat:
www.breastfeedingnetwork.org.uk/chat

THE ASSOCIATION OF BREASTFEEDING MOTHERS

0300 330 5453

Phone lines are open 9.30am–10.30pm. You can also access web chat, send an er____
of your local gr____
abm.me.uk/get-b____
support

LA LECHE LEAGUE GB

0345 120 2918

Phone lines are open 8am–11pm. You can also submit a help request online or find details of your local group at www.laleche.org.uk/get-support

NCT

0300 300 0700

Phone lines are open 8am–midnight, 365 days a year.
www.nct.org.uk/about-us/contact-us

LACTATION CONSULTANTS GREAT BRITAIN (LCGB)

You can find a local, qualified lactation consultant at lcgb.org/find-an-ibclc

DRUGS IN BREASTMILK SERVICE

The Drugs in Breastmilk service was set up by BfN in response to the number of calls received concerning medication. The drugline is run on a voluntary basis by a pharmacist who is also a BfN Registered Breastfeeding Supporter. They have ____lence-based factsheets ____te and you can ____via email or Facebook. ____edingnetwork.org. ____ormation/drugs-in-

ABOUT THE AUTHOR

Professor Amy Brown is based in the Department of Public Health, Policy and Social Sciences at Swansea University in the UK where she leads the MSc in Child Public Health. With a background in psychology, she first became interested in the many barriers women face when breastfeeding after having her first baby. Three babies and a PhD later she has spent the last twelve years exploring psychological, cultural and societal barriers to breastfeeding, with an emphasis on understanding how we can better support women to breastfeed and subsequently raise breastfeeding rates. Her primary focus is how we can shift our perception of breastfeeding as an individual mothering issue, to a wider public health responsibility, with consideration to how we can make societal changes to protect and encourage breastfeeding.

Professor Brown has published over 100 papers exploring the barriers women face in feeding their baby during the first year. She is a regular *Huffington Post* blogger, aiming to change the way we think about breastfeeding, mothering and caring for our babies. Her books include:

Breastfeeding Uncovered (2016, 2nd edition 2021)
Why Starting Solids Matters (2017)
The Positive Breastfeeding Book (2018)
Informed is Best (2019)
Why Breastfeeding Grief and Trauma Matter (2019)
Let's talk about the first year of parenting (2020)
Let's talk about feeding your baby (2021)

BREASTFEEDING UNCOVERED

Who Really Decides How
We Feed Our Babies?

AMY BROWN

For YOU

Breastfeeding Uncovered: Who Really Decides How We Feed Our Babies?
First published in the UK by Pinter & Martin Ltd 2016
This 2nd edition published 2021

Copyright © Amy Brown 2016, 2021

All rights reserved

ISBN 978-1-78066-715-7

Also available as an ebook

The right of Amy Brown to be identified as the author of this work has been asserted by her in accordance with the Copyright, Designs and Patent Act of 1988

Edited by Susan Last
Index by Helen Bilton

British Library Cataloguing-in-Publication Data

A catalogue record for this book is available from the British Library

Printed by TJ Books Limited, Padstow, Cornwall

This book has been printed on paper that is sourced and harvested from sustainable forests and is FSC accredited

Pinter & Martin Ltd
6 Effra Parade
London SW2 1PS

pinterandmartin.com

CONTENTS

FOREWORD

There is a single lecture from medical school which, 20 years later, still stands out from the general blur of knowledge being forced into me. It was about breastmilk and it was given by a midwife called Chloe Fisher.

The first slide was a simple picture, a crude line drawing made at the end of the 15th century by Annibale Carracci. The Madonna suckling the infant Christ.

It shows a baby sitting on Mary's lap sucking hard at her swollen breast. His cheeks are puffed out, ridiculously full of milk, as if he can't swallow fast enough. And the child is immense. I mean really vast. I remember Chloe pointing out the thighs, the creased rolls of fat. Somewhere in Italy 500 years ago, in a city crawling with disease and rife with malnutrition, Carracci had found a child that looked enough like this to model for him. A child nourished exclusively on human milk.

Chloe used this idea to launch an extraordinary lecture about the liquid gold, living fluid miracle that is breastmilk: the only substance on earth that has evolved to be perfect nutrition. Think about it – everything else we eat is a compromise. Animals don't want to be eaten, a few plants make fruit as a treat to disperse seeds but they're fun, not nourishment.

I went home with my twin brother that weekend and we told our mum about the talk; about mammals and how breastmilk isn't just food it's also an immune system; about how, since the first proto-mammal licked a nutrient slime from its mother's skin, lactation has been crucial to survival for creatures like us.

Mum was defensive then tearful. It had never occurred to us to ask about the choices she made.

Of course I'm a formula baby. Born in London in 1978. But there's no evidence that my mum made the wrong choice. We have a great relationship; I love her very much. I certainly never feel that I would have been better off if she'd made a different choice. She had twins and a phenomenal career. She went back to work quickly and created the financial security that has enabled so much freedom in my own life.

So I don't care how you choose to feed your child but I really care that you have a choice. For many people in this country the choice to breastfeed is like choosing to go university. Fine in theory but in reality totally unrealistic because of the structure of the world around us.

If you've bought this book you're most of the way there – it is as near perfect as can be. You just need to read it and if you have a partner make them read it too. Also highlight some of your favourite bits and send them to your siblings, friends and in-laws. You need allies in the fight. And it is a fight because there is an opposition. You'll read more about them in chapter 16 but there is an industry, literally an entire industry, devoted to reducing rates of breastfeeding. Ideally to zero.

They use the same techniques as the tobacco industry to create confusion and doubt. They create narratives of guilt, failure and blame. They fund many of the doctors you see on television and many of the institutions that you might expect to protect children around the world. They fund the discussion groups in online forums and the conferences your midwives are educated at.

There will be times when you are struggling and at those times remember who is really to blame. The fact that you didn't get much support in hospital or when you got home? That's industry. The eyeball roll from an in-law? Industry marketing. The suggestion from your GP that formula would be easier and just as good? That's the industry-funded research.

But we know from research on smoking that focusing on the industry is useful for you as an individual. It shifts the blame away from the individuals in your life and onto the structures in your world. It gives you a realistic sense of the opposition (literally the most powerful food companies on earth) and a sense of being a hero in your own struggle (at least that's what I felt – though it's perhaps easier to feel heroic when you're not the one with sore nipples).

If it helps then focus on industry when you're down but mainly focus on the good stuff in this book. It is as much about mothering as it is about infant nutrition. It's full of science and wisdom about sleep and ancient tribes and normal infant behaviour. For us it was a much needed non-judgmental family member, in the small hours when things seem tougher than they really are.

Now get on with reading the actual book – and know that you do so with all my love and support wherever you are.

Chris van Tulleken
Doctor, TV presenter and father of two

BUILDING A SOCIETY THAT NORMALISES AND NURTURES BREASTFEEDING

In the UK breastfeeding is viewed by many as difficult to achieve and largely unnecessary because formula milk is seen as a close second best. Combined with pressures to return to work, worries about public feeding and few government initiatives to support breastfeeding, this misconception means that the UK now has some of the lowest breastfeeding rates in the world, and eight out of ten women stop breastfeeding before they want to.

We know that breastfeeding saves lives and has a huge impact on the welfare of both baby and mum, from cognitive development to immunity from infection to longer-term disease prevention. To ensure best outcomes for babies, we must remove the myriad of barriers to breastfeeding – social, cultural, economic, physical and practical.

The first step is to acknowledge the pain of those families who have not breastfed – those who didn't start because they believed it wasn't important, and those who tried but couldn't continue. We need to shift the conversation away from guilt and blame; it is not individual mothers' responsibility to tackle an entrenched public health issue. Instead, we need to recognise all the societal factors that have contributed to the UK's low breastfeeding rate, and call for systemic change. This book will support us to make a start by explaining why the UK is in this situation and what could be done to sort it out.

Together, we can build a society that normalises and nurtures breastfeeding, to improve the life chances of children in the UK.

Sue Ashmore
UNICEF UK Baby Friendly Initiative

'The success or failure of breastfeeding should not be seen solely as the responsibility of the woman. Her ability to breastfeed is very much shaped by the support and the environment in which she lives. There is a broader responsibility of governments and society to support women through policies and programmes in the community.'

Dr Nigel Rollins, World Health Organisation, 2016

'The reasons why women avoid or stop breastfeeding range from the medical, cultural, and psychological, to physical discomfort and inconvenience. These matters are not trivial, and many mothers without support turn to a bottle of formula. Multiplied across populations and involving multinational commercial interests, this situation has catastrophic consequences on breastfeeding rates and the health of subsequent generations.'

The Lancet breastfeeding series, 2016

'We need to change the conversation around breastfeeding by stopping laying the responsibility for this major public health issue in the laps of individual women and acknowledging the role that politics and society has to play at every level. The goal of our Call to Action is not to put pressure on women to breastfeed, but to remove the barriers that currently stop women who want to breastfeed from doing so.'

UNICEF Baby Friendly Call to Action, 2016

INTRODUCTION

Late 2020. Five years after writing the introduction for the first version of this book I'm sat here writing again. Contemplating what has changed, what hasn't and what still has a very long way to go. Time is a funny thing. When you're in it, you can't see things slowly changing, but take a step back and look at how things are different to five or ten years ago and you can see that two things are true: we have made progress, but we still have a long way to go.

I remember raising the idea of writing an update of this book I think a year after publication. We sensibly discussed that many book updates happen somewhere around the 10-year mark. I think we agreed to look at it again at seven. And well, here we are. The thing with writing about breastfeeding is that it's both the gift and curse that keeps on giving. You manage to raise awareness, gain support and move forward in one way, only for the opposition to pop back up again, dressed in a different disguise. The main problem of course is that when you are fighting to make things better for mothers, babies and families, you are fighting a complex web of history, patriarchy and of course a billion-dollar industry. We spend a lot of time thinking about who wins if we ensure all families get the breastfeeding support they really need, but to understand why this is such a fight you just need to look at who loses.

So, what is this book about and what am I trying to do? It's simple really. It's about highlighting the multiple and complex influences that stand between a mother deciding she wants to breastfeed her baby and the chances of her reaching her breastfeeding goal. If you've never breastfed a baby or supported a family to breastfeed then you might be a bit confused right now. Why on earth would something that is a biological norm and has kept us alive since mankind began be difficult? Sadly, if this is you, sit down and buckle up, there's a lot of information (and potentially rage) coming your way. If you're a mother grieving (and yes, I mean grieving) the end of breastfeeding before you were ready or it even got going, or a health or lactation professional trying to support women, you're probably very aware of the difference between the positive messages telling you to breastfeed and the reality once a baby is here.

The UK and Ireland regularly battle it out for the dubious honour of having the lowest breastfeeding rates in the entire world. This isn't to be mixed up with intention; we have plenty of women who really want to breastfeed. But their hopes and dreams for feeding and caring for their baby in a certain way seem to get rapidly dashed. During pregnancy they're urged to breastfeed and probably told 'breast is best' (I hate that phrase, more on that later) but after the birth they find that support, possibly from the health service, partners, family, workplaces and society in general just isn't there or is even actively working against their intention. They end up with complications, confused about what to do, or simply finding it all too much, and end up stopping, often before they are ready. In fact, at least 80% of mothers who stop breastfeeding in the first six weeks are not ready to do so.

And when they do? They often blame themselves... 'I couldn't breastfeed' or 'I just should have tried harder' or 'I failed'. Nonsense. Every woman I have ever spoken to who stopped breastfeeding before she was ready tells me a story where someone could have done something, or something could have been different. But instead, our society deflects responsibility and leaves women blaming and even hating themselves for their decision.

These feelings can last a long time. The oldest 'baby' a mother ever told me about, explaining that she was not able to breastfeed and still felt terrible about, had just retired. He was off planning days of golf and his mother, in her late 80s, was still grieving her tiny baby and not being able to feed him how she wanted. *It's not just about the milk.* Yes on a population level breastfeeding protects both maternal and infant health, but that's not actually the only reason why so many women feel terrible when they stop. It's so much more complicated than that. Women are affected by their experiences of trying to feed. Pain and exhaustion. Not being supported by others. Wanting to use their body in a way they had been told to expect and it not playing ball. Their preferred way of mothering and caring for their baby vanishing. Spiritual, religious or cultural ties being severed. Breastfeeding has always been so much more than simply providing milk to a baby, yet we act as if every breastfeeding problem is simply fixed by giving formula.

And then there's the anger. The countless debates over whether breastfeeding matters or whether we should be promoting it at all. 'Stop picking on women who couldn't breastfeed' they say – 'you're pressurising them, making them feel guilty'. 'My baby is fine. I couldn't breastfeed but he's fine'. All of this misses a massive herd of elephants crammed into a room. Wanting better support for women who want to breastfeed is not the same as saying all women should breastfeed. Wanting the barriers placed in the way of breastfeeding women to be removed is not the same as saying all women should breastfeed. Recognising that for some women breastfeeding was really important and mattered to them is not the same as saying all women should breastfeed.

Looking back at my introduction to the first edition, I'll repeat what I said back then – this has to stop. We have to change things. We shouldn't have to fight back against inaccurate or scaremongering media articles designed to turn women away from breastfeeding. We shouldn't have to jump to the support of yet another mother criticised for breastfeeding in public. We shouldn't need to justify why we don't breastfeed. We shouldn't be fighting against an industry that is actively trying to dissuade women from breastfeeding. We shouldn't need to argue with each other or write newspaper articles debating it. We shouldn't feel the desperate need to justify how we fed our baby to strangers. We shouldn't be feeling guilty about factors outside of our control. Breastfeeding should just be how we naturally feed our babies. Our society should be set up for that. Breastfeeding should be what every mother who wants to can do. And it should be a straightforward choice for most. Not a battle. No guilt. Not something that gets criticised. Just feeding a baby in the way nature intended.

We need a new approach to feeding babies. One in which we get rid of the barriers that many new mothers face, recognise that some women are never going to be able to breastfeed and support all new mothers to meet their individual feeding goals. One in which breastfeeding becomes a more common choice because barriers are removed, we get rid of guilt and breastfeeding is just normal. Boobs shouldn't be news. Or debate. Or anger. Or regret.

But we can't leave responsibility for this to families. Or health professionals. Or those who give up their time voluntarily to deliver the support that the government doesn't fund. If we want to raise breastfeeding rates (for the sake of our population health, our national bank balance and simply for the sake of women), we all need to work together. Breastfeeding is ultimately physically done by the mother, but that does not mean it is entirely her responsibility. Rather, breastfeeding is society's responsibility and if we want to raise breastfeeding rates we all need to think about the role we play. Even if you simply *do no harm* you will be doing good.

The three quotes at the start of this book sum up the challenge. We have the worst breastfeeding rates in the world, yet such high levels of *intention* to breastfeed. Many women are miserable about their decision to stop. So what is going on? Why are so many women deciding to stop breastfeeding before they are ready? And, more importantly, how do we change this?

1. THE ISSUE

Breastfeeding is a physiologically normal way to feed a human baby. This is not to be confused with a social or moral imperative that women *must* breastfeed their babies, but from a biological standpoint it is how our species has evolved and fed our babies since the dawn of man (and woman) kind. Although nature never has a 100% success rate and a small proportion of women will have physiological issues preventing breastfeeding (more on this in the next chapter), you would expect this complication rate to be pretty much similar across populations. However, starkly, we have a complete lack of similarity across populations, not so much in terms of how many women start breastfeeding, but how many continue and for how long.

Back in 2016, the prestigious *Lancet* journal highlighted that, despite clear recommendations from the WHO that babies should be breastfed for up to two years and beyond, many countries across the world are not meeting, or even coming close, to these targets. In a series of papers, the journal published statistics from countries around the world, detailing both their initiation rates and how long women typically breastfed for. Most countries had an average initiation rate ranging from around 80–99%, although variation was seen. For example, for initiation alone (which can sometimes count as just one attempted feed), rates were lowest in regions such as the UK (81%), South Africa (81%) and the USA (74%) and higher in regions such as Bangladesh (98%), Brazil (97%), Turkey (97%) and Malaysia (95%). I couldn't find any countries with rates lower than the UK, South Africa and the USA. Most countries had initiation rates well over 90%.[1]

But it was the huge variation in what happened next that rang major alarm bells. While mothers in some countries, such as Malawi, Senegal and the Gambia, continued feeding well into the second year and beyond, other countries such as the UK and USA started to rapidly drop. In fact, looking at the data, the UK and Ireland were found to have the lowest breastfeeding rates in the world by 12 months old, with less than 1% of mothers still breastfeeding at that time. Just 1%! Personally, I think that figure is a little low and after conversations with numerous breastfeeding researchers over the years we think more women are indeed breastfeeding. We'd probably put the figure at around 5–8%. But basically, we still have among the lowest, if not the lowest, breastfeeding rates in the world at that stage.

Let's look at the UK picture in a little more detail. To do that, we need to look at our latest comprehensive UK data on breastfeeding initiation rates, which comes from… 2010. Yes, 2010. Here we have our first problem: our data on breastfeeding at a UK level is over 10 years old. Historically, from 1975 onwards, the UK Department of Health collected data on breastfeeding initiation, continuation and context every five years in a survey known as the 'UK Infant Feeding Survey'.[2] This involved sending out a questionnaire to every mother who gave birth within two specific months of the year. In 2010 this was August and October. Mothers were sent questionnaires when their babies were around 4–10 weeks old, 4–6 months old and 8–10 months old. Note that feeding data past 10 months was not collected. A report was then produced looking at initiation, duration, exclusivity, timing of solids and any other drinks and foods and so on, comparing the findings with maternal age, education, occupation, ethnicity and location.

However, in 2014 this survey was cancelled, supposedly to save money (it didn't cost *that* much).[3] This means we don't have comparative data for the UK anymore. We do have data at local authority level, but it is collected in very different ways and is not as detailed or useful as the survey data was. This is problematic for many reasons, not least the lack of useful data. Not collecting something means you do not have data against which to measure progress (or a lack of said progress). It signals that the data, and by association breastfeeding and mothers, are not considered important enough to measure and invest in. At the time of writing we are hoping the survey will be reinstated; COVID-19 put a stop to progress on this issue. Meanwhile, Scotland went ahead and did its own infant feeding survey in 2017, recognising the value of both collecting the data and making improvements to better support breastfeeding.[4]

So what did that 2010 data show us? Mainly that alongside having some of the lowest initiation rates in the world, we also had some of the worst drop-off rates. It showed that by one week in the UK only 69% were breastfeeding, by six weeks it was 55% and by six months just a third. Looking at the patterns in previous surveys, although we have seen a rise in the numbers of women who initiate breastfeeding at birth, the drop-off in the first few days remains as steep. In the 2010 data, of those mothers who started breastfeeding, 6% stopped within 48 hours and 14% by the end of the first week. In terms of exclusivity rates are even lower. Although 81% of women breastfed at birth, before the first day was out exclusive breastfeeding had dropped to 69%. By the end of the first week, less than half were exclusively breastfeeding. And at three months, about 15%. By six months? A whole 1%.[2] And I would bet that those figures are actually slightly better than what is actually happening. The data from the survey relied on sleep-deprived mothers sending back a detailed paper questionnaire. If you were breastfeeding you might have been more likely to send back a questionnaire that asked a lot of breastfeeding questions. Put it this way: I was part of the 2010 cohort of participants and I, with a PhD in breastfeeding research, nearly forgot to send it back.

But the most important statistic in that whole report for me is not simply how many mothers breastfed or not, but rather how many were happy about their decision. Out of those mothers who stopped breastfeeding in the first six weeks, 80% were not ready to do so, stopping for reasons outside of their personal control. This suggests that something fishy is going on. This isn't a physiological issue with breasts in the UK stopping them working, or even a lack of desire to breastfeed: a large proportion of women want to and try to breastfeed, but feel they have to stop before they are ready.

You might ask whether these findings are simply an artefact of living in a developed country where we have access to everything: we can formula-feed babies if we want to. You might also argue that women in developing countries have far less choice about whether they breastfeed or not, and that for some breastmilk may be the only food resource a child has. This is true to some extent, but is certainly not the full picture. First, the '80% not being ready to stop' statistic challenges this. But secondly, it isn't just a developed versus developing countries issue: breastfeeding rates differ vastly between countries that are very similar from a cultural, economic and social perspective. For example, in Iceland, 98% of mothers start breastfeeding at birth, with 74% breastfeeding at six months and 27% at one year. In Finland, 34% of mothers are breastfeeding at twelve months. However, Norway beats both of these countries; at six months 80% are breastfeeding, with 46% breastfeeding at 12 months. Breastfeeding rates are also much higher in Australia, New Zealand and even the USA,[1] despite many women being forced back to work when their babies are very young due to a lack of paid maternity leave.[5]

What is also interesting is that in these countries, exclusive breastfeeding status is also maintained far longer. In the UK only 15% of babies are still exclusively breastfed at 12 weeks old. However, at the same time point, 67% of Icelandic babies and 63% of Norwegian babies are exclusively breastfed.[6] Likewise, in New Zealand, 15% of babies are breastfed exclusively until six months[7] compared to just 1% in the UK.[2] I regularly put that 1% figure on presentations, and am regularly asked whether it is a typo because it's so low. No, it is not a typo. Most babies have had formula by six months old, or have been introduced to solid foods before the six-month recommendation. Which as an aside completely destroys the idea of two camps of women, breastfeeders or formula-feeders, battling it out as the media likes to suggest. Your average baby in the UK is breastfed at birth but receives at least some formula in the coming weeks and months. Most women mix-feed over the weeks and months of giving their baby milk feeds. There are no camps. They are a figment of the imagination of formula industry marketers. More on this later before I get distracted.

So are British breasts different to Norwegian breasts? American to Swedish? Perhaps don't answer that, but stepping aside from any raised eyebrows and winks, the answer is no. There is no biological reason why breastfeeding rates should differ between countries. Yes, you could argue that in developing countries with no access to formula, sanitation or indeed a safe and reliable water supply, breastfeeding is more important. However, that doesn't change the fact that theoretically, from a biological perspective, country of birth should not determine a woman's ability to produce breastmilk and breastfeed. If high numbers of women are breastfeeding in particular regions, whether they 'have to' or not misses the point, because in other regions, high numbers of women are feeling like they 'have to' stop – and this makes no sense. Ultimately this is the key issue for this book: when does 'I couldn't breastfeed' truly reflect a biological issue, and when does it reflect a combination of societal forces that make breastfeeding the difficult or even seemingly impossible option?

Differences within countries

As well as significant differences between countries, there are also notable differences when you start exploring who breastfeeds *within* countries. Even in countries where breastfeeding rates are high, there is still variation between different groups. And when rates are low, these differences tend to be even starker. These differences cannot be explained, or fully explained, by biological factors. Instead, different women are affected differently by these complex societal influences. So what are they?

Maternal age

Mothers who are younger are far less likely to breastfeed than mothers who have their baby at an older age. For example, in the 2010 UK Infant Feeding Survey, 87% of mothers aged over 30 breastfed at birth, compared to only 20% of those aged 20 and under.[2] Given that from a biological perspective the female body is most fertile and well prepared to have a baby at a younger age, this strongly suggests that wider psychosocial factors are exerting an influence. Indeed, as will be discussed further, many of the barriers to breastfeeding are more strongly felt within the younger age group. Coupled with a seeming cultural expectation that younger mothers will not even want to attempt to breastfeed their baby, mothers in this age group can find it challenging to overcome the societal hurdles that appear to be put in their way.[8]

Parity

First-time mothers are more likely to breastfeed at birth than second-time mothers, but second-time mothers who breastfed their first baby past the early days are more likely to breastfeed their second baby. To some extent there may be a biological influence at work. First-time mothers are more likely to report that their milk production is delayed (and this is based on examination of milk production rather than simply perception). Some kind of 'breastmilk-producing memory' may be responsible. One study found that second-time mothers produce around a third more milk by the end of the first week than first-time mothers, and studies of mice show that the breasts wait in a 'state of preparedness' in between babies (I'm not sure when they realise they've been retired and give up waiting for their next turn!).[2]

However, first-time mothers also experience a range of other pressures, such as a longer labour and greater anxiety, that can impact on breastfeeding (more on this in a bit). What this shows is the importance of getting breastfeeding established right from the very beginning, with the first baby and subsequent babies.

Maternal education, socioeconomic status or income

Looking again at the UK Infant Feeding Survey data, 91% of mothers who left full-time education after the age of 18 initiated breastfeeding at birth, compared to only 63% of those who left education aged 16 or younger. Closely tied to this, socioeconomic status, or income, closely predicts breastfeeding. In the UK in 2010, 90% of women in managerial and professional jobs began breastfeeding, compared with

74% of those in routine and manual occupations and 71% of those who had never worked.[2] Similar patterns are seen in the USA, Australia and Europe, and even in countries with very high breastfeeding rates such as Sweden.[1] Again, this is situational. Gaining a degree or working in a corner office does not affect the composition of your breastmilk or the functionality of your breasts! But it can affect your job, your disposable income, your confidence and your social circles, which in turn affect your chances of breastfeeding.

Ethnicity

This is a really complex one, which perfectly illustrates the nuance of the issue. Breastfeeding rates not only differ by ethnic group, but also interact with the country a woman resides in. For example, in the UK women from non-white British backgrounds are significantly more likely to breastfeed than those from white backgrounds. In the UK, while 79% of white mothers breastfed at birth, 97% of women from a Chinese background, 96% of black women and 95% of Asian women did so.[2] In Ireland 49% of women from white Irish backgrounds initiated breastfeeding at birth, compared to 86% of those from other white backgrounds. Meanwhile African or black women had a 92% initiation rate, while Chinese and Asian women a 92% rate.[9]

Conversely, in the USA, women from black American backgrounds are significantly less likely to initiate or continue breastfeeding than both white Americans and those from Hispanic populations.[10] This leads to something known as the 'Hispanic paradox', where despite similarities in economic and other structural influences on health, on average Hispanic babies have better health outcomes than black babies. It is thought that the longer duration of breastfeeding contributes to this. Why do women from black American backgrounds have lower breastfeeding rates? Again, this is not physiological but due to experiences within society, with current and historical perspectives affecting breastfeeding.

A central issue is the horrific history of slavery, particularly in the USA. This continues to play a role, particularly for older generations. It was not that long ago that black women were forced to nurse white women's babies, and the association between breastfeeding and slavery has remained. Older family members in particular, some of whom may have been wet nurses themselves, may hate the idea of breastfeeding and see formula-feeding as a freedom.[11]

Racially biased healthcare is also a major issue. Research has shown that black Americans do not get access to the same support, or quality of information, as white populations.[12] This includes breastfeeding support. One study found that African American women received poorer attitudes, information and support for breastfeeding from the Women, Infants and Children (WIC) service.[13] Other research with black mothers reveals that they felt that unless they initiated a conversation with health professionals about breastfeeding, no one would talk to them about it because of a presumption that they would not want to do it.[14] A growing body of other work highlights similar perceptions that black women, particularly in the USA, simply won't want to breastfeed.[15-17] This unconscious bias therefore impacts the support mothers receive.

Black women as a population are also more likely to experience health problems that can make breastfeeding more difficult, including an increased risk of poor perinatal health, chronic illness, depression and stress, all of which can make the experience of breastfeeding more difficult.[18] Poverty, or low-paid long hours jobs, which disproportionately affect black mothers, also plays a major role. Black mothers are more likely to be back at work six weeks after birth compared to other groups, with greater job insecurity.[16] For more discussion on this and other issues to do with infant feeding, I recommend you get hold of a copy of Kimberly Seals Allers' book *The Big Letdown: How medicine, big business and feminism undermine breastfeeding*.

There is also an impact of acculturation: individuals adapting to the society in which they live. Some of the highest breastfeeding rates in the UK and USA are seen among immigrant populations, but as groups settle in different countries, their breastfeeding rates slowly start to drop. For example, Polish women have higher rates of breastfeeding when living in Poland compared to when they come to live in the UK. Likewise, in the US, women born outside of the US have higher breastfeeding rates than those born in the US. In fact for each year a foreign-born mother lives in the US, the odds of her breastfeeding decrease by 4%.[19]

Interestingly, this does not appear to be a direct impact of ethnicity, but more the experiences of living within that ethnic community. In the UK, white women who have a partner from a different ethnic group are more likely to breastfeed than if their partner was also white. Breastfeeding rates are also higher among white single mothers when they live in diverse communities.[20] So it is about community and cultural beliefs about breastfeeding. For example, in one study of Somali women who had moved to Norway, one mother noted that the concept of not having enough milk was alien back in Somalia, but many of her new peers in Norway were worried about it.[21]

Location

Even within the UK breastfeeding rates differ. The 2010 Infant Feeding Survey showed that in England 83% of women breastfeed at birth, but in Scotland it's 74%, Wales 71% and 64% in Northern Ireland. I know it rains a lot in Wales, but I don't think that directly affects your chances of breastfeeding.

Of course there are variations within all these patterns, and exceptions to the rules. I'm sure many readers have acquaintances who have breastfed despite the statistical odds. After all, we are the sum of our experiences rather than labels that society puts on us. But when you start to explore the experiences of women who did breastfeed, despite everyone assuming they would not, their wider situation is often revealed to be conducive towards breastfeeding. Typically, those who breastfeed despite the societal barriers in their way tend to have the tools at their disposal to help them overcome those barriers.

So what's going on?

As we will see in upcoming chapters, there will always be a small proportion of women unable to breastfeed, or breastfeed exclusively. But, as evidenced above in the data from countries with much higher breastfeeding rates, most women, given the right support, should be able to if they want to. We wouldn't be seeing such vast disparities in rates if it was all purely physiological. So despite public health messages encouraging women to breastfeed, the investment needed to create an environment that enables them to do so is lacking.

As I'm writing this update, Boris Johnson is prime minister in the UK and we're in the middle of the global COVID-19 pandemic. Johnson has decided that one way to fix this is to encourage more people to cycle, the logic not being that we're going to run the virus off the cycle path in the style of a MAMIL (Middle Aged Man in Lycra) on a bike, but rather it will apparently help us as a nation to lose weight. This announcement has met with mixed reactions (yes, I'm being polite) but one stark point I did notice is that cycling and weight experts immediately pointed out that you can't just encourage more people to cycle without creating an enabling and safe environment for them to cycle in.

Right. So in this instance we appear to recognise that just telling people to do something does not mean that they will immediately do it. Why isn't it the same for supporting breastfeeding, which needs the exact same enabling approach? What's needed in both cases is a public health approach, whereby we encourage the behaviour, be it cycling or breastfeeding, but more importantly we support it by creating the right conditions, be it cycle paths or well-trained health professionals. At the moment we don't have that environment for breastfeeding. We don't even have a pretty diagram of that environment on the wall. Instead, on the one hand new mothers are told, half paternalistically, half patronisingly, that breastfeeding is extremely important and they really must do it. This raises mothers' expectations, desire and to some extent anxiety about breastfeeding. And on the other hand, society simultaneously places numerous barriers in mothers' way. Although society tells women that they must breastfeed, insinuating that it is a simple and straightforward choice, it sets them up to fail at the same time. Although breastfeeding is superficially welcome, it really isn't and women can face many psychological, social and political challenges when it comes to feeding their baby.

These barriers might be direct: a partner stating that they want to bottle-feed his or her baby, a workplace that doesn't allow a mother time to express, or derogatory comments from a stranger in public. Or they might be more subtle: others' opinions about when babies should sleep through the night, when a woman should 'get her pre-baby body back' and promotion of formula. Infant feeding has become more than simply giving a baby milk; it is bound up with views of how babies are cared for, love and emotions, and mothers in the workforce. We moralise it. Infant feeding becomes not just about nutrition, but about being a 'good' mother.

This isn't to say new mothers are helpless, bowing to the views of society or giving formula simply because their partner tells them to, but often the pressures aren't obvious. It's the subtle messages, day after day, drip, drip, drip. Carrying on breastfeeding can seem just too difficult, at a time when women are already dealing with adjusting to life as a new mother (and all that brings). And there is always, always someone telling you it doesn't matter anyway.

Many people don't understand the barriers to breastfeeding and hold mothers wholly responsible for their 'choice' of how to feed their baby. They see it as black and white, a simplistic choice. Surely if you stop breastfeeding, it's just because you couldn't be bothered any more, right? *No*. As with any human choice or decision, it's far more complex than that. New mothers are often those who perceive this responsibility most clearly – 'guilt', 'failure' and 'regret' are words that women who stop breastfeeding before they are ready use to describe their feelings.

So the aim of this book is to examine the barriers to breastfeeding in our society, describe how they affect breastfeeding and, more importantly, to look at how we dismantle them. It's not a book about how to breastfeed. And it certainly isn't telling women that they must. Don't want to breastfeed? Fine. Fed up of hearing about it? Then quietly pass the book to someone who isn't. This is a book for anyone who has ever struggled with breastfeeding or wondered why there is so much emotion and 'fuss' around it. It is a voice for those who feel others are judging them for their decisions and, most importantly, it is a call to action that demands a change in our society.

Unfortunately, at this point I feel I have to write some kind of disclaimer. How babies are fed has become highly politicised. A lot of emotion goes into what should be a fairly simple discussion. You can consider the 'debate' from numerous angles, but I do not want to add fuel to the fire by suggesting that all mothers *should* breastfeed. Nor am I suggesting that mothers who couldn't or didn't should feel guilty about that choice. I believe that mothers (actually, families) should decide how their baby is fed within the wider context of their family situation.

I do not believe in telling mothers they should breastfeed, or that their decision about how to feed their baby is somehow a reflection of their worth as a mother or person. Nor should mothers who choose not to breastfeed have to defend themselves or go without support. We also need to recognise that some mothers will never be able to breastfeed. Even if percentage-wise few mothers technically cannot breastfeed, even 1% of the maternal population is a lot of individual mothers. However, I do not want this to be misinterpreted. It is important for the health of the population that babies are breastfed. We want more of it. But it is not always possible for everyone. What we need is a situation in which every woman who wants to breastfeed is supported to do so, and no one has needless barriers in their way. A society in which breastfeeding is the easy choice. A society in which more mothers breastfeed and fewer mothers feel guilty about not doing so, because their breastfeeding experience has been made so straightforward.

So what do we need?

If we recognise that no mother makes an infant-feeding decision in isolation, we need to understand the factors that influence her decision. Throughout this book I will explore the evidence around the factors that affect mothers' breastfeeding decisions, and look at what we need to do, as a society, to change things. I'm also going to highlight *why* all this is our collective responsibility. I will be looking at the factors in depth, but I want to start by listing the goals I think we need to achieve if we really want to improve the experience of breastfeeding for women:

1. Invest in woman-centred, one-to-one care during pregnancy and birth to get breastfeeding off to the best possible start.
2. All hospital, neonatal and community services should adopt UNICEF Baby Friendly standards and practices.
3. Invest in expert support for all breastfeeding women right from the start of breastfeeding.
4. Tell all new parents and those around them about normal feeding and sleep, and support them in other ways to get more rest.
5. Tell parents and those around them about normal patterns of weight loss and weight gain in breastfed babies, and why this doesn't mean that they are underweight.
6. Bin all the rubbish baby care books.
7. Give new mothers the emotional and practical support they need, every step of the way.
8. Stop the ridiculous body image pressure on new mothers and come to terms with our own illogical sensitivities and prejudices about human milk and the female body.
9. Educate partners and family to be the breastfeeding supporters they can be.
10. Educate the public to stop being idiots, or at least to do no harm.
11. Support employers to be breastfeeding friendly.
12. Regulate industry to prevent the promotion of unnecessary and potentially harmful products.

That's quite some challenge, isn't it? Now consider this – if all these factors affect a mother's decision to start and carry on breastfeeding, is it really any wonder that we have such low breastfeeding rates? Intention is one thing, but continuation is a completely different ball game. Now let's get started.

2. WHY DOES BREASTFEEDING MATTER ANYWAY?

THE PHYSICAL, EMOTIONAL, ENVIRONMENTAL AND ECONOMIC IMPACT OF INFANT FEEDING

So, we know that breastfeeding initiation and continuation rates vary dramatically around the world. The next obvious question is... so what? Why does it matter if we see low breastfeeding rates? What's it got to do with us?

Plenty.

Supporting more women to breastfeed should be a collective responsibility because it affects us all. Not simply because we were all babies once and many of us will go on to have children, grandchildren, great-grandchildren and beyond, but because it affects our everyday existence. Sound too dramatic? Well, no. How our babies are fed doesn't just affect individuals, it affects our health services and our environment. It should matter to us all. Breastfeeding matters because:

- It affects the health of infants, now and as they grow and develop
- It affects the health of women, particularly in terms of reproductive health
- It affects maternal mental health and therefore family wellbeing
- It impacts our health service: as a population group formula-fed infants require more medical treatment
- It affects our environment: producing, distributing and preparing infant formula has implications

But most of all it matters because we are seeing so many women in countries such as the UK, USA and Australia unable to breastfeed their babies as long as they want to, compared to other regions around the world. It matters because this, for many women, is fixable with the right environment and support. And that's what we need to work together to achieve.

Breastfeeding and health

The scientific literature examining the health impact of infant feeding is vast. If you go to Google Scholar and do a search for 'breastfeeding' it returns 749,000 academic papers (apparently it was 426,000 when I did this back in early 2016). 'Breastmilk' offers 2 million papers (1.5 million in 2016) and 'infant feeding' also 2 million (again 1.5 million in 2016). Apparently in 2016 I didn't do a search for 'human milk' but that offers 3.2 million. That's a lot of papers. Not all are perfect (by a long way) and not all show exactly the same thing, but overall what they describe is a general pattern: babies who are formula-fed and mothers who do not breastfeed have higher levels of illness than breastfed infants and their mothers.

This information is important, particularly if we want to look at overall population health and why breastfeeding is promoted, but it also needs to be understood in context. As the phrase 'lies, damned lies, and statistics' goes, we know statistics and research can be misused and misinterpreted (for much more on this, check out my book *Informed is Best*). What the evidence for breastfeeding shows overall is that on a population level – multiplied over hundreds of thousands of babies – breastfeeding prevents illness, and saves the costs of treatment. This shows why supporting breastfeeding should be a societal responsibility, and if we all work together we stand a chance of achieving much higher breastfeeding rates.

But my baby wasn't breastfed and he's fine

Excellent. Contrary to what sometimes seems to be popular belief, we don't actually want babies who are not breastfed to be ill. We don't want babies, mothers or families to be affected by decisions that are sometimes out of their control. We don't want feelings of guilt and regret, or arguments between different infant feeding 'camps'. We want all babies who are formula-fed to be OK. And their mothers to be okay with that decision too.

But just because a baby who is formula-fed doesn't get ill, this doesn't invalidate the arguments for breastfeeding. Firstly, health is complex and we can't tick a box to say that someone is absolutely 'healthy' or 'unhealthy'. Formula-feeding has been shown to increase the risk of many different illnesses. The important word is 'risk'. Risk is not a definitive. Just because breastfeeding protects against ear infections, doesn't mean that all babies who are formula-fed will suffer repeat ear infections while their breastfed peers will never have any trouble with their ears. It means that more babies who are formula-fed will experience an ear infection than those who are breastfed.

For example, if 10% of babies who are breastfed get a certain illness, and 20% of those who are formula-fed get it, statistically this means that twice as many formula-fed babies experience the illness. Ten per cent of babies are essentially experiencing the illness because they are not breastfed. This is a large increase. However, 80% of babies who are formula-fed will still *not* get it (which again is great). But just because a baby falls in that 80% category doesn't mean that formula-feeding didn't increase their risk of illness – they just avoided that risk. One baby falling into the 80% category doesn't predict what will happen with the next baby, or the one after that. So if a baby isn't ill, that's great. But encouraging breastfeeding remains the least-risky option, the best bet as such because, although many babies may be 'fine' in hindsight, we don't know that in advance.

Further, although we can look at how many babies tend to get an illness and compare them by how they were fed, we know that illness is more complicated than that. Lots of things, such as genetics, poverty, parenting and just bad luck will determine whether a baby actually gets an illness. Or, indeed, is even exposed to that illness. To develop meningitis we know that you have to be exposed to the virus or bacteria responsible for it, and this is thankfully very rare. But we also know that if a baby is unlucky enough to be exposed to meningitis, that being breastfed will reduce their risk of contracting it, and then affect how they deal with the illness.

How a baby is fed is part of an important jigsaw puzzle of factors; it is not the only factor. But it is important, and potentially more important for some babies than others. We know that health and illness are socially patterned. By that I mean that those living in deprived circumstances are more likely to become ill than those who are more privileged. Protecting breastfeeding for all babies is important, but protecting breastfeeding for those babies born into the most challenging circumstances is especially so.

But I thought breastfeeding protected against illnesses?

Nothing we do can definitively protect against any illness. We can reduce risk, but we can't stop it happening altogether. A mistake often made when interpreting breastfeeding research is applying population statistics directly to an individual. Population statistics, which look at patterns of data across large numbers of individuals, cannot be used to predict individual risk. Sometimes breastfeeding research is wrongly cited (and often it is deliberately misinterpreted by the media to stir up argument) by those who say things like 'You bottle-fed so your baby will get an ear infection'. Population statistics can only really give you a relative risk based on what we know about the bigger population.

Most health statistics are like this, but are publicised in more general ways. Smoking kills, right? No, actually there is a 15% risk of dying from lung cancer if you smoke all your life. Eating five portions of fruit and veg per day stops you getting heart disease, doesn't it? No, eating five portions a day, compared to one portion, reduces your risk of heart disease by 6%.[1] This doesn't mean we should immediately eschew all health advice! Most of us try to do a number of things on a day-to-day basis that give us the best chance of being healthy. And anyway, as I will discuss below, it's not actually all about health.

So what's the value of population-level statistics? Look at it this way. In the UK, around 700,000 babies are born every year. If out of every 100 babies born, 10 of the breastfed ones get an illness and 20 of the formula-fed ones get it, then that's a difference of 10 babies for every 100 born (the individual formula-fed baby's risk is still 20%, as we've seen above). If all 700,000 babies were breastfed, that would mean 70,000 babies not experiencing this illness every year. That's a lot of healthy babies! More cynically, it's a lot of money saved. Imagine it costs £200 to treat the illness (a visit to the GP and a prescription). That's 1.4 million pounds saved each year that could be spent on other things. But actually, for you and your baby, there's an 80% chance you'll be OK.

But my friend's baby was breastfed and she got ill!

Again, looking at those population statistics, a certain proportion of breastfed babies will still experience the illnesses that breastfeeding protects against. If 10% of breastfed babies get an illness and 20% of formula-fed babies do, then the formula-fed babies' risk is doubled and 10% of breastfed babies will still experience it. This certainly doesn't mean that breastfeeding 'doesn't work'. The breastfed babies that did get the illness were unlucky. This may not be much consolation on an individual level, when you are awake at night with a fractious baby, but the population statistics show that many thousands of babies will not have had the illness because of breastfeeding. And there are other factors at work too: even within the same family, where all babies are breastfed, there can be one child who seems to succumb to illness for reasons other than how they were fed.

Also, although breastmilk is an amazing substance, it can't overcome all pathogens and circumstances all of the time. Stuff like genetics can be having an effect too. Sometimes, the main way in which breastfeeding protects is through strengthening the immune system. This can reduce the chances of a baby getting ill, but may not always stop it. So on paper – and for the data of a study – the baby has the illness, but do they have it as severely?

Breastfeeding can often affect a baby's experience of an illness. Until we discover parallel universes, or develop the ability to go back in time and change history, we will never know what would have happened to a baby if they had been fed differently. If a breastfed baby catches a cold, we will never know how many colds breastfeeding prevented them getting, or what their experience would have been like if they hadn't been breastfed. Similarly, for illnesses that have a strong genetic component such as eczema, no one should be surprised if a baby develops it if both parents and other family members suffer too. Breastfeeding may not prevent the baby from developing eczema, but may well affect how badly the baby suffers or how frequently.

But isn't it down to who breastfeeds, rather than being breastfed?

A common criticism of breastfeeding research is that mothers who breastfeed tend to have a different background to those who do not breastfeed. On the whole, breastfeeding mothers are more likely to be older, have a higher level of education, be in a professional job and earn more money. These factors in themselves are significantly linked to child health. Critics of breastfeeding research therefore often suggest that it is this background that protects against child health, rather than breastfeeding itself. They argue that mothers who are more likely to live in a healthier neighbourhood, be able to afford better quality food and who read to their children will have healthier children anyway, whether they breastfeed or not. This problem is known as confounding and to some extent the critics have a valid argument.

However, most decent (and certainly most recent) studies have acknowledged this problem and controlled statistically for the impact of maternal background. Some use what is called a 'matched samples design', in which mothers in the breastfeeding and formula-feeding groups are paired by age, education and income. Others restrict their samples to mothers with a professional background. Others add maternal age, education and occupation to their statistical models. Very few studies are now published which don't consider these factors.

In addition, we also know *how* breastfeeding protects against health and *which* elements of formula-feeding increase risk. We can thus show logically how the method of feeding, or the content of the milk, protects against or increases the risk of certain illnesses.

But there are studies that show breastfeeding doesn't have a long term impact on X/Y/Z

Yes, there are. Breastfeeding does not protect against every illness or enhance every aspect of human nature. And that's OK. Eating apples doesn't either. But your mother was still right when she told you that they keep the doctor away.

But different studies come out with different numbers!

This is because we are human beings and not machines. Studies of any human behaviour always return slightly different figures. It's just how it works. In all areas of health, not just infant feeding. However, one of the issues with breastfeeding research is that different studies use different measures of breastfeeding. Some look at any breastfeeding, others at exclusive breastfeeding only. Some might look at initiation or the rate of any breastfeeding at six or 12 weeks. Some look at longer duration. Some even group women as not breastfeeding if they don't exclusively breastfeed for a set duration of time.

Understanding these differences in methodology is key, but often overlooked when the research is reported. Sometimes research studies are reported as showing 'no difference' between methods of feeding, but when you look more closely it turns out that the study only considered whether babies were breastfed in the hospital or not at birth. The best studies are careful to look at defined measures of breastfeeding, over longer periods of breastfeeding duration.

These nuances in data collection are actually a major part of the whole issue. In other areas of public health – say exercise, how much fruit and veg you eat or smoking – measures of these behaviours tend to be more complex (although not in all studies). People aren't generally lumped into 'ever had a cigarette' (including all those who had that one puff behind the bike shed when they were 15 that sent them into a coughing fit, through to those who smoked 40 a day for 40 years) versus 'never'. But in breastfeeding research, the actual measures of breastfeeding are often quite frankly a mess.

Specifically, a lot of breastfeeding research is problematic because it fails to fully measure breastfeeding. 'Breastfeeding' somehow becomes a yes/no dichotomy, so everyone whose baby licks a nipple briefly through to those who are breastfeeding toddlers and pre-schoolers is lumped together in one homogenous group. Sometimes it feels as though studies have been designed by someone who has never encountered a baby, and is no expert in feeding. If I was being suspicious, I'd say that some researchers don't *want* to find an impact of infant feeding.

Breastfeeding research often fails to measure duration or exclusivity, meaning it often vastly underestimates the protection breastfeeding may bring. But duration and exclusivity really matter. One study in Greece, for example, which properly measured how long babies were breastfed for and how, found that exclusive breastfeeding was more protective than mixed feeding against infections, but that mixed feeding was more protective than not breastfeeding at all.[2] Likewise, the longer a baby was breastfed, the fewer infections.

However, lots of studies don't look at duration of feeding, and if they do, they often stop at about six weeks, sometimes six months. Yet when research looks fully at the impact of longer-term breastfeeding, or accumulative breastfeeding over subsequent babies, it shows an increase in protection the longer breastfeeding continues. For example, a systematic review paper published in 2015 looked at breast cancer risk by duration of feeding. The researchers found a 17% reduction in risk for breastfeeding for six months or less, 28% for 6–12 months and 37% for 12 months or more.[3]

In research I did a few years I ago, I looked at duration of breastfeeding and appetite regulation – basically how well toddlers could control their appetite and stop eating when full.[4] Breastfeeding helped appetite control, but only if babies were breastfed for at least six weeks. This makes sense. One of the theories for why breastfed babies are less likely to be overweight is that they have greater experience of learning to regulate their own appetite. You cannot see how much milk is in a breast, so the baby is more in control of deciding when they have had enough. But if we had just measured breastfeeding at birth we probably wouldn't have found that link.

But issues with exclusivity and duration are unfortunately not the only problems. Some breastfeeding research uses simplistic measures, such as whether babies were breastfed at birth or not. This is essentially just a measure of whether mothers intended to breastfeed, or perhaps as little as the impact of one feed of colostrum. It could include babies who pretty much just sniffed or licked a nipple. It could have some effect, through transferring antibodies or populating the microbiome, but it's really not going to give the full picture. Yet sometimes researchers use this as a measure of 'breastfeeding' and conclude that breastfeeding doesn't protect babies.

For example, there is a much-talked-about sibling pairs study, which measured outcomes for families where one baby was breastfed and the other baby formula-fed.[5] The idea of a sibling study is that it may remove potential bias from outcomes because everyone grows up in the same family. This means they are likely to be exposed to the same education and income level, and so on. So if you are measuring differences for one baby who is breastfed and another who is formula-fed, you could more confidently say that the differences (or lack of them) are down to the feeding method, rather than socio-economic factors.

This study declared that there was no difference in health and development outcomes for babies based on whether they were breast or formula-fed, and declared it was all down to who chooses to breastfeed, not the actual breastfeeding. But the problem with the design of this particular study is that there is no detail on how long babies were breastfed for. They are grouped into 'ever breastfed' versus 'never breastfed', which could mean that the ever-breastfed babies received just one feed.[5] I have read the paper numerous times but cannot find any details on duration of breastfeeding. The fact that the duration details are missing is problematic. If we knew that we were comparing one baby who was breastfed for six months with one who was not breastfed at all, we would be making a more meaningful comparison.

Occasionally research has the reverse issue and babies are only counted as breastfed if breastfed for longer, which means the 'not breastfed' group could include breastfed babies. In one study that claimed there was no difference in health outcomes between breast and formula-fed babies, babies were classified as formula-fed unless they were breastfed exclusively for two months or more.[6] So babies who were breastfed for a long time but not exclusively were grouped as formula-fed.[6] Babies who had 10 weeks of exclusive breastmilk – which is more than 80% of babies in the UK get – were classed as formula-fed. No wonder no differences in outcomes were found! This didn't stop the media claiming there was no impact of breastfeeding on health.

Sometimes researchers ask mothers to indicate how their baby was breastfed in the last week. This can be detailed, including whether the baby is breastfed, if any formula is given, and any other foods or drinks. However, it completely fails to account for the fact that what is happening this week doesn't necessarily accurately describe the past. For example, exclusive breastfeeding refers to receiving breastmilk only with no additional formula milk or other foods. By those measures a baby could be exclusively breastfed this week and maybe even for many weeks. But it doesn't mean they always have been.

This design doesn't capture early milk feeds such as formula top-ups in the hospital, pre-lacteal feeds or perhaps a mother who was mixed feeding moving over to exclusive breastfeeding. An accurate infant feeding history cannot be measured in one or two simple questions. It's like asking someone how much alcohol they have drunk in the last two weeks and determining from that they are teetotal, but completely ignoring the fact it's the beginning of the year and they are participating in dry January.

Yet another issue is that, particularly in randomised controlled trials, some babies get grouped into a particular way of feeding, even if they do not follow the guidance given to that group. For example, one trial with babies who had lost a lot of weight split mothers into those giving a little formula, compared to encouraging exclusive breastfeeding. They looked at weight outcomes, the microbiome and whether babies continued to be breastfed.[7]

However, this particular study used what is known as an 'intention to treat' design, which means that they measured the outcomes for babies based on their randomisation at the start and not whether they were actually exclusively breastfed or not. When you look at the details over one-third of the 'exclusively breastfed' group had used formula in the last 24 hours at one month old. In fact, at one week old, over a third of 'exclusively breastfed' babies (37.3%) had received some formula, compared to 22% of the formula top-up babies in the last 24 hours, with the exclusively breastfed babies actually receiving more formula on average per day than the formula top-up babies (13.7oz per day versus 10.2oz per day). If the supposedly exclusive breastfeeding group were having on average more formula per day than the formula group, what were the researchers comparing?

Why does all of this matter? Well, it matters not only because the impact of breastfeeding is underestimated (and that is then used to fail to invest properly in supporting it), but also because it is so illustrative of how we as a society treat breastfeeding. It appears it doesn't really matter and it isn't valued enough for science to accurately measure it. Without good data we face a much tougher battle in getting a real-life mother and baby the support they need.

Breastfeeding is really only important in developing countries, isn't it?

I often hear that breastfeeding is only needed in developing countries where infant feeding can really be a life or death decision. And it is true that babies born in developing countries with little access to safe sanitation, clean water or adequate formula milk have significantly greater risk of illness and death if they are not breastfed. A recent review showed that exclusively breastfed babies in low-income countries had 12% the risk of death compared to those never breastfed.[8] Another study suggested that of babies under six months old who were never breastfed, boys were 3.5 times more likely to die and girls 4.1 times more likely to die, compared to those who received breastmilk. Translating this into lives means that over 800,000 babies would be saved every year in low-income countries if nearly all mothers breastfed. That's almost 15% of deaths prevented.[9]

Other research suggests that if all babies in low-income countries were breastfed, around half of all incidences of diarrhoea and a third of respiratory infections could be avoided. This would prevent 72% of hospital admissions for diarrhoea and 57% for respiratory infections.[10] Women who are breastfeeding often do not ovulate or have periods, sometimes for many months. In areas with no contraception, but high levels of breastfeeding, the birth rate might increase by 50% if breastfeeding rates fell.[11]

So no one would argue that breastfeeding means the same in developed countries and developing countries. Luckily in Western society our health and welfare systems mean that babies do not have to starve and families do not have to search for clean water (although sadly for some living in significant poverty, facilities for safer formula preparation may not be available). However, the evidence from developed countries does show similar patterns in risk of illness, although at a lesser level.

The impact of breastfeeding upon infant health in developed countries

One of the most useful papers to explore the impact of breastfeeding using data only from developed countries is a systematic review published about 10 years ago.[12] For a systematic review authors analyse data that has already been published (and its quality), bringing together papers on a topic to see whether they agree. If they do, this adds weight to the findings of the individual papers.

Overall the authors looked at over 9,000 papers before reducing them to the ones they considered to be best conducted, using good methods, big enough samples and taking into account things like mothers' education and income. In the end they had 43 studies looking at babies' health, 43 studies on mothers' health and a further 29 systematic review papers (which themselves considered 400 papers – so this was a review of reviews!). They then conducted a series of 'odds ratios', looking at how much more likely it was that a baby would get an illness depending on how they were fed.

Another interesting study in this area is the PROBIT study.[13] This used a randomised controlled trial to see whether length of breastfeeding affected child health outcomes. Randomised controlled trials are usually considered one of the best types of evidence you can get, because they reduce the influence of background on behaviour. Everyone who signs up to the study is randomly assigned to one group or another. However, this is often difficult to do with breastfeeding from an ethical perspective. Because we know breastfeeding is important for health, it's not ethical to tell a woman to formula-feed for the purposes of a study. And given the barriers women face to breastfeeding, it's also quite difficult to tell a woman to breastfeed! So randomised controlled trials are very rare in breastfeeding research.

This study took the health advice in Europe at the time (to breastfeed exclusively for four months) and randomised women to either breastfeed exclusively for four months, or to breastfeed exclusively for six months. They used a cluster approach, whereby women in certain areas were randomised to the four-month group and women in other areas to the six-month group. They then gave the six-month group lots of additional support to try to naturally encourage them to breastfeed for longer. They could then measure outcomes for the two different groups.

In reality there was actually a lot of overlap between the two groups and remember that all mothers in the study intended to breastfeed. At three months 73% of babies in the intense support group were receiving any breastmilk, compared to 60% in the control group (and 19.7% versus 11.4% by 12 months). This meant, in fact, that at three months the majority of babies were breastfed, but at 12 months, the vast majority of babies were not breastfed. The intervention also increased exclusive breastfeeding until six months, but again the differences were not huge: 7.9% in the intense group compared to 0.6% in the control group. A significant difference in *exclusive* breastfeeding was seen at three months – 43.3% versus 6.4%.

This means that any difference in health outcomes between the two groups is weakened, as most babies got some breastmilk for quite a while. It is not, as is commonly misreported, a trial comparing breast and formula-feeding. If this had been the case you would expect any of the differences in outcomes to be even bigger. So what did they find?

They found that lower breastfeeding rates were linked to higher levels of lots of different types of illness, but there was much stronger evidence for some of those illnesses than for others. These included respiratory infections, gastrointestinal infections and ear infections. Babies in the intense support group – with the higher rates of any and exclusive breastfeeding – had fewer occurrences of gastrointestinal infections (9.1% versus 13.2% of babies) and atopic eczema (3.3% versus 6.3%). Or in terms of those babies that developed those illnesses, roughly 60% of gastroenteritis cases were in the lower breastfeeding group and 65% of the eczema cases.

Below I summarise some more of the findings, alongside results from other good-quality studies conducted in developed countries.

Respiratory infections

Compared to babies who are exclusively breastfed, babies who are partially breastfed (given both breastmilk and formula milk) are three times more likely to get a respiratory infection, with babies who are formula-fed nearly four times more likely.[14] For respiratory infections, breastfeeding can be protective. For example, the risk of respiratory syncytial virus, a respiratory infection that leads to mild symptoms in adults but can be more serious in babies, increases from 5% in breastfed babies to 8% in babies who are not breastfed.[15] Another study found that babies with pneumonia were 22% less likely to be breastfed.[16] Finally, babies who are exclusively breastfed for at least four months are 72% less likely to be hospitalised with a serious respiratory infection.[17]

Gastrointestinal infections

Generally, the longer a baby is breastfed, the less likely they are to have a gastrointestinal infection in the first year of life.[18] Looking at the increased risk for formula-fed babies, those who have never been breastfed have 2–3 times more infections than those who are exclusively breastfed.[19] Partial versus full breastfeeding has an effect too. In the trial of breastfeeding, those exclusively breastfed for three months were around one and a half times more likely to get an infection than those exclusively breastfed for six months.[13]

37

Ear infections

The longer a baby is breastfed, the lower their risk of getting an ear infection. This really is a case of 'the more the better'. In fact, if a baby is breastfed exclusively for six months, the data suggests that they will have one less ear infection than if they were mix fed.[20] In the review paper above the researchers found that never being breastfed increased the risk of ear infections by 50% compared to at least three months of breastfeeding. However, any breastfeeding helped and those who had been breastfed even for a short time had a 23% lower risk than those formula-fed from birth.[12] Finally, if a breastfed baby does get an ear infection, it's less likely to be serious. The chance of a baby having an ear infection that lasts over 10 days is 80% reduced if they are breastfed.[21]

Overweight

Lots of studies have explored whether breastfeeding could prevent against obesity, and overall the findings seem to cautiously suggest that it can. A study in Australia looked at whether infants were exclusively breastfed, partially breastfed or formula-fed and found that exclusive breastfeeding for at least four months was associated with a reduction in overweight up to 14 years old. Introducing formula milk, either alongside breastfeeding or stopping breastfeeding entirely, was linked to an increased risk of overweight.[22] Another study in the Netherlands found that each additional month of breastfeeding up to 12 months old was associated with reduced risk of overweight at age one.[23]

Interestingly, one study looked at the combination of milk type and timing of introduction to solid foods. If a baby was breastfed, the timing of solids had no impact on their weight. However, if a baby was formula-fed and introduced to solid foods before four months, they were more likely to be overweight at three years old.[24]

Another study shows that there may be a specific impact for mothers who are overweight, or have significant weight gain during pregnancy. Mothers who are overweight are more likely to have an overweight child at five years old. However, when overweight mothers breastfed for longer and introduced solid foods later, their child's risk of overweight was reduced.[25]

However, remember when considering anything to do with weight that it is really complicated. Breastfeeding tends to put babies on the right track and helps them develop positive eating habits.

If, for whatever reason, an older child ends up eating a really high calorie diet, then breastfeeding is not going to miraculously 'save' them from becoming overweight. Thus most studies show protective effects in the early years, but less clear effects later on.

For example, one study found that babies who were breastfed for more than 16 weeks had a lower BMI at age one. BMI at age one then went on to predict BMI at age seven, but breastfeeding alone didn't directly predict it.[26] Another review looked at all the factors that affected child weight and found that not breastfeeding was a 'top predictor' of overweight, alongside maternal diabetes, maternal smoking, rapid infant growth, short sleep duration, less than 30 minutes a day of physical activity and drinking sugared drinks.[27] This is really interesting, as it shows that obesity is affected by a number of factors in a jigsaw-like effect.

Cardiovascular health

Blood pressure is lower in children and adults who have been breastfed compared to those who have never been breastfed. However, the difference is usually very small – around 1–2 mmHg. Other studies found no difference.[28] So is a small difference really beneficial? Maybe not for an individual, as it is a fairly small reduction. It has been estimated that each increase of 20 mmHg in blood pressure doubles the risk of stroke.[29] However, at a population level it may have a bigger impact. One study worked it out across the US population and found that a 2 mmHg drop in blood pressure would result in 17% fewer individuals with high blood pressure, 6% fewer with heart disease and 15% fewer strokes.[30]

Cholesterol levels have also been shown to be lower in adults who were breastfed.[12] This was confirmed by another study that suggested that any breastfeeding reduced cholesterol levels in adulthood. However, again the effect was quite small.[31]

Allergies and asthma

The research around allergies, asthma and breastfeeding is more mixed. Some research suggests that for babies with a family history of allergies, exclusively breastfeeding for at least three months almost halves their risk of developing allergies.[32] Another study found that three months of breastfeeding reduced the risk of asthma by 40% for babies with a family history, and by 27% for those who didn't have a family history.[33] Other research showed no difference, with some researchers even suggesting breastfeeding could exacerbate the risk, although that paper was controversial and the methods widely debated when it was published.[34] Lots of research is going on in this area.

IQ

IQ is always contentious in breastfeeding research, with critics arguing that mothers with a higher IQ are more likely to breastfeed. However, a few studies that control for maternal background do suggest a small impact on IQ. One study, for example, found that babies who were exclusively breastfed for at least three months had on average 2.1 more IQ points than those who were mix fed, with six months' exclusive breastfeeding associated with a leap of 3.8 points.[35] In the PROBIT trial, in which mothers were randomised to be given support to exclusively breastfeed for six months compared to four months, children who exclusively breastfed for longer had higher scores at six years old of 7.5 points for verbal IQ, 2.9 points for performance IQ and 5.9 points for overall IQ.[13]

Another study explored developmental milestones at 18 months, finding that compared to those breastfed for less than one month, any amount of breastfeeding above this was associated with an increased chance of meeting milestones at 2, 3, 4, 5 and 6 months old.[36] Another found greater language ability at 5 and 10 years old in those breastfed for more than four months compared to those breastfed for shorter periods.[37]

Finally, some recent studies are starting to suggest that babies who are breastfed for longer may have differences in brain development, although it is difficult to separate this from the influence of wider family environment. For example, research has shown that breastfed babies have larger volumes of white matter in certain areas of the brain responsible for cognitive and behavioural development compared to formula-fed babies.[38] White matter helps our brains function faster, passing messages between different areas at a quicker pace and enabling us to do 'higher order' stuff like thinking logically, processing emotions and doing maths puzzles. Babies who are formula-fed also have greater wave latencies relating to vision and hearing, suggesting these pathways are less well developed. In English this means that messages are sent at a slower pace between areas of the brain.[39]

Rarer disorders and illnesses

Breastfeeding may also protect against a number of less common illnesses. Some studies suggest that being breastfed might reduce a child's longer-term risk of developing diabetes. One study, for example, suggests a 24% reduction in risk.[40] However, others find no direct link. What may be happening is that breastfeeding can reduce the risk of overweight, which in turn can protect against diabetes.

One systematic review of six studies totalling nearly 5,000 babies found that breastfeeding reduced the risk of coeliac disease. Notably there was a further reduction in risk if the baby was being breastfed when gluten was introduced.[41] This adds weight to the idea that breastfeeding while introducing solids may be protective.

A few studies have suggested that breastfeeding for at least six months reduces the risk of leukaemia by 15%.[42] Another study suggested a reduction in risk of childhood leukaemia, Hodgkin's disease and neuroblastoma.[43]

Formula-feeding is also one of the risk factors for SIDS and a few different studies have suggested that not breastfeeding increases the risk of SIDS by around one third to one half.[12] Fortunately, the number of babies affected by these illnesses is very low (fewer than 300 babies per year in the UK die of SIDS). Therefore this is a very good example of how the individual risk of something can be very low (and therefore should not provoke undue anxiety in parents), but on a population level may start to make a difference.

A special note on premature babies

Receiving breastmilk can be life-saving for premature babies. Any illness that a formula-fed baby is at higher risk of is exacerbated in premature babies whose system is still developing. The breastmilk of mothers with premature babies is even different in content to term-baby breastmilk, suggesting that the body tries to compensate for this additional vulnerability. Premature breastmilk has higher levels of protein and a different combination of vitamins and minerals compared to the milk of mothers with babies born at term.[44]

One recent study showed that babies born weighing less than 1250g (about 2lb) who received breastmilk fortified with protein had better outcomes than those fed a cows' milk-based formula. Starkly, whereas 2% of the breastmilk group died, 8% of the cows' milk group died. The breastmilk group also had lower levels of necrotising enterocolitis (NEC) (5% versus 17%).[45] NEC is a condition affecting premature babies in which the tissue of the bowel starts to die. It can be life-threatening, but its incidence appears to be much lower in breastfed babies.

Breastmilk also helps the development of the digestive system of premature babies in other ways. Premature babies receiving intravenous nutrition (via a drip) can tolerate milk fed via a tube into the stomach more quickly if they receive breastmilk rather than formula milk. Breastmilk helps to develop their immature digestive system due to the presence of enzymes such as lipase, which helps with fat absorption. The immune properties in breastmilk also help develop the gut barrier, protecting babies from infections.[46] Premature babies who are given breastmilk have lower incidences of sepsis, urinary tract infections, diarrhoea and respiratory infections compared to those who receive formula milk.[47] Infections are much more serious for premature babies, so these statistics are vital.

There is also a significant difference in IQ scores between premature babies fed breastmilk and those fed formula milk. Estimates suggest a difference of around 8 points, with an increase the more breastmilk the baby gets.[48] Another very recent study showed that premature babies who were fed breastmilk had bigger and stronger hearts as adults compared to those who had been fed formula milk.[49]

Overall, breastmilk is an incredibly important choice for premature babies, which is why breastmilk banks have been set up to allow premature babies, whose mothers cannot provide breastmilk, to receive donor breastmilk. Dr Natalie Shenker co-founded the Hearts Milk Bank with Gillian Weaver, a long-time campaigner for donor milk for premature babies. The milk bank is a not-for-profit organisation, with strong links to research institutions, which will provide safe, screened donor milk to neonatal units across London and the south-east. You can find out more about it at www. heartsmilkbank.com. Natalie explained:

'Strong research exists to show that the use of donor human milk substantially reduces the risk of infants developing necrotising enterocolitis (NEC), a serious gut complication among premature babies. NEC has a mortality rate of 25-40%, and results in major lifelong morbidity as a result of surgery, bowel loss and the need for parenteral nutrition. The estimated cost to the NHS of caring for a severely affected child to adulthood can amount to a seven-figure sum. The care of these infants is extremely complex, and babies that require surgery have a median inpatient stay of 6 months. This places a huge psychological, financial and logistical burden on parents and longer term can have lifelong and life-limiting complications. Donor human milk (DHM) within the first 14 days after birth reduces this risk 8-fold compared to the use of infant formula, along with reductions in sepsis and pneumonia.

However, it is well recognised that many mothers struggle to establish and maintain lactation, especially mothers of babies born before 32 weeks of gestation, those who have medical complications and those who suffer the traumatic experience associated with having an ill or preterm baby. Others may have medical conditions which prevent them from breastfeeding. The short-term provision of DHM is a suitable alternative for their babies, thus supporting mothers as they attempt to establish their own supply. Strong research exists to show maternal breastfeeding rates increase by the use of DHM, as evidenced by the higher rates of breastfeeding on discharge for hospitals with linked Milk Banks. And naturally this increases the wellbeing of mothers too.'

But how? Why?

How breastfeeding might promote health is fascinating. There are lots of ways it might have an impact, either directly through the content of breastmilk, or indirectly in the way it impacts on our bodies or the way in which babies are fed. We are finding out more and more about how breastfeeding protects mother and baby all the time.

Content

Breastmilk contains a number of factors that protect babies, which are not present – or are present in lower levels – in formula milk. Firstly, breastmilk contains a number of active immune factors. These include regulatory cytokines, growth factors, peptides, lysozyme fatty acids and oligosaccharides, all of which help prevent infections and support the development of good bacteria in the digestive system. When breastfed babies get fewer infections, it's not just because they're from healthier families, it's because their milk has immune-boosting properties. Notably, the specific immune properties in breastmilk are different between mothers depending on their environment and previous immune experiences. If a mother is exposed to an infection, she starts to make antibodies to fight it, which are then passed to her baby through her breastmilk.[50]

Breastmilk also has many live components that help with growth and immunity and that are absent from formula milk. For example, it contains growth factors and enzymes such as lipase, which help with the development of the digestive system. It also contains antimicrobial and antiviral factors and a range of cells including macrophages, leucocytes and lymphocytes, which are involved in fighting infections.[50]

Another area of interest is long-chain polyunsaturated fatty acids

(LCPUFAs), which occur naturally in breastmilk. Although some formulas now have added LCPUFA, this may not mirror human LCPUFA or transfer to the baby in the same amounts.[51] Some studies suggest that formulas with added LCPUFA may increase the amount the baby ingests, but there doesn't seem to be any impact on their cognitive development. Even if LCPUFA is added to formula, babies may not be able to absorb it effectively.

Why is this important? LCPUFAs play an important role in many adult diseases, including diabetes and high blood pressure, and may be linked to enhanced cognitive development. These fatty acids are involved in early development and growth. Higher LCPUFAs are linked to lower fasting glucose levels, which can protect against insulin resistance (a precursor of diabetes). In terms of cognitive development, LCPUFAs enhance eye and brain development, particularly during pregnancy and the first three months after birth. Babies who are breastfed have higher levels of LCPUFA than those who are formula-fed.[52]

Another difference is that breastmilk contains insulin-like growth factor. Growth factors help optimise brain and cognitive development and support the healthy functioning of organs like the liver and kidneys. Breastfeeding may boost levels of this growth factor. Adults who were breastfed were more likely to have high IGF-1 levels later in life,[53] and higher levels of IGF-1 are linked to lower blood pressure in later life.[54]

The cholesterol content of breastmilk is also important, in a way that might seem surprising. Breastmilk is actually higher in cholesterol than formula milk, but animal studies have shown that early exposure to high cholesterol actually leads to lower cholesterol levels later in life.[55]

Breastmilk may also have an important influence on the way babies put on weight. Breastmilk has lower levels of protein than formula milk. Formula milk is based on cows' milk, which is far higher in protein than breastmilk. This is because growth is the most important thing for calves, whereas cognitive development is most important for human babies. However, formula milk has too much protein for human babies, which means that growth can be artificially increased (not in a good way) in formula-fed babies. Research is ongoing that suggests that if formula is modified to have lower levels of protein, babies might not put on as much weight. Additionally, breastmilk contains hormones that help to regulate appetite, such as leptin, ghrelin and adiponectin, which are not found in formula.[56]

Protecting the digestive system

Emerging research is showing that the types of microbes and bacteria in our digestive systems can affect our health and development. Essentially, 'good' bacteria are associated not only with our digestive health, but also with much of our functioning. The wrong bacteria – which can proliferate due to diet, stress and medications such as antibiotics – can increase our risk of all sorts of physical and mental health problems. The type of microbes that we have might affect brain development, with the wrong type increasing the risk of allergies, inflammatory conditions and obesity.[57] Fascinating research is happening that shows that our very early experiences – birth and milk feeding – may set up our microbe system for life. For a brilliant and more detailed account of the importance of this critical period, read *The Microbiome Effect* by Toni Harman and Alex Wakeford. It'll turn you into one of those people who disturbs everyone around them by reading sections out loud, in disbelief.

How does this relate to infant feeding? Breastfed babies have far more of the 'good bacteria' than formula-fed babies.[58] Breastmilk also provides the 'right' microbes for a healthy digestive system, which have been shown to change over time according to the infant's needs. There are different good bacteria in colostrum than in milk at one or six months.[59] On top of that, human milk has a wider variety of sugars than formula milk, which act as prebiotics, supporting the growth of good bacteria.[60] Overall, breastmilk leads to healthier digestive systems than formula milk.

Finally, one study has speculated that the melatonin content in breastmilk may help to improve infant sleep and reduce colic. The researchers found clear rises and falls in the melatonin content of breastmilk, but there is no melatonin at all in formula milk. Melatonin can have a relaxing effect on muscle within the digestive system, and also make people feel sleepy, both of which potentially help babies to sleep more soundly.[61]

Are you sure the content of breastmilk has this much impact?

I cannot stress enough how important these pathways between the type of milk a baby receives and its immediate and later health are. Equally importantly, researchers are finding new connections all the time. There is simply not the space in this book to list all the consequences milk feeding can have, but Maureen Minchin, author of *Milk Matters: Infant Feeding and Immune Disorder*, which I highly recommend, argues that to ensure normal development, breastmilk is the necessary bridge between the womb and the world. She considers that the use of infant formula over time has resulted in compounding intergenerational epigenetic and genomic damage, which makes it difficult to see the negative effects of artificial feeding, as they have become 'normal' in Western populations. She points to emerging and deeply worrying biological differences between breastfed and formula-fed children, such as differences in reproductive tissue development evident at 4 months (identified by ultrasound), differences in brain white matter development shown by MRI, and a greater number of chromosomal breaks found by cancer researchers curious about higher rates of cancer in artificially fed infants. For her, microbiomic differences in artificially fed infants are proof of harm that will resonate in many ways through a lifetime and beyond, affecting subsequent generations. Epidemics of obesity, inflammatory and auto-immune disease can be expected, as susceptibility is communicated vertically from parents to children and compounded by postnatal dysnutrition. This is mind-blowing stuff, but the evidence for it is growing all the time.

How babies are fed

Aside from the differing content of breast and formula milk, differences in the feeding process might affect weight gain in babies. It is very difficult to encourage a breastfed baby to take more milk than they want. Breastfeeding is a sequence of actions, as the infant latches onto the breast and manipulates it with their tongue and jaw. The baby must open their mouth widely and place the tongue under the areola in order to suckle efficiently. The baby is in control of the latch, and if the baby doesn't want to feed, milk is unlikely to flow. Conversely, milk from a bottle is consumed by sucking and, if the bottle is held upright, to a certain extent by gravity. It is much 'easier' to drink from a bottle than the breast, and it is far easier to consciously or accidentally encourage a bottle-fed baby to consume more milk because of this.

Two studies of formula-fed babies in the 1960s show how easily a bottle-fed baby can be encouraged to over-feed. In one study researchers carefully bottle-fed babies until they showed subtle signs of being full and did not cry when the bottle was taken away. Babies consumed on average 168ml/kg/day.[62] In a second study researchers bottle-fed babies the largest possible feed they would consistently accept. Babies in this study consumed an average of 189ml/kg/day.[63] This small difference over time can add up to a lot of additional calories over the first few months.

Indeed, in comparison to bottle-feeding mothers, breastfeeding mothers show greater sensitivity to their babies' signals to feed, letting the baby determine when the feed is over rather than initiating a stop. Breastfeeding mothers have also been shown to interact more with their infants during feeding, including touch and gaze. Gazes are longer and mutual touch during feeds increases at a faster and earlier rate than in formula-fed infants.[64] Breastfeeding mothers are more likely to be responsive feeders, feeding their baby on demand and not thinking about schedules or how much the baby might have drunk.[65]

Babies who are bottle-fed are more likely to finish everything in the bottle. Breastfed babies, on the other hand, are more likely to 'leave' milk in the breast. One study asked women to feed their babies normally and then express milk until the breast seemed 'empty'. They could then compare how much the baby drank and how much they left. They found that the amount drunk wasn't related to the amount left – even babies who took low levels of milk still had milk left over, so it wasn't a case of there not being enough milk.[66]

A recent study in the USA decided to trial this, considering whether the size of bottle a baby was given contributed to weight gain. Babies were randomised at two months to receive their milk either in a 6oz bottle or a larger bottle. Those that had a larger bottle gained more weight by six months – around a quarter of a kilogram. That might not seem like a lot, but bear in mind that six-month-old babies probably weigh only around 10kg, so it's an extra 2.5% in weight. If you keep multiplying that small increase in energy intake over time you can see how bottle-fed babies can end up heavier.[67]

Another study showed that babies who are bottle-fed are more likely to drain a cup in later infancy, with that likelihood increasing as they had a greater proportion of feeds via a bottle. This relationship was still found when babies were given expressed milk in a bottle, suggesting it is something about the feeding action that produces this result.[68] Meanwhile, breastfed babies naturally cut down the amount of milk they consume when introduced to solid foods, but formula-fed babies do not.[69]

Overall, formula-fed babies are at a higher risk of a number of illnesses, particularly in relation to infections and obesity. There are plausible physiological pathways for this, which refute the suggestion that these effects are down to who breastfeeds rather than the milk babies receive. At a population level breastfeeding protects against many illnesses, with considerable cost implications for health services.

The impact of breastfeeding on maternal health

When we talk about the health impacts of breastfeeding, the impact on maternal health is often overlooked. However, some of the strongest effects of breastfeeding on health are actually for the mother, often having a cumulative protective effect the longer she breastfeeds, and for each subsequent baby she breastfeeds.

Why? There are a number of different pathways to explain why this happens, but a core idea focuses on our history as a species and how we have evolved. From an evolutionary perspective, women were never designed to have so many periods and such fluctuating hormone levels over their lifespan. We would have been pregnant from an early age and then breastfed our babies before falling pregnant again. This is in no way to say that our more modern approach is 'worse' – contraception, greater power and more egalitarian societies have led to women having fewer babies and greater choice about the number of babies they have. Moreover, in countries where women have less power and fewer health services, we know that childbirth is inherently risky. Contraception and having fewer babies can be lifesaving. However, this reduction in number of pregnancies and time spent breastfeeding over our reproductive lives is a major change from a hormonal perspective, and it is thought that our bodies spending more time in a non-pregnant/lactating state increases the risk of health problems.

So how does breastfeeding protect mothers?

Breast cancer

One of the strongest protections for maternal health is for breast cancer. For each year a mother breastfeeds, she lowers her risk of breast cancer by around 4%. In real terms, this means that if she never breastfeeds, her breast cancer risk is 1.4 times greater than that of a mother who breastfeeds for over 55 months.[70] Another study suggested a reduced risk of about a quarter for breastfeeding for 12 months or more.[71] Altogether this has a serious impact upon maternal mortality rates. An analysis of the impact of sub-optimal breastfeeding rates in the US attributed 838 maternal deaths each year to not breastfeeding.[72]

Why does breastfeeding reduce breast cancer risk? Several reasons have been proposed. Levels of oestrogen are lower during breastfeeding; high oestrogen levels have been implicated in the growth of cancer cells. Although more research is needed, breastfeeding appears to protect the cells in the breast from mutations that can lead to cancer, strengthening them. Breast tissue is also shed during the act of breastfeeding, which is thought to remove cells that have mutated or have the potential to mutate. [73]

Ovarian cancer

Mothers who never breastfeed have 1.5 times the risk of ovarian cancer compared to those who breastfeed for at least 18 months.[74'] Again the effect is cumulative, with one study suggesting that breastfeeding for less than six months reduced risk by 17%, 6–12 months by 28% and 12 months by 37%.[75] Fascinatingly, one study showed that women who have had mastitis have a lower risk of ovarian cancer than those who have not! This is thought to be due to the presence of antibodies that are produced when you have mastitis.[76] The link between ovarian cancer and breastfeeding most likely occurs due to ovulation being suppressed among breastfeeding women. Every time ovulation occurs, cell mutation is possible. Therefore fewer ovulations reduce the risk of such mutation.[77]

Diabetes

Not breastfeeding may increase a mother's risk of diabetes. One study suggested that compared to those who breastfed for at least two years over their lifetime, those who never breastfed had 1.7 times the risk of developing diabetes.[78] Diabetes can be a serious disorder. The analysis of sub-optimal breastfeeding in the US report attributed 473 diabetes-related deaths each year in the US to not breastfeeding.[79]

How does breastfeeding impact upon diabetes risk? Metabolic changes during pregnancy can increase the risk of insulin resistance. However, during breastfeeding maternal insulin-sensitivity appears to improve, with lasting effects, which helps explain a lower risk of diabetes in women who initiate and continue breastfeeding. This is known as the 'reset hypothesis', in which breastfeeding appears to work to reverse risky changes during pregnancy.[80]

Cardiovascular health

Breastfeeding may reduce a mother's risk of high blood pressure, with one study suggesting that for every 29 women who breastfed for over a year, one case of post-menopausal high blood pressure would be prevented.[81] A similar study in Korea suggested that mothers who breastfed for a year or more had a third lower risk of high blood pressure compared to those who did not.[82] There is also a reduction in risk of heart disease. One study showed that compared to women who breastfed for two years or more, never breastfeeding was associated with 1.3 times the risk of heart disease.[83] The impact of this across populations is significant. In the analysis of suboptimal breastfeeding rates in the US, it was estimated that 986 women die each year from myocardial infarction attributed to not breastfeeding.

Again, one pathway to explain this is changes that occur during pregnancy and lactation. During pregnancy, levels of cholesterol and triglycerides rise in the mother, but this is reversed during lactation. Breastfeeding women have lower blood lipid levels than those who are not breastfeeding.[80]

Maternal weight

Some studies suggest that breastfeeding can help increase weight loss after birth, with a longer and more exclusive duration leading to the greatest loss.[84] However, not all studies are conclusive, probably because weight gain and eating behaviour are complex.[85] It has been proposed that breastfeeding uses up to 500 calories per day,[86] but criticism of this suggests that some women's metabolism adapts to account for this. Anecdotally some women appear to retain weight until they stop breastfeeding, perhaps as an evolutionary response to protect the mother and milk production. Other studies have found that breastfeeding women naturally appear to eat more and move less, at a rate that equates to those 500 calories, negating any impact upon weight.[87]

Autoimmune disorders

There is increasing evidence, although not all studies are conclusive, that breastfeeding may reduce the risk of autoimmune disease, particularly in later life. For example, one study found a lower risk of hypothyroidism amongst postmenopausal women. The risk was lowest when women breastfed cumulatively for at least three years, and/or across three or more babies.[88] Research has also identified a lower risk of rheumatoid arthritis in older women, again with a greater reduction for a longer duration of breastfeeding.[89] There is also limited evidence that breastfeeding may reduce the risk of multiple sclerosis in later life.[90]

Breastfeeding and maternal mental health

This is an often overlooked area, but research shows a strong link between breastfeeding and mental health. When breastfeeding goes well, maternal mental health is protected, but when it does not a mother is at higher risk of postnatal depression, grief and trauma. This relationship is complex, and can be explained by both physiological and psychological factors.

When breastfeeding is going well, on average mothers will feel happier and less stressed compared to women who are not breastfeeding. Conversely, not being able to breastfeed is associated with an increased risk of postnatal depression in numerous studies.[91] There are a number of physiological pathways for this. Increased levels of oxytocin during breastfeeding promote feelings of calm and happiness. Mothers who breastfeed also get increased sleep, aided by melatonin in breastmilk promoting infant sleep[92] and increased maternal prolactin levels promoting maternal slow wave and deeper sleep.[93] It may seem difficult to believe, but research exploring energy levels in new mothers found that breastfeeding mothers reported feeling more awake, energetic and physically healthier than those who were bottle-feeding.[94]

Breastfeeding also reduces the physiological impact of stress on the body, reducing inflammation and its consequences. Stress hormones increase inflammation in the body. Sleep deprivation, caring and associated feelings of isolation or anxiety all increase stress in new mothers. We now know that inflammation increases the risk of depression, so breastfeeding can physiologically help protect new mothers.[95] Stress also suppresses the immune system, but breastfeeding appears to mitigate this. In one study with new mothers, stress and depression were associated with lower immune functioning, but only in mothers who were bottle-feeding. Mothers who were stressed but breastfeeding had no similar decrease in their immune system. And a well-functioning immune system helps reduce the risk of you getting sick and further stressed.[96]

However, the link between mental health and breastfeeding is more than just physiological. As we will see later in the chapter, breastfeeding can be important to women for many reasons. It is then only to be expected that if she cannot meet her breastfeeding goals, or desired way of mothering her baby, her mental health and wellbeing will be affected.[97] Pain, difficulty and a lack of support, especially if this leads to a subsequent decision to stop breastfeeding before she is ready, also increase depression risk.[98] This is unsurprising. We know that pain in general increases depression risk,[99] as does a lack of sleep, which is more likely with a baby who is having feeding difficulties.[100]

But the link between breastfeeding and mental health is more than just postnatal depression. Mothers can feel a whole host of emotions when they are unable to breastfeed. Indeed, in research I conducted in 2016, which led to me writing my book *Why Breastfeeding Grief and Trauma Matter*, over 2,000 women who could not breastfeed as long as they wanted to told me their stories.[101] They didn't just feel a little 'sad' or 'fed up' – they used words like 'devastated', 'shocked' and 'grieving'. They truly mourned their experience, hating their body for seemingly letting them down or even blaming their baby for not being able to breastfeed (and then hating themselves for that). Many felt criticised by others, guilty or that they weren't 'good enough mothers' because they couldn't breastfeed, which is a common feeling across the literature.

Indeed, many, as Miriam Labbok described, were showing signs of genuine grief.[102] As I explored the responses, others were showing signs of psychological trauma, having flashbacks to their experiences, strong and vivid emotions of hurt and neglect and reacting viscerally to seeing others breastfeed or talk about doing so. It was abundantly clear how much breastfeeding meant to women and how much they suffered when they didn't get support or answers about why things were working out. This alone, for me, is the main reason why we should be investing in turning things around so that many more women can meet their breastfeeding goals.

The impact of breastfeeding upon the economy

'Supporting breastfeeding makes economic sense for rich and poor countries … This new research demonstrates huge economic gains for individuals, families, as well as at the national level.'

Lancet *series on breastfeeding, 2016*

Many people who are dismissive of health advice will change their minds when you present them with the financial savings that could be had if people changed their behaviour. Simply put, if breastfeeding protects against illness, but large numbers of babies are not breastfed, healthcare costs increase. However, it is only recently that these costs have actually been calculated. And the results are persuasive.

Why might breastfeeding boost our economy? Well, think about its knock-on effect. Formula-feeding increases our health costs, both directly and indirectly. Directly, if we look at the numbers of mothers and babies who are more at risk of an illness if the baby is formula-fed, then we can start to calculate the costs, which can include medical appointments, clinics, hospitals, laboratories and test fees. However, there are also a series of extra costs – outside healthcare – of a baby being ill. A baby may pass an illness to their parents, siblings and friends. Parents may then need to take time off from work to care for an ill baby (and from a feminist perspective, it is more likely to be the mother who will take that time off). For an individual this may not be a huge cost. Perhaps treatment costs were £200, plus a couple of days away from work, which may be unpaid. However, consider that on a population level, multiplied across all the babies who become ill.

Let's go back to our example, in which 3% of breastfed babies get an illness compared to 5% of formula-fed babies. Although the risk per baby doesn't increase that much (a 97% versus 95% chance of not getting it), at a population level this can have a big impact on the economy. As noted above, over 700,000 babies are born every year in the UK, and if 2% more of them are getting an illness due to not being breastfed that means 14,000 poorly babies. If the illness costs £200 to treat… then that's nearly £3 million! If you apply the principle to illnesses that cost more to treat, or places with far higher birth rates, like the USA, then it is a lot of money indeed.

If individuals were paying for their own healthcare, they might look at the odds of getting an illness and think it worth the risk of formula-feeding. But the NHS, and private health insurers, must consider costs in terms of the general population. When they do so, the benefits of breastfeeding are far more significant. This is why we all need to work together if we want to see improvements in our public health.

How much money could increasing breastfeeding rates actually save?

Health economists work out how much money can be saved by looking at the rates of breast and formula-fed babies who become ill and then how much it costs to treat those illnesses. It sometimes seems a bit cold-hearted, in that it looks at the cost of treating illnesses and doesn't take into account how people feel. However, for now let's just consider the money.

One of the largest economic evaluations of breastfeeding in the UK was conducted in 2013.[97] This study worked out how much money could be saved if more mothers breastfed for longer. It looked at lots of different outcomes, but one of its main calculations investigated how much money could be saved if rates of breastfeeding increased so that 45% of mothers in the UK exclusively breastfed for four months and 75% of babies in neonatal units were breastfed at discharge. The findings were pretty clear. If we could reach this modest level in the UK – less than half of mothers breastfeeding for only two-thirds of the length of time recommended by the WHO (World Health Organisation) for exclusive breastfeeding – we would make significant savings in NHS resources and therefore money.[103]

In real terms, this would mean over 9,000 fewer hospital admissions and 54,000 fewer GP appointments, just for gastrointestinal infections, lower respiratory infections and ear infections. In premature babies, we would see 361 fewer cases of NEC. In monetary terms this would mean, for these four illnesses alone, saving over £17 million a year. An increase in exclusive breastfeeding rates could also save at least three families the devastating emotional consequences of a baby dying from SIDS. Considering the impact of SIDS from a financial basis seems very cold, but if you were to consider that the average individual adds around £1.3 million in monetary value to the economy over a full working life, economists might argue that this is 'lost' if a baby dies.

The researchers then started playing around with the data in different ways. For mothers, they found that if half of mothers who did not breastfeed did so for up to 18 months over the course of their lifetime, there would be 865 fewer lifetime breast cancer cases per annual cohort of mothers. What that means is looking at the mothers who gave birth each year, 865 fewer of them would be diagnosed with breast cancer... year on year on year. This would directly save £21 million for each annual cohort of first-time mothers, and if you add on the cost of women living with cancer, this would add another £10 million. That's another £31 million saved for each round of new mothers.

The researchers went even further. They looked at the IQ of breastfed and non-breastfed babies. Even though there is only a small difference in IQ points, if just 1% of those babies who were never breastfed were to be breastfed at birth, then that small cumulative increase across the whole cohort of babies each year could translate into over £278 million in economic gain.

Finally, if we just managed to get breastfeeding rates up to the point where we reduced childhood obesity by 5%, then 16,300 fewer children would be obese and long term we would save £1.6 million annually in obesity-related treatment costs. All together that is a lot of money. Given recent cuts to benefits in the UK, I'm now envisaging a parliament that tackles breastfeeding instead of trying to strip people with disabilities of their money. Wouldn't that be nice?

Studies in other areas of the world echo these findings. An analysis in the USA explored what would happen if 90% of mothers breastfed for at least a year (compared to the current rate of 23%). Specifically they explored rates of breast cancer, ovarian cancer, hypertension, type 2 diabetes and heart disease, using a longitudinal dataset of 1.88 million women followed from 15 to 70 years of age. The results showed that if breastfeeding rates rose to that level there would be 4,981 fewer cases of breast cancer, 53,847 fewer cases of hypertension and 13,946 fewer cases of heart disease. This would equate to savings of $17.4 billion from reducing premature death, $733.7 million in direct costs and $126.1 million in indirect costs. Overall it was predicted that 4,396 premature deaths (before age 70) could be avoided.[104] Bringing that down to an individual level, it was suggested that for every baby breastfed until six months, $3,430 would be saved.[105]

If we look to countries where health and healthcare systems are poorer, and inequalities are greater, the impact is even higher. In one analysis in Indonesia that looked at the impact of increasing breastfeeding rates on the costs of treating gastrointestinal and respiratory infections in children aged under two years, the researchers calculated that the equivalent of US$118 million could be saved.[106]

Research has also calculated the impact of increasing the number of premature infants who receive human milk in neonatal care. The researchers looked at how many babies are typically born prematurely in the UK, and how many of those babies receive any formula milk during their neonatal stay. By calculating the increased risk of adverse health outcomes among premature infants fed formula milk, they worked out that the NHS would save £30.1 million for the year, with increased savings due to reduced healthcare costs in later life. When considering the 'lost productivity' of infants who died due to neonatal infections or SIDS, they calculated that 238 babies' lives could be saved, which equated to £153.4 million in lifetime productivity.[107]

Pulling all this together, in 2019 researchers designed a tool to measure the global impact of babies not being breastfed. They found that globally, almost 600,000 childhoood deaths from diarrhoea and pneumonia occur each year due to a lack of exclusive breastfeeding, alongside almost 100,000 maternal deaths from breast and ovarian cancer and type-2 diabetes. The impact of not breastfeeding equates to US$1.1 billion each year in health service costs, a potential $53.7

billion in future lost earnings, and US$285.4 billion in cognitive losses. Overall somewhere between US$257 and US$341 billion is lost each year, equating to up to 0.7% of all global gross national income. Those figures all make my head spin, but to put it simply: breastfeeding saves an awful lot of money.[108]

The impact of breastfeeding on the environment

The protection that breastfeeding offers doesn't stop with health and economics. Consider the environmental costs of formula-feeding. Formula milk has an impact on natural resources in its production and preparation, its distribution, and in the disposal of cans and bottles. Breastfeeding mothers may consume extra calories, but the cost of this additional food (in terms of price and natural resources) is not comparable to the costs and resources involved in the production of formula. But what is the impact of all of this?

In 2019, a review of the impact of formula-feeding on the environment was published in the *BMJ*.[109] The findings were sobering. Some specific points included:

- Increased need for water: approximately 4,700 litres of water are needed to produce a kilo of powdered infant formula. This includes the water needed to produce cows' milk in the first place and then the additional water needed to turn that into powdered formula.
- Increased methane: livestock are the second biggest contributor to methane production, which traps heat in the earth's atmosphere.
- Added necessary ingredients: powdered cows' milk cannot simply be given to babies; oils, vitamins and minerals need to be added. Palm oil, including its devastating impact on rainforests, is a common ingredient.
- Food miles: there are fewer than 50 formula-milk processing plants in the world. This means a lot of formula is being transported around the world. Europe, particularly Ireland, is a big exporter. Indeed, the formula-milk industry in Ireland is huge, and is often praised as supporting the Irish economy. Marketing messages around cows being fed on the green grass of Ireland are common. Conversely, China is a huge importer of milk, exacerbated by cases of babies being made sick or even dying due to contaminated Chinese formula. Formula milk, particularly from Australia, is seen as safer and its marketing is strong. If you visit a gift shop in an airport in Australia, among the Australian gifts you will find

numerous formula milks for sale.

- Cost of preparing milk: powdered milk needs water added, at a temperature of at least 70 degrees. This means that many millions of kettles are being boiled each year. Dishwashers are running extra loads. Sterilisers are using resources.
- Increased landfill: approximately 550 million empty cans of infant formula are added to landfill each year.
- The cost of marketing milks: marketing involves paper, plastic waste and transport costs.
- Increased healthcare costs: we saw in the last section that increased rates of illness in formula-fed infants lead to more GP appointments, hospital admissions and healthcare resources. These also have an impact on the environment.

The impact of all of this on the environment is clear. In 2015, the International Baby Food Action Network calculated that for each kilo of infant milk produced, 4kg of CO_2 is created – before any impact from marketing, transporting, preparation or landfill.[110] A more recent study by the World Health Organization and Gates Foundation increased this estimate to 11–14kg of CO_2 per kilo of formula, at the point of feeding it to the baby (so still excluding any impacts of landfill).[111]

...and just 'because'

Having said all of that, you can base arguments on all the statistics you like. But what reasons do mothers give for wanting to breastfeed? Why do we have such high numbers of mothers planning to breastfeed, then feeling so dismayed when they cannot? Is our decision to breastfeed really a health, financial or environmental choice? Or is it something else? In one research study I posed the simple question: 'Why did you want to breastfeed?' Of course, most mothers cited lots of different health reasons, but they often went on to add a 'but'. And that 'but' was simply because they wanted to. They felt it was what they wanted. Their choice.

> 'Breastfeeding is about so much more than health. It is about cuddles, and closeness and bonding. It saves time, costs nothing and you can never forget to take it out with you. Why don't we emphasise these things more?' Research participant

So why is breastfeeding so important to women over and above those health, economic and environmental reasons?

1. It's a reproductive right

We've already looked at the impact of breastfeeding on maternal health, particularly in relation to reproductive cancers. But breastfeeding is more than that. It's part of reproduction and growing and birthing a baby. It's how we are designed to feed our babies from a biological standpoint and a natural expectation that our bodies should simply work as we expect them to.

Breastfeeding can also protect mothers physiologically, both in terms of reducing stress and increasing wellbeing. In countries where women have less choice and power, the protection of breastfeeding from delaying the return of periods can be lifesaving in terms of preventing unwanted pregnancies or spacing out children. So breastfeeding is important and should be protected for all these reasons.

2. It's a way of mothering

Breastfeeding is about more than just the milk; it's a way of caring for and mothering a baby. In a recent survey I asked breastfeeding women how they used breastfeeding in ways other than just giving milk.[101] Looking at the proportion who used breastfeeding in different ways at least once a day, 83% did it for comfort, 64% to soothe crying, 60% because their children were unsettled, 92% to help them to sleep and 85% to help them back to sleep at night. Ninety-three per cent had done it to help their baby after their injections, 92% to help them when they had hurt themselves, 97% to help when they are ill and 87% to soothe them in new situations when they are anxious. Most reported that in these situations their baby latched on quickly and then fell asleep or calmed down. That's a pretty remarkable parenting tool! In breastfeeding circles mothers are often encouraged to follow their instincts to parent in this way: 'if in doubt, latch him on'. So when a mother who wants to mother in this way cannot, she doesn't just lose a way of feeding her baby, she loses a way of caring for them.

3. Breastfeeding can help women heal psychologically

Breastfeeding can help mothers heal and reconnect with their baby. Particularly when mothers have had a very difficult birth, have been separated from their baby, or their baby is sick or in neonatal care, breastfeeding restores faith in their body, gives back their control as their baby's mother and helps restore their connection to their baby. For mothers with a baby in special care, being able to feed them, or express their milk for them, can help in so many ways. They might feel that they have 'failed' their baby because they were born too sick or too soon, but being able to give their milk to their baby to help them grow and get stronger makes them feel that their body is working again.[112] For those with a baby who is wired up to different machines, and where nurses and doctors seem to be in charge, breastfeeding and giving breastmilk can help parents feel that they are 'reclaiming' their baby for themselves. This is especially true if they are able to hold their baby, away from the machines.[113]

But putting these reasons aside, really there is no need to have to justify why we should support breastfeeding. After all, it's a normal biological function. Women should not be expected to justify, explain or provide evidence about why it's important. We don't ask people with hearing loss to justify why they want to hear. Indeed, throughout my research over the years, the concept of 'just because' has been a strong factor. Many mothers just want to breastfeed, without having to justify it or even without knowing the reason why. Many couldn't actually put that 'thing' into words. They simply felt breastfeeding was the right choice for them.

'It was just what I wanted to do. I can't really describe why. It's a feeling not a reason.'

'I just really wanted to. Yes it was about health, but actually, it was just what I wanted to do.'

Indeed, 'just because', or an automatic decision to breastfeed, is a theme that arises in many studies exploring women's decisions to breastfeed. I conducted a huge study once, looking at around 50 different things that affected whether a mother breastfed or not. I put them all into a model, pressed compute and waited for some flash of insight to appear. Two things came out of it: an automatic decision to breastfeed (they always knew they would) and 'because I wanted to'. And this is really rather important. It is this feeling that leads to women feeling miserable after the birth because they feel they have failed. Indeed, a recent study I conducted showed that it wasn't breastfeeding duration that was linked to postnatal depression, but readiness to stop. If women wanted to breastfeed for a week and did so, they were far happier than those who wanted to breastfeed for three months and didn't make it.

If you look at the statistics for breastfeeding and health, yes they are important. If you're weighing up the odds about whether to breastfeed or not, breastfeeding is your best option. But it's not a guarantee for any individual baby. The statistics get much more important at a population level, but I don't think many women base such a significant decision on them. What is important is that women who want to breastfeed – for whatever personal reason they give – are enabled and supported to do so. But we're currently in a situation in which 80% of mothers who stop breastfeeding in the first six weeks are not ready to do so.

So must we really justify it? Add logic and science to it? Rationalise it? Breastfeeding is a normal biological act. It's an instinct for many – just what they want to do. We don't need a rationale or excuse; on a biological level it's what the female body prepares to do after pregnancy. Why do we need to provide an argument to support our decision to breastfeed? Shouldn't all women who want to breastfeed be completely supported in their decision to do so? As one mother put it:

'I just loved it. Even the hard bit. I miss it. I don't like to think that I might never get the chance again.'

And this is really what we are fighting for.

3. LET'S LOOK AT THE BIOLOGY

HOW MANY WOMEN CAN WE EXPECT NOT TO BE ABLE TO BREASTFEED?

There are, and always will be, a very small percentage of mothers who are physiologically unable to breastfeed, either due to an inability to produce sufficient milk no matter what support they receive, or biological or medical factors that make breastfeeding difficult or not advised. This is true across countries and cultures and unfortunately is unlikely to be able to be fixed. The number of mothers directly affected by these issues is unclear, with estimates ranging from 0.1–5%, depending on the data collected. A figure of 98% of women being physically capable of breastfeeding is often quoted, and this fits neatly with initiation rates in countries more reliant on breastmilk or where attitudes to breastfeeding are more positive.

However, the origins of this figure are slightly mysterious. In an article written for La Leche League, Pamela Morrison describes how no one is entirely sure where suggestions of around 5% of women being unable to breastfeed, or indeed 98% being able to, ever came from. She refers to work by Dana Rafael in 1955 and Marianne Neifert in 1983, both of whom mention the figure of 5% of women. Morrison goes on to discuss how Betty Crase, a La Leche League leader, eventually traced the figure back to a remark made in a presentation at the British Medical Association conference in 1938. Everyone else since simply copied it. Morrison herself, through her own extensive practice as an IBCLC (International Board Certified Lactation Consultant) suggests that in her experience the number of women who physically cannot make enough milk no matter what support they receive is around 0.1%. However, there are other factors that make breastfeeding inadvisable for a very small minority of mothers and babies, increasing this percentage to around 1–2%.[1]

So why does that figure differ so significantly from data that shows a steep drop-off in breastfeeding rates after the first few days? One issue is the lack of clarity in the figures themselves. We are mammals. We were all babies once and therefore either breastfed or not. This issue is literally relevant to the whole population, yet somehow we don't have accurate figures about how many women have a physiological complication that prevents them from feeding their baby in a physiologically normal way? We have estimates of how much of the population are affected by other disorders. A quick Google search will give you figures for heart disease, asthma and erectile dysfunction, but breastfeeding complications? Not so much. That latter example is hugely important, as this reflects the way in which some societies and cultures do not value the health experiences of women to the same extent as those of men.

However, a really important point to consider when looking at how many women could be physiologically unable to make sufficient milk and why is important to define what we mean by this. One of the most common reasons for stopping breastfeeding in the UK and similar countries is a 'lack of milk', but this is a complex issue to unpick. Sometimes this lack of milk is a genuine low supply, and sometimes it is simply a *perception* of a low supply, perhaps because a baby is feeding very frequently (more on this later on). Furthermore, when a woman does present with a low supply, this can be broadly split into two main categories: those who would never have been able to make enough milk due to physiological factors, no matter how much support they were offered, and those whose experience has meant that they have a low milk supply. It's this latter group of women that this book is predominantly about.

There are three main stages in the production of breastmilk, known as lactogenesis one, two and three:[2]

- Lactogenesis one: this starts approximately midway through pregnancy and is automatic and driven by hormones. Breasts typically enlarge and colostrum starts to be produced in small amounts. Some women will leak small amounts but mature milk production will not start until after birth.
- Lactogenesis two: after birth the delivery of the placenta leads to a large drop in progesterone and oestrogen. This drop, combined with high levels of prolactin that rose during late pregnancy, signals to the body to start full milk production. This will typically take around 1–2 days post-birth, with a noticeable increase in milk from around day three onwards, although this may be delayed by some birth complications (more on this in chapter 5). Again this stage is automatic and controlled by hormone levels.
- Lactogenesis three: this refers to milk production after the birth. Although levels of milk production will be affected by things like

breast function and hormone levels, for the majority of women milk production at this stage is driven by removal of milk from the breast: the more milk that is removed, the more milk that is made in replacement and vice versa.

When structural or hormonal factors impede sufficient breastmilk production this is known as primary lactation failure (a term that I dislike due to the word 'failure', which can be emotive and feel accusatory). Women who experience primary lactation failure are unlikely to be able to be able to change this, even with all the right support. They may be able to increase their milk supply output, but not produce a full supply (more on this in a bit). Women with primary lactation failure may be able to spot signs during pregnancy or after birth (i.e. during lactogenesis stages one and two) that breastmilk production is not gearing up: their breasts may not change in pregnancy and little increase is seen in milk production over those days after birth.

However, for *most* women, it is at the stage of lactogenesis two or three that milk production goes right or wrong.[3] Numerous factors ultimately determine how much milk is removed from the breast and how often, and therefore how much milk their body makes. These factors are varied and complex, some more subtle than others, but account for many of the cases of low milk supply that we see in the UK and similar countries. It is vitally important that we recognise and are able to identify when this is happening to women. How often is a low milk supply genuinely a case of primary insufficiency, and how often does it simply look like one?

What factors can lead to primary breastmilk insufficiency?

So, what factors can lead to a woman being at risk of not being able to produce a full breastmilk supply, no matter how much support she receives?

Hypoplasia

One group of women who can find it difficult to produce significant amounts of breastmilk are those whose breasts have insufficient glandular development, known as hypoplasia. This can happen either in one breast or both, and can be identified by a lack of changes to the breast during pregnancy or after birth, coupled with low milk production despite frequent attempted feeds in the post-birth period.[4] Also known as 'tuberous' or 'tubular' breasts, women with these condition will have breasts that lack fullness both vertically and horizontally. Often the areola is enlarged. The breasts are often widely spaced and lower, but shorter in length. In one study of mothers with hypoplastic breasts, 45% reported little breast growth in pregnancy, with 30% reporting none at all. After birth, 42% had no engorgement at all, with 21% reporting very minimal changes. Looking at the volume of breastmilk produced, 85% produced less than half of the milk needed for their baby during the first week (compared to controls who produced 100%). Only one mother produced all the milk needed. However, over time this did increase. In the first month, while 55% produced less than half the milk needed, 39% produced all of the milk for their baby.[5]

Breast surgery

The impact of breast surgery on breastmilk production depends on the procedure that was performed. Breast reductions typically involve the removal of glandular tissue; the more that is removed, the more difficult it can be to produce a full milk supply, although this can vary from woman to woman. The method of surgery can also have an impact. If the nipple and areola were removed fully to be repositioned, then this tends to have more of an effect. When they are only partially severed and the blood supply, ducts and tissue remain attached then this has less of an impact. Cuts and tissue removal around the areola can affect the nerves in the region which can interfere with letdown, as suckling is not so clearly felt, which can mean the pituitary gland does not get the signal to produce and let down milk. However, in some cases milk ducts do regenerate and reconnect and nerves heal, particularly during pregnancy.[6]

Conversely, breast implants tend to have less of a direct impact in themselves, particularly if they were placed under the muscle wall, as less pressure will be placed on the ducts and tissue. Pressure on these could lead to deformities or reduce milk flow. Incisions under the arm are also less likely to interfere with signals or production compared to incisions around the nipple.[7] Moreover, there is no evidence to suggest that implants are harmful to infants. One study in the 1990s reported instances of oesophageal dysfunction in children whose mothers had implants,[8] but no further clinical problems have been reported. Of course, dysfunction after implants will also depend on why the procedure was conducted. If it was to alter the appearance of hypoplastic breasts, this will not change the underlying issue of lack of glandular tissue.

Maternal illness

There are a small number of maternal health issues that can impact upon milk supply. Note that this is typically about a reduction (or in some cases an increase) in supply, and not about a total inability to produce any milk at all. The most common disorders that can affect milk supply are:

Hypothyroidism

Some women with hypothyroidism may experience delayed onset of full milk production or produce a lower level of milk.[9] One mechanism for this is thought to be lower levels of prolactin when thyroid levels are not managed well, although more data is needed.[10] However, if their thyroid is being well managed with the correct dose of medication, then the risk is much lower. Some research suggests that thyroid levels must be supported to be in the upper regions of normal, rather than just within the accepted boundaries, as some medics may suggest. There is some evidence that a diet low in iodine during pregnancy can increase the risk of iodine deficiency, which in turn can impact thyroid function and breastmilk production.[11] However, mothers with hypothyroidism can be supported to maximise their milk supply.

Diabetes

A number of studies highlight a link between maternal diabetes, low milk supply and breastfeeding cessation.[12] Women who experienced gestational diabetes may also be at increased risk of low milk supply. One study specifically looked at mothers who reported low milk supply but no latch or nipple problems, finding that 15% of these mothers had diabetes during pregnancy compared to around 3–5% of all pregnant women.[13] However, mothers who have had gestational diabetes can be supported to boost their supply.

It is important to disentangle any physiological impact of diabetes on breastmilk production and the postnatal experiences of breastfeeding women with diabetes. As we shall see in the next chapter, birth interventions and complications increase the risk of low milk supply and feeding difficulties. Mothers with diabetes may be at more risk of interventions and complications due to concerns about infant macrosomia (large babies).[14] Mothers with diabetes are at an increased risk of having a high BMI, which in turn can increase the risk of low prolactin levels, as progesterone is stored in fat tissue.[15]

However, diabetes can have a direct impact too, predominantly when it is not under control. Research has found that when mothers have elevated fasting insulin, insulin resistance or elevated fasting plasma glucose, they are more likely to report insufficient milk supply.[16] Lower oestrogen levels during breastfeeding can increase the risk of hypoglycaemia, which in turn increases production of adrenaline, which can inhibit letdown.[17]

Polycystic ovary syndrome (PCOS)
Some women with PCOS can experience a reduced milk supply. Again, it can be difficult to identify the exact pathway. There is a strong correlation between overweight, obesity and PCOS, meaning that physiologically it could be obesity that impacts on breastmilk production rather than PCOS directly.[18] However, women with PCOS often have higher levels of circulating androgens prior to pregnancy, which can impede milk production by down-regulating oestrogen and prolactin receptors.[19]

It has also been hypothesised that lower levels of progesterone and oestrogen during adolescence (which are lower among women with PCOS) may affect breast growth, particularly in terms of ductal and alveolar growth development. In one case study, a mother with PCOS and insufficient glandular tissue who struggled to breastfeed her first baby was treated with progesterone therapy and increased her milk supply with her next baby.[20]

When is breastfeeding contraindicated even though possible?

A second group of women will be advised not to breastfeed due to health issues with themselves or their baby. Again, these situations tend to be rare, although as we will see later in the book, it appears to be more common for a woman to be *told* she must not breastfeed her baby due to an illness, procedure or medication than it is for her to actually be taking a medication or have an illness that is contraindicated. So when is breastfeeding not advised?

Infant factors

In infants, rare disorders such as galactosaemia (when infants are missing the enzymes needed to digest lactase and galactose in milk) mean that a specialist diet is needed. In other disorders such as phenylketonuria, when individuals can't break down a certain part of a protein, partial breastfeeding can be continued with monitoring, as breastmilk is naturally low in phenylalanine.[21] Conversely, while special circumstances such as cleft lip and palate, or Down's syndrome, can make breastfeeding more challenging, they should not preclude all affected infants from being breastfed.[22]

Maternal illness

There are a small number of typically rare maternal illnesses that contraindicate breastfeeding, including human T-cell lymphotrophic virus, untreated brucellosis, and Ebola. One illness that causes a lot of debate is HIV, as there is a risk of the virus passing to the infant. In countries where there is no safe water supply, sanitation or a guaranteed ongoing supply of formula, the risk from HIV and other viruses is lower than the risk of not being breastfed and mothers should breastfeed exclusively (as reflected in international guidelines).[23] In developed regions, where there is access to formula and safe conditions to sterilise bottles and teats, women are usually advised not to breastfeed, unless their baby is known to already be infected with HIV. For example the British HIV Association states that HIV positive mothers should exclusively formula-feed from birth. However, they, alongside the American Academy of Pediatrics, also stipulate that if mothers do decide to breastfeed then they should be supported to do so, as long as the mother takes antiretroviral therapy (ART) and is regularly tested to make sure her viral load is low.

Research has shown that when a mother takes ART the risk of her passing HIV to her baby is almost negligible. Women should also be given high-quality support to reduce risk of complications. Open sores such as those caused by thrush or cracked nipples can increase the risk of transmission. Breastfeeding should also be exclusive as formula can lead to small lesions in the gut wall, which can mean the HIV virus can cross into the bloodstream. Evidence around continuation after six months (or when solids are introduced) is unclear. Research suggests around a 2% transmission rate if breastfeeding is continued to one year and beyond.[24]

For other illnesses, although mother and baby might be separated or direct breastfeeding not advised, infants can safely be given expressed milk. For example, active untreated tuberculosis or chicken pox infection dictates a mother's separation from her baby for infection control, although the rate of transmission through breastmilk is actually quite low. Herpes infection, although very serious in infants, does not stop babies being breastfed unless there are active lesions on or near the nipple.[22] Separation in hospital has been recommended for active flu infection, although critics argue that the risk of separation may outweigh the risk of infection.[25]

Viruses which sound like they would prevent breastfeeding are often not contraindicated, as they do not enter breastmilk to a sufficient degree. These include rubella, hepatitis B and C, cytomegalovirus and West Nile virus. Likewise, evidence emerging during the COVID-19 (coronavirus) pandemic indicates that the virus does not pass into breastmilk.[22] Indeed, for many infectious illnesses, such as COVID-19 or flu, breastfeeding or breastmilk feeding is strongly recommended, as although the infection may not be detectable in breastmilk, antibodies from maternal infection are likely offering infants protection.[26]

Medications and medical procedures

Certain medications are also contraindicated during breastfeeding. However, it is not as many as you might think, and often women are advised against taking medications during pregnancy and lactation based on general warnings because of a lack of testing due to ethical implications of testing on pregnant or breastfeeding women, rather than proof that the substances will have an effect on the baby. Although the majority of medications (prescribed, over the counter and illicit) will pass to some extent into breastmilk, only a few are actually deemed unsafe for infants in terms of how much passes through and whether it will affect the infant. The impact can also depend on the age of the infant; smaller infants will be affected by lower amounts and younger infants will be consuming more breastmilk compared to those also eating solid foods.[27]

Medications that should be avoided include lithium, atropine, bromocriptine and iodides, but usually a safe alternative can be found. Some (but not all) immunosuppressive and anti-inflammatory drugs should not be taken. Chemotherapy is unsafe for infants, as its action is to stop cells growing and dividing, meaning it could impact upon infant growth. Radiotherapy is also contraindicated. However, duration and type of treatment is important. Indium, for example, is only present in milk for 20 hours, whereas gallium can be present for two weeks. Mothers may wish to temporarily stop breastfeeding but continue expressing and discarding breastmilk to maintain their supply, with the aim of recommencing once treatment is finished.[27]

In terms of painkillers, paracetamol and ibuprofen should not impact the infant. Breastfeeding mothers should avoid aspirin, as there is a small risk of bleeding, circulatory problems and Reye syndrome in infants who ingest it. Recent research has also indicated that codeine should be avoided unless other pain relief options have not worked. Codeine is converted into morphine in the liver by the enzyme CYP2D6, but some people have different variations of that enzyme meaning they metabolise the drug differently and therefore have different levels of morphine in their system. Some people will find the drug provides strong relief and may make them drowsy, while others feel no effects. Infants whose mothers have high levels are at risk of becoming drowsy or experiencing respiratory depression. Opioids are potentially linked to an increased risk of sudden infant death syndrome (SIDS), although the impact is not clear.[28]

Debate continues surrounding psychotropic drugs such as those taken for anxiety, depression or epilepsy. Often results are based on small case studies of women who did not inform their prescriber that they were breastfeeding, or continued to take the medication alongside breastfeeding. Some further medications need to be treated with caution, particularly those that might have a sedative effect, as they can cause heavy sedation and even withdrawal symptoms in infants. However, despite these caveats the vast majority of antidepressant and anxiety medications have no reported or possible effects on infants (although for some (e.g. fluoxetine) infant irritability or slow weight gain has been reported. Generally medications appear in breastmilk in low concentrations, although they may remain in the infant's system for quite a long time, which might cause problems for very young infants with developing renal function. However, where there is no significant evidence of harm, the best approach may be to weigh up the protection of being breastfed against the potential unknown risk to the infant. Maternal mental health is no minor factor either. If a mother wants to breastfeed, continuing to do so while taking medication may protect her wellbeing and ensure she interacts positively with her infant.[29]

Finally, the impact of any medication upon milk supply should be considered. For example, although decongestants are safe for the infant, evidence suggests that they can reduce milk supply, particularly when mothers have older infants who are feeding less frequently.[30]

Maternal lifestyle

Finally, there are a number of lifestyle factors that might affect the safety of breastmilk or breastfeeding. The evidence for recreational drugs is mixed. Impact can come both from the effect of the drug passing into milk, and the effect on caring for the infant. The safety of street drugs and how they are prepared is also an issue, as the content and safety of whatever has been taken will be unknown. Specifically, women who have taken cocaine are advised not to breastfeed, as it passes into breastmilk. However, for a one-off event, the drug will also leave the milk after around 72 hours, meaning she can recommence feeding. Conversely, prescribed methadone appears to have no impact.[31]

For cannabis, the evidence is less clear. The active ingredient tetrahydrocannabinol does get into breastmilk and can affect infants. Infants may be very sleepy, which can affect feeding and weight gain. They are also at higher risk of SIDS. Animal research suggests it may adversely affect brain and motor development, although little research has been conducted on human infants. Ingesting cannabis removes the impact of associated second and third-hand smoke upon the infant, but leads to greater amounts being ingested and therefore potentially impacting the baby more harshly. Cannabis is also stored in body fat and released slowly into the bloodstream and therefore breastmilk. Some evidence suggests breastmilk can end up with up to eight times the level in the mother's body.[32]

For smoking cigarettes, nicotine does enter the breastmilk in small amounts, increasing the risk of infants being unsettled or suffering from colic. Mothers who smoke have lower levels of prolactin, which can lead to a lower milk supply and poorer letdown, making breastfeeding more difficult. However a main effect of smoking is the increased risk of second and third-hand smoke for the infant and therefore if mothers do smoke, it is recommended that they continue breastfeeding. Smoking around infants increases the risk of respiratory and ear infections, alongside the risk of SIDS. However, breastfeeding may reduce the impact; research with mothers who smoke shows that infants who were breastfed had lower levels of respiratory infections than those who were formula-fed. Nicotine replacement patches are safer than direct smoking due to an absence of smoke and chemicals and a lower level of nicotine in the bloodstream.[33]

Alcohol is considered safe for infants in lower amounts. The level of alcohol in breastmilk will match the mother's *blood* alcohol level, not the level in the alcohol she consumes. For example, a 175ml glass of 11% wine is approximately two units. For an average-sized woman, that would lead to a blood alcohol level of 0.04. Drinks that have an alcohol level of 0.05% and lower are considered alcohol free, while those between 0.5% and 1.2% are considered low alcohol. Limited research suggests that alcohol consumption can make infants sleepy, weak and slow to gain weight, as it may interfere with the milk ejection reflex. However, this effect is only seen with regular maternal blood levels over 300 mg/dl, which equates to around a whole bottle of wine for an average-sized woman.[34]

Caffeine does enter breastmilk but at a low level; a level of 1% of caffeine ingested can be found in breastmilk. However, different infants may react in different ways, with smaller and younger infants most affected. It can take over 80 hours for a newborn to metabolise the caffeine they ingest, but older infants will do so within 2–3 hours. Research suggests that mothers need to ingest over 750mg a day for any significant impact on the infant (approximately five standard-sized cups of coffee, although caffeine is also found in tea, sports drinks and chocolate). However, the main impact on infants will be increased fussiness and shorter sleep duration rather than any significant long-term impact.[35]

Finally, things like using fake tan or face cream, teeth whitening and getting a tattoo are fine. They do not reach the breastmilk, although many practitioners will not tattoo breastfeeding women because of the potential infection risk and need for antibiotics.[27]

If in doubt, there are several useful resources for checking medications, procedures and other substances:

- Pharmacist Dr Wendy Jones – her books include *Why Mothers' Medication Matters*, *Breastfeeding and Medication* and *Breastfeeding for the Medical Profession*.
- Breastfeeding Network Drugs in Breastmilk Service – for factsheets and one-to-one support for medications and procedures: www. breastfeedingnetwork.org.uk/detailed-information/drugs-in-breastmilk
- LactMed – for medications information: toxnet.nlm.nih.gov/ newtoxnet/lactmed.htm

Overall, there are a limited number of factors that can prevent mothers from breastfeeding, alongside physiological issues that can lead to primary lactation failure. The central issue, however, is the frequency with which these events occur, in comparison to the high numbers of women presenting with real or perceived milk insufficiency or inability to continue breastfeeding. Combined with the significantly different levels of breastfeeding initiation and continuation rates around the world, the finger strongly points at broader variations in environmental influences affecting women's ability to continue breastfeeding. Ultimately barriers at the social, cultural, political and economic levels are impeding women's ability to breastfeed, not their primary biology.

But those figures are so different? What's going on?

You'd be right in thinking at this point that something strange is going on. If we take any of those estimates from 0.1–5% of women unable to physiologically breastfeed, even if we add a bit of wiggle room, there is still a huge difference between those figures and the number of women who have to stop breastfeeding before they are ready. The Infant Feeding Survey only asked mothers who stopped breastfeeding in the first six weeks whether they were ready to stop feeding or not. Of those, 80% were not ready, suggesting they were experiencing issues outside their control. That gives me a figure of approximately 40% of women who start breastfeeding stopping before they are ready in the first six weeks.

Then you have those who weren't ready to stop after that date. And that's before we tie ourselves in knots trying to work out what percentage of the women who formula-fed from birth would have had difficulties if they had started. Let's just say that *a lot* of women in the UK are not able to breastfeed for as long as they want. We could go for at least half for simplicity's sake. Whatever the number, it does beg the question – what on earth is going on?

To answer that we have to look to our society. This is made up of a complex web of factors that influence women's feeding decisions in a million and one different ways. At the heart of it, we simply have a poor understanding of how breastfeeding works. Think about it. The majority of babies in the UK have had some formula milk by the end of their first week of life. A third have had it by the end of their first day. Formula is actually our normal, even if we don't say this in health promotion campaigns.

This means that although many people may be outwardly supportive of breastfeeding, their actual experience, which they can share with others, and which drives their attitudes and knowledge, is of formula-feeding. If fewer than 1% of mothers exclusively breastfeed for six months in the UK, this means that nearly all of them have experience of bottle-feeding, compared to only half who have experience of any breastfeeding past six weeks old. And if you trace that back through the generations, we're likely talking far fewer.

Now add to this the fact that although both are used to feed a baby, breastmilk and formula milk, and indeed breastfeeding and formula-feeding, are actually quite different in all sorts of ways. Milk differs in content and digestibility, the method of feeding varies and ultimately baby behaviour can be different. However, given the normality and visibility of formula-feeding in our culture, it is very easy to see why formula-feeding is viewed as the 'normal' behaviour – after all, it is the most common behaviour after a few weeks of life. Industry and 'experts' facilitate these beliefs. Older family members, who likely fed their babies at a time when breastfeeding was even less common, lack knowledge of breastfeeding too. And mothers can get really anxious when their breastfed baby isn't acting like their friend's formula-fed baby. Consequently, many mothers find that they 'didn't have enough milk' or 'couldn't breastfeed'.

But this knowledge is only half the story. Research has shown that many different factors are involved in whether a woman decides to start or carry on breastfeeding. These include physical events, pressure from others, lifestyle issues and pressure from society to act in a certain way. Many of these issues affect a woman psychologically, but many can also have a physical impact on her ability to breastfeed. As we saw earlier, breastfeeding works best when done 'responsively' – whenever the baby wants. Skipping, replacing or stretching out the time between feeds can damage a woman's milk supply because her body thinks milk is not needed and adjusts supply accordingly. In the end this can lead to a reduced milk supply and mothers feeling that they 'couldn't breastfeed'.

In cultures that are completely removed from the day-to-day norms of Western life, reasons for stopping breastfeeding are typically physiological. One study that explored influences on stopping breastfeeding in a rural, impoverished tribe in East Africa found that all babies were breastfed for at least six months, 90% breastfed for at least a year and 75% breastfed until two years. Reasons for stopping breastfeeding before two years included maternal illness, pregnancy, needing to go on a long journey or the child being able to eat the diet of the tribe.[36] Not once did a mother mention that their mother-in-law suggested the baby was waking too frequently, or that someone had commented on how inappropriate it was to breastfeed in public. Or told her to go on a diet. Or get back to work.

Compare this to our experience of trying to breastfeed a baby in Western culture. Feeding on demand is crucial to good milk supply, but babies are often not fed on demand. How often does a baby not feed because there is biologically no milk for him? Rarely (although not never). Compare this to how many a times a breastfeed is delayed, replaced or skipped because…

- Your mother tells you that she fed you every four hours and you

are fine
- Your mother-in-law insists on holding the baby a little longer and not giving him back
- Your partner wants to bond with the baby and sees feeding as the only way
- You buy a book that tells you when babies should be fed (and it's not now)
- You feel so exhausted your health visitor suggests your partner does a feed
- A mother at baby clinic asks if your milk is enough because he's feeding so much
- Society can't handle a woman using her breasts in public so you use a bottle
- A difficult labour meant that you were exhausted and sore
- Society insisted you needed to 'get your life back' by being out and about
- Your employment contract or pay meant that you had to be back at work
- Your friends without children want you to go out for a 'break from the baby'

None of these things directly say 'you must not breastfeed' or directly physically damage your milk supply. But all of them mean that the baby isn't breastfed *when they need breastfeeding*. A feed is missed, or delayed, or a bottle of formula is given in place of breastfeeding. A drop in milk supply can happen. And thus breastfeeding ends. And mothers feel guilty that they were 'unable' to breastfeed when in fact so many obstacles were thrown in their way.

The problem with the list above is that many people do not realise that this is happening, or that it is a problem. Many people are immune to the subtle messages that breastfeeding women receive every day, which suggest that they are not 'acceptable' in public. Many do not realise the practical impact such messages can have on a mother feeding her baby. Many think that a woman can simply 'feed her baby before she leaves the house', or 'just give a bottle in public'.

In a society that understood, encouraged and protected breastfeeding, none of these things would happen. All of those things should be avoidable and – importantly – avoidable by *other people*, not the woman who is trying to feed her baby. All of these things make life for a breastfeeding mother a daily challenge. Something else she has to fight against. Another straw on the camel's back. What if we lived in a society in which a mother's role is to feed her baby when it needs feeding, and the rest of the world supports her in doing that? What if…

- Rather than wanting to feed the baby himself, dad cooks a lovely meal for everyone (which kind of feeds the baby anyway)?
- Your mother passes the baby back to you and makes you a cup of tea (with biscuits)?
- Society just gets on with their coffee, cake and gossip and doesn't even notice a mother breastfeeding her baby as it's so normal?
- Friends come round to the house, tidy up a bit and hold the sleeping baby for you while you have a moment hands-free?
- Someone writes a parenting manual that simply says 'Feed and cuddle your baby whenever you both want. The End' (short book maybe, but priceless).

And this is the essence of what this book is about. Exploring the factors that conspire against a mother's ability to feed her baby. Exploring the complexities of how normal patterns of breastfeeding become damaged and thinking about what we can do about it. Yes, 'we' – because this is not just about new mothers. As we have seen, it's not only mothers who should be shouldering the blame for the low breastfeeding rates in many Western countries. If we want more babies to be breastfed, we need to figure out how we make the world a breastfeeding friendly place. And stop telling mothers that 'breast is best', then tripping them up at the first hurdle.

4. HAVE THINGS ALWAYS BEEN THIS WAY?

A BRIEF HISTORY OF INFANT FEEDING

To understand where we are now, it helps to look back at what has happened to shape our attitudes, expectations and understanding of how babies are fed. If we understand the influences and messages women have been given over the past century, it is much easier to see why breastfeeding rates, attitudes and support are as dire as they are now.

Obviously, things have not always been this way. We are mammals and therefore evolved to feed our babies using our mammary glands. This seemingly obvious fact appears to be one that some people have forgotten or choose to ignore. And if you look back through historical texts and records, it's clear that breastfeeding was once normal, encouraged and even recognised as supporting health. For example, in both the UK and USA breastmilk was considered to have medicinal properties, curing infections. References can be found to it being used to cure eye infections – something we still often recommend today. Breastfeeding was very much seen as more than simply providing a baby with nutrition, and was in fact seen as the ultimate expression of love and care for an infant.[1]

Many references to breastfeeding exist in religious texts and scriptures. For example, the primary sacred text of Hinduism, the Vedas (1800 BC) consists of four texts – Rig Veda, Sama Veda, Yajur Veda and Atharva Veda, which have many references to breastmilk, the breast and wet nursing. This is also reflected in other Ayurvedic writings including that by Acharya Charak who is considered the father of medicine.[2] Breastmilk is seen as a nectar, providing life and longevity. For example, when the god Shiva creates Parvarti a baby boy out of her dress, he only comes to life when she puts him to her breast. Many references are also made to caring for breastfeeding women and increasing breastmilk production through special foods such as dahl, eggplant and dried fish, and supporting her to rest, recover and take care of her baby.[3]

Reference to breastfeeding, and support for it, is also seen in Islam. For example, the Koran states that mothers should be encouraged to breastfeed for two years and it is a responsibility of the father to care for her and enable that. Breastmilk is seen as belonging to the baby – it is God's gift and a way of passing on the mother's wealth onto the baby. Some Muslim women believe they will be punished if they do not breastfeed and fulfil this obligation.[4] Support is also evident for breastfeeding through explicit permission to be exempt from fasting during the month of Ramadan.[5]

Outside of religious texts, other historical documents also contain references to breastfeeding, including supporting breastfeeding mothers or ways to increase breastmilk production. For example, Aristostle viewed breastfeeding as a maternal duty, while the Papyrus Ebers, written by the ancient Egyptians, is the earliest known medical encyclopaedia, dating from around 1550BC. It includes this suggestion for increasing milk supply:[6]

> 'To get a supply of milk in a woman's breast for suckling a child: Warm the bones of a swordfish in oil and rub her back with it. Or: Let the woman sit cross legged and eat fragrant bread of soused durra, while rubbing the parts with the poppy plant.'

Any takers for the swordfish bones? No? What this does show, though, is that breastfeeding was supported and encouraged and that effort was made to solve problems. Now that isn't to say it was perfect. Some women still wouldn't produce enough milk, some babies still wouldn't latch and of course many women died in childbirth. It wasn't all idyllic. Many babies were fed inappropriate substitute foods such as 'pap' (essentially flour and water). Many babies died. In some ways therefore, the invention in later years of formula milks prevented the unnecessary deaths of these babies, while simultaneously creating more lower-level issues in others. Of course, this was only true in developed nations where families had access to formula milks, clean water and the ability to prepare bottles safely – as noted previously, the introduction of formula milks into areas without these resources has been catastrophic.[6]

Historically it was more common to use a wet nurse: another woman who would breastfeed a baby. Sometimes a family member or caregiver would act as a wet nurse if a mother died or could not breastfeed. Some babies were sent to a wet nurse who would be responsible for feeding a number of babies, even caring for them in her home. Conversely, among affluent families a wet nurse was often employed to live with the family – a relatively well-paid position for the times. References can be seen to infants being wet nursed in the Papyrus Ebers, texts from the Roman Empire and throughout the Middle Ages and Renaissance. Wet nurses were employed to allow the affluent wife to rest, or because feeding and childcare was seen as 'work', but often commonly because the contraceptive effects of breastfeeding were recognised even back then. Fertility and the ability to produce numerous children was seen as a sign of vitality and success and some men wished to impregnate their wives as often as possible, which would be made less likely by breastfeeding.[7]

However, wet nurses may also have nursed poorer women's babies when they had to leave the baby to seek work. We also know that wet nurses were not always employed or cared for. Particularly in American history, as noted earlier, some black African slaves were forced into wet nursing for their 'master', either for his own children or those of other slaves so he could profit from their work.[8]

However, even among more affluent families, wet nursing wasn't always fully accepted and during the 16th and 17th century questions started to be raised about the bond between a woman and a nursing child, suggesting that love and connection could exist between them. Some also believed that a woman's 'character' was passed to the nursing child and saw this as risky or unacceptable, especially if the woman was of a lower class or a servant. There were also concerns around infections or illnesses being passed on.[9]

At around this time historical records start to show an increase in feeding artefacts made from clay, wood, ceramics or even animal horns. Some were more open, others had more of a spout and all were most likely used to feed a variety of animal milks. Some of these items were found buried alongside the remains of young infants, suggesting that animal milk was used from a young age, potentially contributing to their death. Of course, there would likely have been issues with the safety of the milk used, and the ability to clean these vessels. We know now that milks from other animals are not directly suited to the needs of human infants; mammalian milk varies significantly in terms of fat, energy and protein content (alongside other factors) to meet the needs of the growing infant it was designed for.[10]

By the 19th century scientists were starting to look at the differences between animal and human milk and realised that infants who were breastfed were more likely to survive and thrive. It was also clear that when infants could not be breastfed and a wet nurse could not be found, that this could be catastrophic to health. A consequence of this, alongside growing industrialisation of food, was the creation of the first infant formula milk. In 1865, a chemist called Justus von Liebig created the first infant milk – first in liquid and then in powdered form – which consisted of cows' milk, wheat and malt flour and potassium bicarbonate. He called it 'Liebig's formula' and it was thought to be the perfect infant food. In 1810 Nicholas Appert had worked out how to sterilise food in steel containers, and by the end of the 19th century there were around 27 different types of patented infant formula, consisting of cows' milk with various added sugars, starches and dextrins. Numerous feeding bottles, teats and other apparatus were also developed alongside infant formula.[11]

By the start of the 20th century, marketing of these milks had become hugely successful. One key element was that these formula milks were seen to promote weight and growth in infants. It is understandable why; many had added cereals or other carbohydrates and were based on cows' milk, which contained significantly more protein than breastmilk. Both encourage rapid growth in infants, which at the time was seen as the main indicator of health (and is an irritating legacy we are still battling now). These milks started to gain the support of various physicians and childcare 'experts' who promoted them as the ultimate nutrition for infants. Further improvements in technology led to increased production.

However, this proliferation of formula milks proved devastating for some infants. Many babies died unnecessarily, particularly in the summer months, as there was little understanding of how bacteria proliferated. Families would use unclean receptacles to feed their infants, or leave milk out for hours in hot weather. Once germ theory was developed and understood, the safety of formula milk improved: milk was chilled in iceboxes and washable rubber nipples were designed. Infant mortality rates declined. This meant that by the 1940s formula milk was seen as safe, scientific and by some even better than breastmilk. Doctors advised mothers to use it not only if they could not breastfeed, but instead of breastfeeding. Science was seen as superior to anything the human body could produce.

The medicalisation of childbirth in the 1940s and 1950s further exacerbated the issue. Many women were now giving birth in hospitals and remaining there for up to two weeks to recover after birth. This meant that the influence of doctors and hospital routines was extremely strong.[12] Advertising of formula milk brands directly to hospitals and doctors was common, and later on milks would be directly advertised to parents (more on this in chapter 16).

When women were breastfeeding, they were often recommended to feed to a strict four-hourly routine (for more discussion see chapter 10). For example, the so-called childcare expert physician Walter Sackette, who published a book in 1953 called *Bringing up babies; a family doctor's practical approach to child care*, believed that babies should be breastfed around hospital routines. Specifically, he believed they should be breastfed only at 6am, 12pm, 6pm and 12am, as those times were *'the most workable ones in keeping with hospital routine'*. However, by three weeks he advised that the 12am feed should be dropped *'...having fully served its purpose, which was not to pacify the infant but his parents, grandparents, neighbours and doubting friends'*. He also believed infants should be starting on solid foods within days after birth.[13]

Somewhat unsurprisingly, by the 1970s in the UK very few babies were breastfed; only around 25% by the end of the first week, with just 18% exclusively breastfed by the time they were discharged from hospital.[14] Although rates have been steadily climbing since that point, is it any wonder we are where we are? When we stopped breastfeeding, we lost generations of embodied knowledge and skill passed down from woman to woman over time. Our knowledge was replaced by how to use formula and bottle-feed – which is very different to breastfeeding. And not only did we lose our knowledge of breastfeeding, we stopped seeing it too. It became unusual, something rarely seen, and as is so often the case we then stopped accepting it. We had also, consciously or not, passed responsibility for how our babies are fed to an industry that profited enormously from mothers.

The remainder of this book will explore what is currently influencing breastfeeding in the UK and what we can all do to bring things back to where they need to be.

5. OUR BIRTH EXPERIENCES CAN INTERFERE WITH GETTING BREASTFEEDING OFF TO A GOOD START

In 2015 my friend recently had kittens (or rather, my friend's *cat* had kittens). When it was time for the cat to give birth, she disappeared, as many cats do, only to be found somewhere safe and warm (in the wardrobe). She went on to give birth there and stayed cuddled up with her new kittens for some time. The kittens latched on after birth and stayed close to mum, feeding whenever possible for the next few weeks.

Compare this to the experience many mothers have of birth, particularly first-time mothers. Birth, for many women, is *not* in a warm, familiar and comfortably lit place. Women usually go into labour at home and then need to travel to hospital, where there are bright lights, noise and general hustle and bustle. Some will feel anxious about going into a hospital that they associate with ill health. Stress levels rise and levels of the good hormones that help labour along fall. Our modern lives may have evolved to let us google cats in boxes at a moment's notice on our phones, but essentially we are still animals with instincts underneath it all. And when animals are disturbed during labour, their labour slows down or stops, as they think it might be unsafe to give birth. The same happens for women in labour. If we feel stressed our body slows things down and we often need intervention to speed it back up again.

Where am I going with this tale of kittens? I am not suggesting you give birth in the back of a wardrobe, but start to think about how our experiences of giving birth affect our ability to breastfeed. Normal birth is known to set both mother and baby up for the best start in their new lives, but it can also have a pretty big impact on their breastfeeding experience. Of course, interventions during childbirth can be lifesaving. But childbirth is getting more and more complicated. Only 45% of women in the UK now give birth vaginally with no intervention to speed up labour or get the baby out. Far more have some kind of pain relief in childbirth. And this can have a knock-on effect on breastfeeding, both physiologically and psychologically. How the baby is delivered, any interventions during labour, and medications that a mother might receive can all interfere with breastfeeding. Getting birth right is not only important for mother and baby's initial health, but also what happens to them in the longer term. A normal birth is a very positive step in getting breastfeeding off to a good start.

To begin thinking about labour, birth and breastfeeding we need to go back to thinking about breastfeeding from a hormonal perspective. The hormones prolactin and oxytocin are the good guys. They are involved in the progression of birth and breastmilk production. The stress hormones cortisol, epinephrine and adrenaline are not. Stress hormones not only make labour more difficult, but can also interfere with the production of prolactin and oxytocin, which in turn interferes with the production of breastmilk. Stress in labour is unfortunately very common, made worse by a long labour, a lot of pain, interventions and anxiety.

Caesarean section

Around a quarter of babies in the UK are now born by caesarean section. In the USA it is around a third. Many studies have shown that if a baby is born by caesarean section they are less likely to be breastfed.[1] Why depends in part on the reason why the caesarean was performed in the first place. Some babies can be distressed, particularly if they have become so during labour. Breathing difficulties are also more common among babies born by caesarean. In turn mothers may be ill, experiencing further complications or simply exhausted after a traumatic delivery. All of this means that perhaps babies do not have immediate skin-to-skin, or are not fed straight away. They may even be taken away from their mother, needing medical assistance. When babies are born by elective caesarean they are more likely to be breastfed than those babies born by emergency caesarean.

A caesarean section can also make it more difficult for a mother to breastfeed effectively after birth because she may have restricted movement or be in pain. This can make her more reluctant to pick the baby up, or she may need someone else to pass her the baby, meaning that perhaps her baby isn't fed as frequently, or has to wait a little longer for a feed. This can mean that the baby becomes more distressed as he thinks he isn't going to be fed, so when he is, it is more difficult to latch him on. When a mother can pick her baby up she might find it more painful to hold the baby in a comfortable position to get an effective latch, meaning feeds are longer or the baby seems unsettled. She may be more likely to feel exhausted after the birth (especially if there were complications) and others, well-meaning or otherwise, may leave her to sleep, giving the baby 'one bottle' while she recovers.[2]

A caesarean can also have a physiological impact on breastfeeding. Mothers who have a caesarean don't have such a strong release of oxytocin and prolactin after the birth, meaning milk production can be delayed as the body takes a while to realise it has given birth.[3] Likewise, another study found that prolactin levels did not rise as much in response to the infant breastfeeding after birth among women who had a caesarean section.[4]

Skin-to-skin after the birth is less likely, which can also interfere with oxytocin production. Mothers who don't have skin-to-skin with their baby after birth release lower levels of oxytocin than those who do,[4] alongside higher levels of stress hormones (which in turn can block oxytocin).[5] And indeed, when mothers who have a caesarean section do have opportunity for skin-to-skin straight after delivery, research shows that they have higher rates of exclusive breastfeeding in hospital, which extend to six months and beyond.[6] However, one study found that levels of oxytocin during skin-to-skin were low among women who had a planned caesarean before labour started, suggesting the importance of the physiological process of labour in supporting oxytocin release after birth.[7]

This is particularly true during an emergency caesarean, when stress levels are likely to be high. One study that took blood samples during pregnancy, birth and breastfeeding found that women who had an emergency caesarean delivery had far higher levels of stress hormones in their blood. In turn these women were more likely to experience breast fullness later than other women, and when they measured milk volume on day three, these women were producing less milk than the less stressed women.[8] Another fascinating study suggested that mothers who had high levels of cortisol postnatally were more likely to have infants reported to have a difficult temperament than those with lower levels. However, the effect was only seen when breastfeeding, suggesting that cortisol might possibly affect the infant through the milk, making them more restless.[9]

Babies who are born by caesarean may also have more difficulties latching on to the breast. In one study that visually assessed the feeding behaviours of mothers after birth using the LATCH criteria (Latch on breast, Audible swallowing, Type of nipple, Comfort breast/nipple and Hold) found that mothers who had a caesarean section found latching their baby on and holding them more difficult compared to those who had a vaginal birth.[10] Another study used ultrasound to see what was happening with the babies' tongues and suckling during feeding. Babies who had been born by caesarean section showed less variation in tongue movement and faster suckling compared to babies born vaginally, suggesting they find it more difficult to latch effectively. An incorrect latch means milk is not removed efficiently, meaning less milk will be produced.[11] Indeed, studies that have controlled for the impact of fewer feeds and latching difficulties find that once these are taken into account, the impact of a caesarean section on breastfeeding is much less. This suggests that with enhanced support, mode of birth should not have a large impact upon feeding experience.[12]

Babies may also be sleepier if born by caesarean section, as they don't experience the pressure of being pushed through the birth canal. This experience might 'wake them up' a little, making them more responsive to feeding. One experimental study of rat pups showed that this might be the case by attempting to simulate a vaginal birth during a rat caesarean section. They pulled half the rat pups through a rubber ring while still in the womb, before delivering them by caesarean section. The pups that were pulled through a ring started feeding sooner than those not pulled through a ring.[13] I have absolutely no idea how you come up with that design for an experiment, but it shows that birth experience may be more important for breastfeeding than we realise.

Assisted delivery

Babies who are born by assisted delivery (forceps or ventouse) are also less likely to be breastfed at two weeks.[14] Around 12% of babies are now born this way. Many babies have some bruising to the head. This can interfere with their ability to latch on effectively at the breast and suckle because they are so sore.[15] Women who have had a traumatic delivery may also be sore and find certain positions uncomfortable if they have had lots of stitches.

Assisted delivery can be traumatic for the baby. One study measured cortisol levels in umbilical cord blood and found that those born by assisted delivery had higher levels than those born by normal delivery.[16] Another study looked at babies' stress response – in terms of duration of crying and amount of cortisol produced – to inoculations at eight weeks, dependent on their mode of birth.[17] Baseline cortisol levels before the injections were the same in all babies, but the babies who had been born by assisted delivery had the greatest rise in cortisol and also cried for longer after inoculation. It is possible that these higher stress levels make babies more unsettled and trickier to feed, or it may simply be the case that their restless temperament is blamed on breastfeeding.

Pain relief

Medications that babies are exposed to during labour can impact on their ability to feed. Around a third of women in the UK have an epidural during birth and around a quarter use opiate-based medications such as pethidine. Both epidurals and pethidine are linked to lower breastfeeding rates for a number of reasons.

Pethidine

Pethidine is given as a pain-killing injection. It can pass to the baby and make them very sleepy at birth. Mothers who receive pethidine are less likely to breastfeed at birth or be breastfeeding at three days.[18] Babies who have been exposed to pethidine tend to take longer to first latch onto the breast, and when they do latch on, they can find it very difficult. Their suckling seems to be weaker, and they are less likely to root around trying to find a nipple. This weaker suckle can still be present at five days old.[19] The knock-on effects on breastfeeding take many forms: babies may be removing less milk from the breast due to a poor latch or weak suckle, or may take longer or seem more difficult to feed. This can increase a new mother's anxiety levels and concerns about her ability to produce milk. Formula top-ups might be suggested, which can further reduce supply and interfere with latch.

Remifentanil

Remifentanil is another opioid painkiller but has a short half-life. Rather than being injected as a one-off by a health professional (as pethidine is) it is controlled by the patient. A small tube is placed in a woman's vein (although sometimes it is delivered intranasally – through the nose) and she can then press a button to receive a small amount of the drug. Although research is sparse as yet, being able to control their own levels of pain medication appears to promote feelings of control and satisfaction in women.[20]

One study compared breastfeeding outcomes for mothers based on whether they received pethidine or remifentanil. No differences were seen in initiation of breastfeeding within an hour of birth, but by six weeks after birth, 47% of women in the remifentanil group were breastfeeding compared to 26% in the pethidine group.[21] Another small study in Australia found fewer breastfeeding difficulties among those using remifentanil compared to pethidine.[22]

It is unclear why such a difference is occurring. One reason is that women seem more satisfied with the pain relief from remifentanil, and are less likely to go on to have an epidural. However, it is difficult to disentangle the effects of the drug from the effects of being in control of your own pain relief.[23] A Cochrane review of limited data also found a reduced occurrence of assisted delivery among those who had remifentanil compared to pethidine.[24]

Epidural

Women who have had an epidural are also less likely to breastfeed.[19] This may be because they had a difficult birth and are in more pain afterwards; indeed, the rate of assisted deliveries increases with an epidural which is in turn associated with feeding difficulties.[25] However, epidurals may also have a physiological effect. Mothers who give birth by caesarean, as we have seen, have a lowered oxytocin response. An interesting study also showed how oxytocin given during the birth affected women's behaviour. The researchers looked at whether mothers had oxytocin to start labour or after birth, and their behaviour on day two. Oxytocin is often known as the hormone of love and tends to make people more relaxed and friendly. They found that women who had received oxytocin had lower levels of anxiety and aggression and felt more sociable than those who didn't. However, if they had received an epidural, this effect wasn't seen.[26] Given we know that oxytocin is an important factor in breastmilk production, these results show how epidural use may impact on breastfeeding by blocking oxytocin. In animal studies, when oxytocin is blocked mothers typically don't show bonding behaviour, spending less time touching their babies and feeding them.[27] Women who have an epidural have lower levels of oxytocin circulating in their body during labour.[28] Additionally, epidural pain relief is associated with a lower level of prolactin release in response to feeding after birth. [29]

It is possible that the anaesthetic used in epidurals may interfere with the release of oxytocin after the birth. Epidurals work by injecting anaesthetic into the epidural space between the vertebrae in the lower back, blocking impulses and nerves that lead to pain. It is possible that the epidural may also block the nerves that trigger the release of oxytocin. The Ferguson reflex, which stimulates contractions during labour, is caused by the baby's head pressing on the cervix and leads to the release of oxytocin. Women who have had an epidural may be unable to feel this pressure, meaning less oxytocin is produced.[30] Women who have received an epidural have lower levels of oxytocin after birth, and are more likely to stop breastfeeding in the early days.[31]

Another study found that babies had poorer suckling behaviour when their mothers had an epidural.[32] Babies who have been exposed to epidural anaesthetic are less likely to latch on within the first hour and show less rooting and a poorer latch. This may lead to a delay in full milk production. Another study found a significant difference in infant sucking behaviour and subsequent breastfeeding depending on the dose of epidural used. When a lower dose was administered, infants had better muscle tone and sucking behaviour and were more likely to be breastfeeding at six weeks compared to those who received a higher dose.[33]

Other birth complications

The number of women experiencing complications during labour (such as needing to have their labour sped up, babies becoming distressed during labour or mothers losing a lot of blood after birth) is increasing. In one study we explored the different types of complications women had and whether they were breastfeeding at birth and two weeks. What we found was that the more complications a woman experienced, the less likely she was to be breastfeeding at two weeks. Somewhat unsurprisingly, the more complications mothers experienced, the bigger the impact on breastfeeding. And many mothers did experience more than one complication, in a good illustration of the 'cascade of interventions', in which one complication leads to another. Typically, mothers would be diagnosed as 'failing to progress', which led to their labour being sped up, foetal distress and an assisted or caesarean birth. You can imagine the knock-on effect, both physical and emotional, on these mothers.[14]

However, complications didn't seem to affect whether mothers tried to breastfeed at birth, suggesting that these women wanted to breastfeed, but something about their experience stopped them from continuing to do so. Of course, if a mother has a complicated delivery it is more likely that she will be separated from her baby after birth. This may be as simple as not holding the baby and missing out on skin-to-skin, or it might be more serious, with either mother or baby needing special care. There may also be hormonal forces at play.

However, in this study we didn't just look at whether she stopped breastfeeding or not, but also why she did so. Reasons were split into categories such as difficulty (baby won't latch), pain, pressure from others, body image, embarrassment and convenience. What we found was that certain complications were associated with stopping breastfeeding in particular because it was difficult or painful, rather than for other more social reasons, suggesting there was a biological explanation. Below are some of the complications we found were associated with increased breastfeeding difficulties and stopping breastfeeding.

Induction and augmentation of labour

There are a number of reasons why induction or augmentation of labour may increase breastfeeding difficulties. Some of these are related to the interventions that may follow; we know that when labour is induced, other complications can increase. We know labour can sometimes be more painful, increasing maternal stress and therefore reducing oxytocin. However, the medications used to induce or increase labour can interfere with natural hormone levels. For example, it is thought that artificially increasing oxytocin levels may interfere with the amount of oxytocin mothers naturally produce after the birth, or stress hormones may interfere with oxytocin production.[34] Likewise, prostaglandins, often used to induce labour, block the release of dopamine, reducing prolactin levels.[35]

In our research we found that women who needed to be induced or have their labour augmented were more likely to stop breastfeeding because of pain and physical problems.[14] Other research confirms these patterns, although not all research is conclusive. In one retrospective study of birth records in Wales, women who had been induced were less likely to be breastfeeding at day two.[36] Another study in Spain found that mothers who had their labours induced or augmented were less likely to be breastfeeding at three months.[37]

Further research questions whether induction and augmentation of labour may be associated with reduced suckling after birth and long-term feeding behaviours. A number of observational studies have found increased feeding difficulties among those who were induced or had their labour augmented, but both studies have serious limitations, either due to small sample size, or almost complete crossover with having an epidural during labour. However, it would make sense that the impact of synthetic hormones on future oxytocin and prolactin response would increase risk of feeding difficulties, especially because these medications can pass to the infant.[38]

Postpartum haemorrhage (PPH)

A PPH has also been associated with reduced breastfeeding in a number of studies. For example, we found that women who had a PPH were less likely to be breastfeeding at two weeks. Another study of women who had a PPH found that although 85% had intended to initiate breastfeeding, just 63% ended up doing so. An effect was also seen for amount of blood lost; 70% of those who lost less than 2,000ml were breastfeeding during the first week compared to 50% of those with a loss greater than 3,000ml.[39] Severe maternal anaemia or the need for a blood transfusion after birth has also been associated with the introduction of formula milk in the days after birth.[40]

If a mother has a severe bleed after the birth, this can affect milk supply. Blood loss can lead to low blood pressure, which in turn can affect hormone release, particularly prolactin. A PPH appears to affect functioning of the pituitary gland, which is responsible for prolactin release.[41] To stop a haemorrhage, mothers are usually given a high dose of oxytocin to contract the womb and stop the bleeding – this is essential to treat the mother. However, large doses of oxytocin might interfere with the body's ability to naturally go on to produce its own. Large doses of ergometrine may also block dopamine receptors and again reduce prolactin.[42] Increased stress is also likely to affect oxytocin levels. This can all interfere with milk production, with long-lasting effects. In one study of infants presenting with neonatal hypernatraemia, a quarter of mothers had a PPH.[43]

However there are also non-hormonal pathways. In the study of mothers who experienced a PPH, many were separated from their baby after birth, with feeding delayed for up to several hours; only half could feed within an hour after birth. Others talked about the psychological impact of being unwell, being separated from their baby and generally losing breastfeeding confidence.[44]

The role of the placenta

How the placenta is delivered (or not) may also affect breastfeeding. The placenta is delivered in one of two ways. Either 'physiologically' – no drugs are given and the mother waits to deliver the placenta naturally – or mothers are given an injection of oxytocin or ergometrine, which speeds up the delivery of the placenta. Injections are often given as they reduce the risk of a post-partum haemorrhage. However, for women who have had a normal birth and have no risk factors, this might not be needed, as the risk of haemorrhage is low.[45]

Research has found that giving an injection to deliver the placenta appears to be linked to shorter breastfeeding duration. In one study women who had an injection were less likely to be breastfeeding at 48 hours after birth.[31] In another, we found that mothers were less likely to be breastfeeding at two weeks, but also that mothers who had the injection were more likely to report physical difficulties and pain when breastfeeding.[46]

These injections contain high levels of oxytocin. We think that giving large doses of it blocks, interferes with or reduces the body's natural production of the hormone after birth and reduces milk production. The hormones oxytocin and prolactin are essential for milk production, but if the body 'thinks' there is already enough, it might not produce more. We also know that if ergometrine is given in this injection, it will block or reduce the production of prolactin. This may lead to reduced milk supply, but also pain as the baby tries hard to get milk out or feeds very frequently. It might lead to mothers worrying about their milk supply and thinking they need to give formula. Even a small drop in milk production might make a mother who is already more anxious after the birth worry that she is not making enough milk.[47]

However, at present this has not been tested in a randomised controlled trial. It may be that women who are more motivated to breastfeed are less likely to have an injection to deliver the placenta, perhaps because they are aware of this initial research or generally like to avoid intervention when possible.

There is also the issue of what happens when a retained placenta occurs. Although production of breastmilk begins in pregnancy, it is the removal of the placenta and subsequent drop in oestrogen and progesterone that triggers a rise in prolactin and the beginning of full milk production. Therefore if the placenta is not removed, or fragments remain, milk supply is unlikely to significantly increase despite a baby suckling. Indeed, a link between retained placenta and a lack of milk production (ranging from very little at all to a low supply) has been identified in case studies and reviews of records in a number of research articles.[48]

A word on IVF

In recent years, research has started to explore the association between IVF and ICSI and experiences of breastfeeding. Overall the evidence is very mixed. Some studies suggest that women who undergo fertility treatment have no greater difficulties breastfeeding than women who don't.[49] However, other research suggests there may be additional challenges.[50] One reason for this is the higher level of birth complications and interventions in assisted pregnancies. Women who have undergone fertility treatment are more likely to have a multiple pregnancy, a lower birth weight baby or a caesarean section, therefore experiencing the additional complications this can bring.[51]

However, other barriers can be more psychological. A common anxiety is that because a woman may feel her body didn't 'work properly' in conceiving, she won't be able to make enough milk for her baby either.[52] She may also place even more value on breastfeeding and feel under a lot of pressure to make it work because of the challenges of becoming pregnant.[53] When breastfeeding works, it can help heal her previous experiences around difficulty conceiving, but when it does not it can make things feel even worse.

Psychological experience of labour

Women who have a long labour, or find it more painful, are less likely to be breastfeeding at two weeks.[7] This may be because they are exhausted after the birth and feel unable to breastfeed. However, one study showed a physiological impact. Length of labour, duration without sleep and ratings of stress and pain during labour were all negatively correlated with breastfeeding. In other words, the more difficult your labour and the more stressed and exhausted you feel, the less likely you are to breastfeed. However, what was interesting was that these factors were not just psychological; they were also linked to less breast fullness, with babies having lost more weight by day three.[54] It is likely that the stress hormones released as part of a long and painful labour interfere with oxytocin, in turn affecting milk production.[55]

Feeling very stressed during the birth can mean that higher levels of cortisol are released. In turn, mothers who release higher levels of cortisol are more likely to have a delay in their milk coming in, because cortisol stops oxytocin from being released properly.[16] Holding her baby after birth, particularly in skin-to-skin contact, reduces the level of cortisol in a mother's body. Unfortunately, it is often the women who have the most stressful experiences who don't get this opportunity, yet need it the most.[56]

In more recent years, research has considered the relationship between psychological birth trauma and breastfeeding. The likelihood of a woman feeling traumatised after birth is associated both with physical complications and interventions during birth and how she was made to feel during it. Higher lasting feelings of trauma can be found amongst women who felt dismissed, ignored or out of control, despite on paper having a 'straightforward' birth. Associations between birth trauma and breastfeeding may therefore be a consequence of a more difficult labour and birth from a physiological perspective, but also the impact upon her wellbeing.

Indeed, research has shown that both are associated with breastfeeding. For example, in one study physical events during labour and perceptions of feeling traumatised were both associated with lower breastfeeding rates at three months and reduced feelings of breastfeeding self-efficacy.[57] For others, birth complications exacerbated breastfeeding difficulties, leaving women dealing with both the trauma of birth and then the additional trauma of not being able to breastfeed.[58] Conversely, a positive birth experience can support breastfeeding. In one study, women who had positive recollections of their birth were more likely to have high breastfeeding self-efficacy in the days after birth.[59]

'But you have a healthy baby... that's all that really matters'

'Of course the consultant knew best. You should be grateful for his intervention'.

'Who cares how you were spoken to. I'd rather they did their job properly than worried about my feelings'.

'It's what millions of women do, stop thinking you're so special.'

How many women have heard these phrases? Possibly some of the most damaging and demeaning phrases a new mother can hear. Phrases that in a few seconds imply that mothers are somehow selfish, stupid and ideological for wanting the best start for themselves and their babies. Of course we want healthy babies, and of course interventions during labour are sometimes life-saving. But we also know that it is possible to approach labour and delivery in a way that minimises a woman's chances of intervention and protects her wellbeing wherever possible.

A woman's experience of childbirth can have a lasting impact on her psychological wellbeing, including her confidence as a mother.[60] It can also affect breastfeeding. A difficult birth can also increase a mother's risk of anxiety and depression, which in turn can make it more difficult to breastfeed (more about that later).[61] It can also ruin her confidence in herself. She may think that her body has let her down physically during labour, so why would it work during breastfeeding? To a mother who is doubting herself, breastfeeding can seem like a step too far.[62]

How does this affect breastfeeding? Well the medications, interventions and levels of stress a woman experiences in labour can interfere with her ability to breastfeed, both through her baby being reluctant to latch on, and physiologically through her delayed milk production. She can also find feeding more difficult due to any pain or mobility issues.

Formula milk is often seen as the solution. Some believe it will be temporary, but feeds replaced by formula milk in those early days can have a damaging effect on milk supply. They can also exacerbate how helpless a woman might feel after the birth. However, if the mother is ill or exhausted after the birth, health professionals might offer formula, especially if mother and baby have been separated. Partners or family might think the best solution is to give the baby a bottle, even if they believe it is 'just for now' while the mother recovers.

It is important that those supporting new mothers consider how the birth might be affecting the experience of breastfeeding and work with mothers to find ways to establish and continue feeding. It's also important that new mother's know how their birth experience can affect their baby. Of course, if they need a caesarean section, they need a caesarean section, but it's important for them to be aware that this may delay their milk coming in, and not to panic.

A difficult birth certainly does not mean that a mother cannot breastfeed, nor does it mean she should avoid necessary interventions. It does mean she might need more support, both physically and emotionally. It is possible that the mother may face pressure from others to stop breastfeeding, especially if she appears to be having physical difficulties, or there is a feeling that she isn't producing enough milk. Helping the mother understand how her birth experience might be making feeding a little more difficult is a really important step in supporting mothers to breastfeed. These problems can be overcome by understanding and support over the first two weeks, while the effects of the drugs wear off.

What is stark here is that we know that with the right investment, training and staffing we would be able to reduce some of the complications and interventions women experience during birth that go on to affect their breastfeeding experience. Experiences during birth don't end the moment the baby is delivered. We know they can have longer-term physical and psychological consequences and an impact on mothers' wellbeing. The impact on breastfeeding is part of that.

We also know what works to help reduce interventions and complications in labour and birth.[63] Woman-centred care. Shared decision-making. Respect. Communication. One-to-one support. None of it is rocket science, but most of it requires greater investment in the healthcare system, rather than taking away training bursaries and grants from student nurses and midwives and stretching staff to the point of burnout. We know what is needed, we know what works and we know how to make that happen. So let's do it.

Action 1

✓ Invest in woman-centred, one-to-one care during pregnancy and birth to get breastfeeding off to the best possible start.

6. OUR EARLY POSTNATAL ENVIRONMENTS ARE NOT ALWAYS CONDUCIVE TO SUPPORTING BREASTFEEDING

What happens after a baby is born also plays a crucial role in establishing breastfeeding. This particularly includes the information and support a mother receives straight after birth and on the hospital ward and, where relevant, if her baby is admitted to the neonatal intensive care unit (NICU). Overall, we know that the best outcomes for breastfeeding happen when mother and baby are together straight after birth, ideally with prolonged skin-to-skin and breastfeeding started within the first hour. Feeds should then be responsive according to the baby's needs, continuing throughout the night, with no substitute feeds (unless necessary) or dummies. Support and care for the mother should be responsive and sensitive to her needs.

Ah. So that's where it goes wrong. How many mothers feed their babies like that? How many are able to? How many know the importance of it? And how many staff have the training and time to be able to support mothers this way? Let's look at what we know can help mothers and babies get off to the best possible start.

The importance of Baby Friendly standards

The Baby Friendly Hospital Initiative (BFHI) was set up in 1991 by the World Health Organization and UNICEF to develop a series of standards and steps by which hospitals and maternity units could best support initiation, continuation and exclusivity of breastfeeding. It has had amendments and changes over the years. A central part of the BFHI is a series of Ten Steps that hospitals must achieve in order to be awarded Baby Friendly Hospital status.[1] These were revised in 2018 and state that every facility providing maternity services and care for newborn infants should:

1. (a) Comply fully with the International Code of Marketing of Breastmilk Substitutes and relevant World Health Assembly resolutions; (b) Have a written infant feeding policy that is routinely communicated to staff and parents; (c) Establish ongoing monitoring and data-management systems.
2. Ensure that staff have sufficient knowledge, competence, and skills to support breastfeeding.
3. Discuss the importance and management of breastfeeding with pregnant women and their families.
4. Facilitate immediate and uninterrupted skin-to-skin contact and support mothers to initiate breastfeeding as soon as possible after birth.
5. Support mothers to initiate and maintain breastfeeding and manage common difficulties.
6. Do not provide breastfed newborns with any food or fluids other than breastmilk, unless medically indicated.
7. Enable mothers and their infants to remain together and practise rooming-in 24 hours a day.
8. Support mothers to recognise and respond to their infant's cues for feeding.
9. Counsel mothers on the use and risks of feeding bottles, teats, and pacifiers.
10. Coordinate discharge so that parents and their infants have timely access to ongoing support and care.

As you can see, the Ten Steps reflect the optimal conditions for getting breastfeeding off to a good start. In the UK, the UNICEF UK Baby Friendly Initiative have an accreditation programme that is based around the concepts of the Ten Steps but with a particular focus on relationships between parents and their baby. It has expanded over the years from hospitals to also include community breastfeeding support (including children's centres and health visiting), neonatal units and universities. It focuses not just on supporting breastfeeding, but also supporting families to develop 'a close and loving relationship with their baby'. The programme consists of a set of standards that services must meet, training and support to enable this and an assessment programme to measure the skills of staff and listen to families' experiences.

The standards include three main stages.[2] These are:

1. Building a firm foundation including: (a) Written policies and

guidelines to support the standards; (b) An education programme to allow staff to implement the standards according to their role; (c) Processes for implementing, auditing and evaluating the standards; (d) Ensuring that there is no promotion of breastmilk substitutes, bottles, teats or dummies in any part of the facility or by any of the staff.

2. An educated workforce – ensuring staff receive the education to implement the standards.
3. Parents' experiences.

This is the most detailed section and consists of a series of steps to ensure that parents have positive infant feeding support and care across different venues.

For maternity services it includes:

*   Support pregnant women to recognise the importance of breastfeeding and early relationships for the health and wellbeing of their baby. This includes conversations about feeding, recognising and responding to newborn needs and support to develop a positive relationship with their baby during pregnancy.
*   Support all mothers and babies to initiate a close relationship and feeding soon after birth. This includes skin-to-skin and feeding as soon as possible.
*   Enable mothers to get breastfeeding off to a good start. This includes skills such as positioning and attachment, hand expression and understanding the signs of effective feeding. It also includes information about responsive feeding. Specialist support should be available, alongside details of community support. A formal breastfeeding assessment should be carried out as often as needed in the first week ensuring effective feeding and to check on the wellbeing of the mother and baby.
*   Support mothers to make informed decisions regarding the introduction of food or fluids other than breastmilk. This includes giving detailed information about why exclusive breastfeeding matters, how to give formula milk safely, responsive bottle-feeding and no promotional material.
*   Support parents to have a close and loving relationship with their baby. This includes aspects such as skin-to-skin, understanding normal newborn needs, responsive feeding and information about parenting support.

For neonatal services it includes:

- Support parents to have a close and loving relationship with their baby. This includes conversations about the importance of touch, comfort and communication.
- Enable babies to receive breastmilk and to breastfeed when possible. This can include conversations about the importance of human milk, expressing, transition to breastfeeding and discharge support.
- Value parents as partners in care. This includes enabling all parents to have unrestricted access to their baby, making the NICU as comfortable and private as possible, supported to be involved directly in care and effective communication between staff and parents.

For health visiting it includes:

- Support pregnant women to recognise the importance of breastfeeding and early relationships for the health and wellbeing of their baby. This includes conversations during pregnancy.
- Enable mothers to continue breastfeeding for as long as they wish. This includes a formal feeding assessment at 10–14 days, specialist support for complex issues, talking about issues such as responsive feeding and return to work, information about peer support and no advertising.
- Support mothers to make informed decisions regarding the introduction of food or fluids other than breastmilk. This includes timely conversations about exclusive breastfeeding and introducing solids, alongside support where needed to safely and responsively bottle-feed.
- Support parents to have a close and loving relationship with their baby. This includes supporting parents to understand their baby's development, encouragement to respond to their baby's needs, responsive bottle-feeding and access to support for parents' wellbeing.

For children's centres it includes:

- Support pregnant women to recognise the importance of early relationships for the health and wellbeing of their baby. This includes support services for pregnant women and partners such as feeding and care information.

- Protect and support breastfeeding in all areas of the service. This includes a welcoming atmosphere for breastfeeding, no advertising and referrals for specialist support.
- Support parents to have a close and loving relationship with their baby. Again this includes support for developing responsive care and understanding baby development

Do the Ten Steps and Baby Friendly accreditation actually improve breastfeeding rates?

In short, yes. A growing number of research studies, each using different methods, has highlighted that when Baby Friendly accreditation is gained, or the Ten Steps are implemented, then breastfeeding rates tend to rise in the hospital and community. Overall, these studies tend to show that the more steps a hospital/community follows, the better the increase in breastfeeding rates. These studies include:

- A review of a number of studies from across the globe exploring the impact of the Baby Friendly Hospital Initiative found that following the recommendations had a positive impact on breastfeeding in the short, medium and long term. Overall, the more of the steps hospitals implemented, the better their breastfeeding outcomes. In particular, support in the community once mothers had left hospital was identified as being one of the most important steps.[3]
- The PROBIT trial in Belarus found that babies born in BFI hospitals had longer breastfeeding and exclusive breastfeeding durations. A follow-up study eight years later found that these mothers were also more likely to go on to breastfeed their second child. Some studies compared babies born in BFI hospitals to those born elsewhere in a range of countries including Taiwan, Brazil, Russia and Canada. Overall they found that women who delivered in BFI hospitals had a longer exclusive breastfeeding duration. Other studies have looked at what happens to breastfeeding rates in hospitals pre- and post-BFI intervention. Studies from Brazil, India, Italy, Spain and Turkey all suggested an improvement in either exclusive breastfeeding or overall breastfeeding duration.[4]
- An American study found that when hospitals had BFI status, more mothers breastfed in the first hour after birth and they were less likely to use formula in hospital.[5]

- Another review in the US of the Ten Steps found that when hospitals had BFHI status, breastfeeding rates increased. Again, the more steps that were followed, the higher the breastfeeding rates.[6]
- A systematic review specifically examining the importance of step three (prenatal education) found that prenatal interventions delivered alone or in conjunction with postnatal care increased breastfeeding initiation, duration and exclusivity. This is a much stronger effect when these interventions focused not just on factual information, but also interpersonal support and involving partners and/or family.[7]
- Another review of step two of the Ten Steps (training of healthcare staff) found that training improved knowledge, attitudes and compliance, but not always breastfeeding rates. In some studies exclusivity increased.[8]
- A whole range of other studies highlight higher breastfeeding initiation, duration and exclusivity rates in hospitals with accreditation compared to those without in numerous regions including Belgium,[9] Italy,[10] Brazil[11] and Los Angeles,[12] to name just a few.

Why do the Ten Steps and BFI standards work so well?

The rationale behind the BFHI Ten Steps and UNICEF UK BFI standards is clear: each of the themes/practices is associated with a better chance of getting breastfeeding off to a good start and keeping it going. Some of them are common sense. If you ensure mothers have more information about breastfeeding, more practical support and more specialist skilled support then it's hardly surprising that breastfeeding rates rise. Responsive care and feeding are also key to supporting breastfeeding, which we have already seen, and will discuss more in chapter 8. Here is some of the evidence behind the steps.

Skin-to-skin

Babies love skin-to-skin. Research comparing those babies who receive skin-to-skin and those who don't has shown how it can have a positive impact on how they adapt to life outside the womb. Babies who have skin-to-skin have better temperatures, steadier heart rates and breathing and better oxygen levels. They have even been shown to put on more weight in the long term. Skin-to-skin has a positive impact for healthy term babies, but is particularly important for those babies born prematurely.[13]

Babies also expect and appreciate skin-to-skin. Imagine being born – one minute you're all wrapped up warm and cosy, listening to your mother's heartbeat, and the next you're out in a bright noisy world, wondering where on earth you are. Being on your mother's chest, in the warmth, listening to her heartbeat and hearing that familiar voice, is rather nice. And babies let us know this. One study compared how much babies put in a cot cried compared to those on their mother's chest and found it was 40 times more![14] If that's not a reason for skin-to-skin I don't know what is.

Mothers who have skin-to-skin with their babies generally report less stress and better bonding and spend more time touching their babies. One study showed that mothers who have skin-to-skin become more confident and less anxious in caring for their baby, and engage in more affectionate touch at one year old.[15] One study in particular looked at the experience of skin-to-skin of mothers with a premature baby. Overwhelmingly, skin-to-skin helped mothers emotionally at a very difficult time. Words such as rewarding, restorative, relieving and regaining control were used when talking about the experience, as mothers felt their bonding as a family was enhanced.[16]

Skin-to-skin also helps with breastfeeding and it is easy to see why. Babies who have skin-to-skin are more likely to initiate breastfeeding and to carry on, perhaps unsurprisingly given that they're right next to a nipple.[17] Babies who have skin-to-skin show better latching behaviour and a stronger suckle, and as a consequence experience less weight loss.[18] Skin-to-skin can also be restorative after a caesarean section, but only if it is done for at least an hour. Mothers who have this length of skin-to-skin are more likely to be breastfeeding at 48 hours, probably, as noted above, because their levels of stress hormones drop and oxytocin levels rise.[19] Skin-to-skin makes babies more settled, which in itself makes them seem easier to feed, giving women confidence.

However, unfortunately lots of things disturb skin-to-skin. Around 80% of mothers in the UK have skin-to-skin within the first hour, but there is no data on how many have a full, undisturbed hour. Anecdotally, many report being rushed through skin-to-skin, particularly if professionals want to give stitches or move her to another room. Pressures on staff make it seem sometimes like a tick-box exercise. One mother reported:

'She was snug and secure on my chest but only for about 10 minutes, but she didn't want to feed so they asked my husband to hold her whilst I had stitches and then they took me straight back to the ward. So it was at least another hour or so before I could hold her again and by that time they'd dressed her so it seemed a shame to make her cold again.'

Mothers who have had a difficult birth or who are in pain, medicated or exhausted are less likely to experience skin-to-skin. As discussed earlier, women who have had a caesarean section are less likely to have skin-to-skin, or only have it briefly. Babies who are born too early, too small or too sick are the ones who need it most, but are least likely to have it. But women who have had a straightforward birth may also be prevented from having skin-to-skin, or for long enough. Someone wants to weigh the baby or give an injection. Clean the baby. Dress the baby. Have photos with the baby. All these can interrupt skin-to-skin. There can also be significant pressure to move a woman to the ward from the delivery suite. So although many women now have skin-to-skin, for some it can be brief and almost tokenistic.[20] If skin-to-skin is disrupted, early breastfeeding is damaged.

Golden hour

Ideally, while skin-to-skin is happening, a baby should be getting to grips with breastfeeding. Globally, initiating breastfeeding as soon as possible saves lives. In fact, delaying breastfeeding until after the first hour doubles the risk of mortality.[21] In developed countries starting breastfeeding as soon as possible is also important. Babies who are breastfed within the first hour are more likely to go on to continue breastfeeding, with the sooner the start the better, although sometimes it is hard to untangle that from the reasons leading to the separation.[22]

However, in an infant feeding report published by the Royal College of Midwives in 2014, only 75% of midwives who took part reported that breastfeeding was usually initiated at their hospital within an hour, and only 61% of mothers said they had been encouraged to breastfeed within the first hour. We're not paying enough attention to ensuring that nothing gets in the way of skin-to-skin.[23]

Keeping mother and baby together

As mentioned before, keeping mother and baby close together with skin-to-skin straight after the birth is important in getting breastfeeding off to a good start. However, the need to keep mother and baby together continues after the early hours. Generally, if mother and baby are separated by placing the baby in a nursery, instead of rooming-in (being next to mum), breastfeeding is less likely to continue.[24]

Separations can be temporary. But even if the separation is short (less than 20 minutes), suckling problems can occur.[25] Women who are separated from their baby for any length of time after the birth are less likely to continue breastfeeding.[26] Obviously separation can be complicated by all sorts of other factors. A difficult birth resulting in the mother being taken to the operating theatre, or the baby needing medical care, means that mother and baby won't be together. Situations like this cannot be avoided (although investing in better maternity care services might prevent some of them). However, when mother and baby are allowed to go to NICU together, breastfeeding outcomes are better.

Sometimes mother and baby are separated for no medical reason. Nurseries on hospital wards used to be the norm for babies in the UK, and in some parts of the world they are still common. Babies were typically taken from their mother after birth and kept in the nursery, being brought out for feeds. Dads could view them at set hours of the day. Gradually this has changed, and rooming in, with baby in a crib next to the bed, has become more common. In countries where babies still go to nurseries, the reasons for the practice include increased security and to allow the mother to rest. It was once believed that infection risk was lower if babies were in nurseries, but we now know that the opposite is true.[27]

In the USA, the practice of taking babies to a hospital nursery is still common. One February 2016 headline read: 'Maternity wards are moving away from nurseries'. The move, aimed at increasing breastfeeding rates, is causing a lot of outrage, as women demand time away from their babies in order to rest and sleep. Some suggest that rooming-in will lead to exhaustion and postnatal depression in new mothers. It has also been postulated that babies will be injured or even die when they are dropped by exhausted mothers. This is a fascinating example of the extent to which the prevailing culture is internalised by those within it, despite a sound scientific and anthropological basis for rooming-in, and its prevalence in other countries.

A number of studies have shown that babies rooming in are more likely to be breastfed. In fact, one study that compared breastfeeding outcomes for hospitals that roomed-in versus those which used nurseries found that rates of breastfeeding in the rooming-in hospitals were 77% at two months compared to 27% in the nursery hospitals.[28] Why the link between rooming-in and breastfeeding? Firstly, it may be down to selection. Women who are very tired after a difficult delivery may ask for their baby to be put in a nursery (or for the midwife to take their baby if there isn't one).

However, one randomised controlled trial that allocated babies either to a nursery or to rooming-in found that 86% of the roomed-in babies were exclusively breastfed on discharge compared to 45% of the nursery babies. Having baby close means that babies are fed more often. Babies who were roomed-in had 20% more feeds than those who were in a nursery.[29] So babies who are separated from their mother, for whatever reason, are more likely to be given formula and less likely to be breastfed by the time they leave hospital.

No formula top-ups (unless necessary)

The importance of feeding on demand without supplements has already been discussed, but research has also shown the importance of not receiving formula in the early days in hospital. One recent study found that if babies had formula supplements in hospital they were 1.8 times more likely not to be breastfeeding at one month and 2.7 times more likely not to be breastfeeding at two months, compared to those who had been exclusively breastfed in hospital.[30]

The reasons for formula supplementation are often based on concerns about milk supply, which shouldn't really be an issue during the short period of time that women are in hospital. One study found that of mothers who supplemented with formula, 18% did so due to insufficient milk, 16% because they believed their baby wasn't feeding enough and 14% due to poor latch. The notable irony is that formula supplementation exacerbates or 'confirms' these concerns.[31]

There appears to be something about feeding with a bottle in particular that leads to stopping breastfeeding. Studies that have looked at different ways of supplementing have found the riskiest option (in terms of likelihood of stopping breastfeeding) to be with a bottle, followed by a syringe and then a cup or finger-feeding. The more passive a baby is in the process of getting the milk, the more of a risk to breastfeeding. Does the baby simply perceive the bottle as 'easier'?

Birth has an impact too. Babies are more likely to receive supplements in the early days if the mother had a long labour, a post-partum haemorrhage or labour was sped up artificially. Babies with a low Apgar score or who needed oxygen are more likely to be supplemented.[32] However, in one study there was no clear clinical need for supplementation in 87% of babies who received it during their hospital stay.[33]

Supplementing is less common in the UK than in the US, where rates are very high. In fact, 78% of US hospitals routinely supplement babies if there is any concern about intake, latch or weight loss.[34] In a US study, 80% of babies who were supplemented received the milk within five hours of birth, suggesting that it is not being used as a last resort for a baby who is difficult to feed or a mother who is struggling.[35]

It may not only be supplementing with formula that impacts negatively on breastfeeding. A number of studies have shown that babies who receive expressed breastmilk in the hospital are less likely to continue to receive breastmilk later. Of course, for some babies receiving expressed breastmilk is a consequence of a difficult delivery or a health problem. But not all women who are expressing do so for this reason. One study explored what happened to babies who were born with a healthy Apgar and no major complications, but were given expressed milk rather than being breastfed. Those babies who were given expressed milk were less likely to be breastfeeding at six months.[36]

One study compared the milk output of mothers of term babies who were feeding directly from the breast, compared to a group of mothers using a pump to express milk. They found that mothers using a pump were nearly three times as likely not to be able to produce enough milk. This was linked closely to physiological factors. Mothers who were directly breastfeeding fed their babies more often than mothers who used a pump. Mothers who used a pump only did so about six times a day, even though they were recommended to do so at least eight times a day. Conversely, mothers who breastfed directly did so around eight to nine times a day. Mothers who breastfed directly had a higher milk output than those who expressed milk, with mothers who pumped also more likely to get mastitis.[37]

There has been some recent research exploring the impact of managing formula top-ups more effectively. In this series of studies, mothers whose baby had lost a lot of weight after birth were either randomised to receive continued breastfeeding support, or for their baby to receive formula supplements alongside breastfeeding. Both studies[38,39] found no impact upon breastfeeding duration for babies who received the top-ups, which sounds like great news. However, it is important to understand the details of this study to be able to extrapolate the findings to consider whether they would apply to other groups of mothers.

First, the study contained mothers who were older and motivated to breastfeed despite difficulties – rates across the study were much higher than population averages. Mothers were also given a lot of support and information about giving the top-ups, with continued enhanced breastfeeding support to build their own supply. Top-ups were also limited to just 10ml of formula after each feed. Many bottles of ready-made infant formula come in 70ml portions at the smallest – a big difference. A specific hydrolysed formula was also used which is different in smell and appearance to many first-stage formula milks, creating a separation between formula perhaps as a medical intervention versus a long-term decision. On top of this a syringe was used for feeds – not a bottle. So while these findings are very interesting, they show us what might be possible in the best possible scenarios – not what may happen on busy postnatal wards, or at home, especially if volume is not controlled.

So formula supplements, often given due to concerns about milk supply and weight loss, can actually exacerbate or cause these problems, leading to cessation of breastfeeding, often sooner than the mother wants.

Nipple shields

This is another ongoing debate. Nipple shields are sometimes recommended if there are breastfeeding problems. In one study of why they were used, 70% reported it was because baby wouldn't latch on, 10% said it was because of pain and 20% said it was both.[40] This makes examining outcomes difficult, as women who use them are likely to be having a difficult time anyway and are therefore more likely to stop breastfeeding.

However, routine use of nipple shields instead of breastfeeding problem-solving in healthy full term babies should be avoided.[41] One study found that oxytocin levels were lower among mothers randomly assigned to use nipple shields, and that their babies received less milk per feed (27g versus 47g) than the babies of those who didn't use them.[42] Another study found that milk output when expressing was six times greater when mothers did not use a nipple shield than when they did.[43] Babies have also been shown to suck differently and less effectively when using a nipple shield.[44]

Saying that, nipple shields might be useful for some mothers and babies. One study looked at premature babies at 33 or 38 weeks who had difficulties latching. They found over half the babies consumed over 50% of a set feed when using a shield, when before they were consuming very little.[45] Another study of babies who had a very poor latch found that among babies whose mothers were using nipple shields (mainly due to poor latch), all babies consumed more than when not using the shields (18.4ml compared to 3.9ml).[46]

Use of nipple shields should therefore be selective. For babies who are having latch problems they might really help, but for those who can feed effectively without they may reduce milk supply. The problem comes when women automatically think they are something that is needed and will help, and use them without advice. The shield makes a nipple shape in the mouth, meaning that babies don't have to suck as hard, and it may then be more difficult to persuade the baby back onto the breast.

Dummy / pacifier use

The debate on whether dummies (also referred to in the literature with the US term 'pacifiers') damage breastfeeding is ongoing. Some studies suggest that they may disguise early signs of hunger and stretch out feeds. Indeed, one study found that the more babies aged 1–6 months used a dummy, the lower their weight.[47]

Some studies suggest that among mothers who are determined to breastfeed, dummy use doesn't make any difference.[48] However, among those who are less motivated, using a dummy might decrease their ability to breastfeed. Other studies suggest babies who have their dummy removed may resort to finger-sucking instead.[49] Generally, though, non-nutritive sucking on a dummy should be avoided, and no study has shown that it has enabled breastfeeding to continue for longer.

No advertising or promotion of bottles, teats or formula brands

In short, research has shown that when hospitals are prevented from advertising specific brands and products, breastfeeding rates increase. This will be discussed in more detail in chapter 16.

But hasn't the Baby Friendly Initiative been criticised?

There have indeed been numerous criticisms of the Baby Friendly

Initiative. Some of these constructively question how the standards affect mothers who want or need to formula-feed (short response – there are numerous resources to support safe and responsive bottle-feeding on the UNICEF UK Baby Friendly website).[50] Others, it could be argued, are driven by more individual beliefs, with an agenda to discredit the initiative. I am not talking about articles that rigorously collect data around outcomes or experiences, but those that use data in the opposite way. Many of these are published as 'position pieces' – essentially opinion-based articles rather than those that have collected new data or reanalysed existing data in a different way.

For example, in 2016 an article was published in the *Journal of the American Medical Association* entitled 'Unintended Consequences of Current Breastfeeding Initiatives'.[51] The main point of the paper was to criticise the BFHI, saying that it had unintended consequences for infant health and mortality. Specifically it critiqued the consequences of skin-to-skin contact, keeping mother and baby together and not using pacifiers. It stated:

'It is important to be certain that the basis for the recommendations has been documented in reproducible scientific studies and that the benefits of the practices recommended outweigh the risks. Unfortunately, there is now emerging evidence that full compliance with the 10 steps of the initiative may inadvertently be promoting potentially hazardous practices and/or having counterproductive outcomes.'

A lot of the focus in the paper was around the risk of 'sudden unexpected postnatal collapse' (SUPC) – or in other words, babies who collapse unexpectedly (e.g. not because of illness or prematurity) in the first few days of life. It specifically claimed that skin-to-skin promotion made this more likely, because *sometimes* it occurs during skin-to-skin contact. This was the headline that many news outlets chose to run with, without considering the details.

SUPC is very rare, affecting an estimated three in 100,000 babies.[52] Occasionally it happens in the first two hours of life (when skin-to-skin after birth may be occurring), but actually only a third of cases happen at this time. Two case studies are listed in the paper of mothers whose baby collapsed on the second day of life, during skin-to-skin contact. However, even the authors of those case studies say they can't think why this would be a causal relationship. There is no reason why skin-to-skin should cause collapse, and nor do we know what would have happened if the baby had been in their cot at the time.

The authors also focused on the issue of mother and baby being kept together, suggesting it caused maternal exhaustion and therefore a risk of dropping her baby. A paper is cited which estimated the risk of babies falling out of bed in hospital at around 1.6–4.1 in every 10,000 births.[53] Again the authors of that paper do not suggest that the solution is to separate mother and baby, but rather to ensure mothers are monitored more closely and that improvements are made to safety equipment. Likewise, research in the UK examining the impact of keeping babies in bed, in a sidecar crib or in a standalone cot, reported no adverse effects, e.g. falls.[54]

Another study picked up on this idea of more babies being dropped in hospital due to Baby Friendly Standards and the practices of promoting breastfeeding and keeping mother and baby together.[55] This study brought together cases of mothers who dropped their baby in hospital after birth. Entitled 'In-hospital neonatal falls: an unintended consequence of efforts to improve breastfeeding', it also caused anxiety in 2019. The first lines of the abstract read '*In-hospital neonatal falls are increasingly recognised as a postpartum safety risk with maternal fatigue contributing to these events*'.

If you simply read the abstract you might believe that there had been a significant increase in falls. It is based on what the authors called 'a cluster' of falls in hospital. This cluster was actually just three falls over a two-year period. When you look at the individual cases there are red flags all over them which would suggest other reasons why the babies were dropped:

1. '*Elective caesarean. Breastfeeding did not start until 15 hours after delivery. Mother reported feeling very fatigued*'. If a baby isn't being fed until 15 hours after delivery this suggests that the birth was extremely complicated or that mother and baby were unwell after birth. This would also likely explain the extreme fatigue.
2. '*14-year-old mother with history of foster care and depression. Mother initially breastfed 4 hours after birth but then stopped breastfeeding. On day 4, she fell asleep when holding the infant and he fell to the floor*'. So in other words, the mother was not a breastfeeding mother when she dropped her baby.
3. '*Mother with significant traumatic experiences including domestic abuse and enslavement. Baby first breastfed after 9.5 hours. Mother reported feeling drowsy from pain medication and she asked for him to be taken to the hospital nursery on day two. On day three, she fell asleep breastfeeding her baby*'. Again, the significant issues around

her birth and previous history may have affected events. It was also unclear as to whether the baby was staying in the nursery around the period she dropped him.

What about when babies are in neonatal intensive care?

Sometimes mothers and babies do need to be separated. Babies who need life-saving treatment in neonatal or special care units won't always be able to follow the steps outlined above. Unfortunately, this means that, despite the increased importance of breastfeeding for special care babies, they are less likely to be breastfed due to numerous challenges.[56]

Depending on the timing and reason for special care, babies may be unable to breastfeed directly at all. The sucking reflex doesn't develop in babies until around 34 weeks, and even then premature babies may have a weak suck or be unable to latch effectively.[57] Expression of milk is therefore recommended for very premature or sick babies, but that in itself has numerous challenges. It can be difficult to express milk at the best of times, but with added stress and anxiety, and potentially the impact of a difficult birth, expressing for a special care baby is not as straightforward as it sounds. Being physically separated from the baby can mean that getting the let-down reflex to work can be very challenging. Many women are also disheartened by the amount they can express, not realising that only very small amounts are made in the early days.[58]

Expressing is also very time-consuming. Of course, breastfeeding a baby is time-consuming too, but the experience of holding a newborn baby is intrinsically more rewarding than having to express milk under pressure. For example, mothers who are expressing for their premature baby need to be doing so for at least a couple of hours a day, which can be a very long time when you're sitting alone with a breast pump. Skin-to-skin enhances the amount of milk produced, but the mothers of the smallest and sickest babies may be unable to have this.[59]

There is also a huge emotional aspect to having a special care baby. One study explored how many mothers of babies in neonatal intensive care deliberately stopped themselves from bonding too deeply with their baby as a self-protective mechanism. Others experienced significant levels of shame, guilt and blame. Many were scared to touch their baby in case they hurt them. A common theme in one study was that mothers felt they were 'on the edges of mothering', rather than having a maternal role. Their lives were dictated by hospital staff and routines, and this, combined with the fear of loss, meant that they held back.[60]

Other studies describe how mothers feel powerless and helpless, and as though they are not in charge. Many come to resent the need to express milk, feeling considerable pressure and duty during a time of such stress. Some mothers, who need pumps that can't be used on the ward, resent the fact that it takes them away from their baby.[61]

All of this can make breastfeeding feel really challenging. Although stress does not interfere with breastmilk production, it can sometimes interfere with letdown.[62] Not being able to hold your baby reduces oxytocin. As we saw, a difficult birth, which is more likely when babies are in NICU, can complicate things. And that's before we get to the psychological impact. It doesn't take a rocket scientist to see how all this combined can have an impact on breastfeeding. Any negative emotions after the birth, and feelings of failure about oneself and one's body, are exacerbated when a baby is in special care. If mothers who feel confident, knowledgeable and supported are the ones who breastfeed, you can understand why mothers with babies in special care may struggle.

This makes investing in support in the neonatal unit so vitally important, not least because research shows that when mothers are able to give their premature baby human milk, or to breastfeed them, this can help them enormously in overcoming a difficult experience. It can help them feel empowered, connected to their baby and it can restore faith in their body.[63] The impact of human milk on premature babies and their mothers were both core drivers for the development of the Baby Friendly Initiative neonatal standards.

Action 2

✓ All hospital, neonatal and community services should adopt UNICEF Baby Friendly standards and practices.

7. A LACK OF INVESTMENT IN SKILLED SUPPORT MEANS THAT TOO MANY WOMEN EXPERIENCE PAIN AND DIFFICULTY

'You'll call me melodramatic but I'd rather give birth again than go through the pain I felt when nursing Alfie. It was like someone was sticking needles in me every time he fed, to the point I often had tears streaming down my face. The midwife checked the latch a few times and told me it was perfect and to carry on doing a good job. Couldn't she see what he was doing to me?'

Pain is one of the most common reasons why women stop breastfeeding. Some studies suggest that up to 96% of new mothers report some form of pain when breastfeeding in the early days after birth, but for some unfortunate mothers, pain is not just short-term or fleeting and can last for weeks after birth and beyond. Pain can be significant enough to cause psychological distress and interfere with sleep, mood and enjoyment of life, and it can impact upon bonding between mother and baby.[1] Indeed, mothers with severe nipple pain are more likely to experience postnatal depression.[2]

Pain can be classified into 'transient' (occurring and resolving during the first week) and 'prolonged' (continuing after this point). Although distressing, transient pain is often considered normal, in that it is a frequent occurrence. However, 'normal' does not mean that it is not distressing, or that it shouldn't be fixed.[3] Pain tends to peak at about 3–7 days, just when milk is coming in, and engorgement adds to the fun of it all.[4] In one recent study of new mothers in Australia, 79% reported nipple pain even before they were discharged from hospital. Over the next eight weeks, 58% reported nipple damage and 23% vasospasm, although by eight weeks this had dropped to 8% experiencing damage and 20% pain.[5]

Just to give you a picture of what nipple pain can be like if you've never breastfed a baby (or were lucky enough not to experience any pain), one study asked mothers to classify the nipple pain they experienced using a series of adjectives. They found the most common were pinching (57%), sharp (54%), shooting (50%), stinging (50%), intense (39%), radiating (36%) and tender (36%). Yeah, ouch.[6] Pain can stem from visible damage to the nipple, the baby sucking the nipple into an odd shape, or deeper breast pain and infection. When there is visible trauma women tend to report greater pain than when there is no visual trauma. However, pain can still be felt when the nipple looks normal.[7]

Pain stops women breastfeeding (who knew?). One study asked women why they stopped breastfeeding and found 29% said pain and 37% said sore, cracked or bleeding nipples.[8] This pain is repeated at every feed, or experienced between feeds. And, as we know, babies feed very frequently. It is pretty obvious why women stop breastfeeding altogether, or are tempted to supplement some feeds with formula, reducing their supply of milk (which in turn makes breastfeeding more difficult and more painful).

However, even though intuitively you would expect women who are experiencing pain to be happy to stop breastfeeding, actually women who stop for this reason are more likely to say that they weren't ready to stop, and are more likely to experience symptoms of postnatal depression.[9] So not only are these women in pain, but they're also miserable about having stopped breastfeeding.

What causes nipple pain?

Nipple pain can arise for many different reasons. Often there is a positioning problem. When the baby is latched on to the breast correctly, the nipple is deep inside the baby's mouth. If the baby has a shallower latch, the nipple might get squished between the tongue and roof of the mouth, compressing the nipple.[10] Issues may be exacerbated by the shape of a mum's nipples. Nipples stretch a lot during feeding. If women have short, flat or very wide nipples they may find this particularly painful.[11]

Pain from incorrect positioning and attachment is the primary cause of pain during the first week. One study that explored the reasons why women consulted with a breastfeeding centre found that 36% were due to nipple pain, with the most common reason for the pain being incorrect attachment and positioning.[12] Sometimes the nipple will be visibly damaged or misshapen after a feed. Ultrasound images taken of babies feeding from mothers who were experiencing pain showed differences in the babies' tongue movement, which

113

could be leading directly to nipple trauma. The findings showed that in the babies of mothers who were experiencing pain, there was a smaller space between the tongue and top of the mouth, and the nipple did not extend as far back as would typically be expected. Babies also tended to suckle harder, probably because they are struggling to remove milk effectively.[13]

Support to fix this pain as soon as possible is important, as solving this issue is a major predictor of continued breastfeeding. One study showed that examining and supporting mothers to improve latch helped to resolve pain in 65% of cases.[14] However, that leaves 35% of mothers still in pain. Another study showed that, even when mothers were helped to get 'correct' attachment, 10% experienced no reduction in pain.[15]

Interestingly, a recent study has shown that babies who are breastfed in what is thought to be a 'good' position, the common cross-cradle hold, may be more likely to cause nipple damage due to poor attachment. Bringing the baby to the breast this way can mean the baby's face is not in an optimal position, and the nipple isn't taken comfortably deep into the baby's mouth. Infection, nipple damage and mastitis can all result.[16]

When an infant causes damage to the nipple tissue, cracks can become infected. Nipple thrush can cause a burning, shooting or stabbing pain deep in the breast. Antifungal treatment (and diet restrictions) can help many women in this situation, but 8% of women have no reduction in pain.[17] Sometimes, infections of the skin on and around the nipple can occur, such as dermatitis and psoriasis, but these can often be treated with topical ointments. Sometimes this can be caused by irritants, allergens or even breast pads.

Another source of breast pain is mastitis. Mastitis is often described as an inflammation of the breast and tends to be accompanied by flu-like symptoms. One study suggested up to a third of women might experience mastitis, although others have suggested occurrence is more like 10%. The most common time for women to experience it is 2–3 weeks postpartum, with around 75–95% of cases occurring in the first three months.[18] Often pain is deep in the breast, which has a firm, red tender area. Cracks in the nipple can mean that bacteria can enter the breast, which can cause mastitis. Blocked milk ducts and thrush can also lead to the condition. Babies who have palate or cleft issues, or difficulty attaching to the breast, may exacerbate it. Missed feedings or pressure from an ill-fitting bra or even seatbelt can increase the risk. Extreme cases of mastitis can lead to an abscess forming, which will need to be drained. Treating nipple damage may reduce the risk of mastitis.

Engorgement can also present a problem. Although normal at around 3–5 days postpartum, if women are unaware of its transience, meaning and how to manage it, this may lead them to stop breastfeeding. However, engorgement can also become more serious and longer lasting, leading to full, hard and painful breasts. Although engorgement can usually be eased through warm and cold packs, expressing and massage, in some cases women may need anti-inflammatory medication. Information and support from knowledgeable professionals and/or supporters is often key to women managing engorgement rather than seeing it as an issue.

Sometimes pain may be caused by the infant's feeding style. Babies who are quite 'vigorous' might cause excessive nipple stretching and movement, which may leave a mother in pain.[19] Back in 1945 an interesting paper reported how babies could suckle so hard that they left marks on the nipples.[20] Indeed, babies who have a very strong suck are more likely to cause pain for their mother, which is difficult to solve.[21] And suckling can be quite strong – vacuums of up to -200mmHG for two minutes in a two-day-old baby were measured in a small study in the 1940s.[22] Given that I'm a psychologist by background and not a physicist or engineer I decided to check what this figure meant. Friend-of-a-friend Christopher Deen, who has a degree in 'aerospace engineering with propulsion', is an engineer and a new Dad. He likened it to 'the force of a good vacuum cleaner'. 'A Dyson?' I asked. 'A little bit under,' he said. Ouch.

McClellan and colleagues collected similar data measuring the power of baby's suck and the pain their mother felt.[23] The strength of the suck was examined during active feeding and pauses. Mothers who were experiencing pain had babies who suckled more strongly, but actually consumed less milk over all. During active suckling, the babies causing pain applied vacuums more than 50% stronger than the babies who didn't cause pain, and it was nearly double during the 'pauses' too. Comparing this to what you might experience with a breast pump, the mean peak vacuum created by infants of mothers in pain was stronger than the maximum comfort ranges allowed with breast pumps. However, breast pumps can cause their own damage, with one study finding that 15% of mothers had experienced a breast pump injury.[24] Again, ouch.

Another physical issue can be the shape of the infant's palate. A high arched palate can mean the nipple becomes damaged, and this can often be reduced by changing the position in which the nipple enters the mouth.[25] Babies who have very small mouths, or chins that are tucked in, may also cause pain for their mothers. Some babies may have developmental difficulties that make it difficult for them to get an effective latch and strong enough suck. They might not be able to coordinate suckling and swallowing, leading to nipple damage and engorgement. Trauma to the face or jaw might make babies bite or clench their jaw at the breast.

A separate note on tongue-tie

Structural issues from the baby's perspective can also cause pain. Ankyloglossia, known as tongue-tie, can mean that an infant struggles to get a good latch or feeds a lot because of an ineffective latch. The tongue is naturally anchored to the floor of the mouth by a strip of connective tissue called the frenulum. In babies with tongue-tie this is too short, thick or tight, meaning that they cannot fully move their tongue. This makes latching onto the breast difficult.[26]

Tongue-tie has always existed, but the rate of diagnosed or suspected tongue-tie has increased rapidly in recent years. Studies have found a rate anywhere between 0.1–10.7% of babies born, which is obviously a significant difference across a population. However not all babies with a tongue-tie will have feeding difficulties.[27] Depending on factors such as tongue length and movement, babies may have different degrees of ability to feed. Those who struggle may try to use their lips to create a vacuum or their jaw to increase pressure. This will usually be ineffective, creating an even more shallow latch and reduction in removal of milk from the breast.[28] This can also lead to pain and nipple trauma, increasing stress levels which in turn block oxytocin production.[29]

So what causes tongue-tie and why might rates be increasing? The role of folic acid supplementation is often central to this discussion. Levels of supplementation in pregnancy are increasing globally with the aim to reduce neural tube defects, with potential further effects on the reduction of oral clefts and hypospadias. These are all considered to be issues linked to cell division and midline structures of the body. Folic acid appears to be involved in essentially 'tightening' the midline, bringing it together, hence the impact on these disorders. However, it has been theorised that such tightening has caused an increase in another midline structure – the lingual frenulum. Indeed, in one study that asked women to self-report folic acid intake, those who had a baby with a tongue-tie were more likely to have taken folic acid in pregnancy.[30]

There is also evidence that tongue-tie might be genetic, specifically in relation to the Tbx22 gene which plays a central role in the development of the mouth and jaw structure, influencing development of the frenulum.[31] Mutations of this gene have been linked to cases of tongue-tie, although there is much debate over the strength of this link.[32] Another gene that has been considered is Lgr5 – a protein-coding gene. However, research on this area is predominantly based on mice, which has obvious limitations.[33] Finally, a more commonly discussed gene is MTHFR. This gene is involved in healthy DNA functioning and needs sufficient folic acid to do so well. Those with a mutation of this gene do not appear to be able to process folic acid well, meaning that, even though they make take supplements, they do not work efficiently. This increases the risk of midline defects in the baby.[34]

Other studies are more critical of the rise in tongue-tie. Some attribute a rise in diagnoses to an increased awareness, while others suggest that as breastfeeding rates and motivation have started to increase again in recent decades, it is only natural that we will start to see more tongue-tie. It has also been suggested that a decrease in understanding of how breastfeeding works, and pressures on health services to adequately provide breastfeeding support, mean that for some women there could be a tendency to blame normal feeding difficulties on something definitive that they believe can be easily solved – tongue-tie.[35]

Research examining the impact of tongue-tie on breastfeeding is complex. Qualitative research with women highlights issues of pain, distress and desperation to find support. It is an increasingly common reason for women to access breastfeeding support.[36,37] However, studies examining the impact on breastfeeding cessation and milk supply are mixed, in part due to variations and limitations in study design.

In terms of what can be done if a baby has a tongue-tie, the evidence is again mixed. 'Cutting' tongue-ties (or frenotomy to give it its formal name) with scissors or a laser, attracts some controversy, but many studies suggest that the procedure improves tongue action, latch scores and maternal nipple pain.[38] Others suggest that the frenulum will naturally stretch over time without surgery, but that of course does not solve pain in those important early days and weeks. Other studies find no difference in feeding behaviour or duration after the procedure, although this is where it starts to get complicated.[39]

One reason why research into the impact of cutting tongue-ties is difficult to interpret is that it is challenging to adequately find a control group. The best type of design for comparing outcomes for dividing or not dividing a tongue-tie would be a randomised controlled trial where babies were randomly assigned to division or not. But a major limitation of this, apart from the reluctance of some women to take part, is that it is difficult to hide from women whether their baby had a division or not. In many randomised controlled trials, the researchers would attempt to 'blind' participants to a medicine or procedure that they had done to prevent knowledge of the procedure affecting perceived outcomes. For example, if a mother knew her baby had their tongue-tie divided, she might be more tempted to report a positive outcome and vice versa.

Researchers sometimes get around this by pretending to do something to the baby, known as a 'sham procedure', but in reality most mothers will be able to guess if their baby has had a division, either because it feels different when they feed or simply by looking. It also seems that even just taking part in a study and having a sham procedure can affect the belief that something has been done and lead to a reported improvement in outcomes. In one study that used this approach for tongue-tie, mothers whose baby had not had their tongue-tie cut reported an improvement in pain because they believed something had been done. However those whose baby did have their tie divided reported a much bigger improvement in feeding and comfort.[40]

Another method of trying to blind participants is to blind researchers to the procedure. In one study researchers who did not know whether a baby had received a division or not rated the baby's feeding behaviour using the LATCH tool. They did not find any difference between babies who had a division or not, but in follow-up interviews with their mothers, women reported less pain and easier feeding, which made them feel more confident about feeding their baby.[41] However, other studies do show a difference in feeding behaviours after frenotomy. One example used ultrasound rather than relying on external observation and found significant improvements in milk transfer, milk intake and reduced pain.[42]

Overall, many of the studies report that mothers say they can feel a difference and are in less pain post-frenotomy.[43] Even if researchers cannot view a difference themselves, shouldn't maternal pain and comfort ratings be what is important here? However, this important point aside, given that frenotomy is not always risk free, we should be cautious and ensure that we are no more over-diagnosing than we are under-diagnosing.[44] More research is needed.

How does this all affect breastfeeding?

I don't think I really need to spell this one out, do I?

If a woman is experiencing pain when she latches her baby on, or if she has lasting damage to her nipples, it is easy to understand why she would stop breastfeeding! Given the frequency with which some studies suggest women experience pain, the frequency with which we know babies feed, and the fact that our government is cutting a load of the support services that help women alleviate pain, it is a wonder that our breastfeeding rates are as high as they are! What this shows is the determination of many women who really want to persevere with breastfeeding.

However, alongside the not-so-minor issue of the mother's pain and distress, a further complication of nipple pain can be poor milk supply. The issue with a poor latch is that it can have a knock-on effect on milk production. If the baby doesn't latch onto the breast efficiently, the baby cannot stimulate milk supply and access the milk available. There is also a link between breastfeeding pain and postnatal depression, although potentially this relationship could work both ways. Mothers who experience pain may be at more risk of depression, but mothers with depression could also be more perceptive of pain. Either way, it's not great.

What is really important is to note that, with the right support from experts, breastfeeding pain should ease for many women. After all, if we think again about breastfeeding rates in Scandinavian countries, pain does not stop breastfeeding there to the same extent. This is highly unlikely to be because all Scandinavian women are battling through despite the pain, or have nipples of steel! But how many women in the UK have someone in their family who can help them with positioning and latch? Or know where to access professional support? Even if they do know where to access help, how many breastfeeding experts do we have in this country, who have enough time to properly support women? Not enough.

The importance of skilled support

'I asked for help picking him up and latching him on as I was still so sore and I swear she rolled her eyes at me. She handled me quite roughly, latching him on for me, said there you go and walked off. I felt such a nuisance.'

'I couldn't have done it without my midwife. She sat with me and helped me work out just what wasn't quite right. She didn't stop trying until he latched on beautifully, all the while making me feel like she had nothing else to do, even though I knew she was so busy.'

Two very different stories. Two very different outcomes for women. One had stopped breastfeeding after a few days. The other was a mother I was interviewing to understand women's experiences of successful breastfeeding. It's not hard to work out which is which. Health professionals, their interactions, attitudes and approach to mothers, play a big role in how a woman feels about breastfeeding. And feeling supported, both practically and emotionally, by a midwife, is a key predictor of whether a mother continues breastfeeding. However, as with everything there are two sides to it: there are professionals who are motivated and skilled in understanding what women want, and those who are, well… less so.

Lots of research has shown that new mothers expect to be supported with breastfeeding, including things like being shown how to latch a baby on. They expect to be educated and value this. Meanwhile, most health professionals value their role in supporting mothers to breastfeed and gain satisfaction from doing so. However, many women postnatally report disappointment in the support they receive with breastfeeding, particularly in the hospital after the birth, and many health professionals are themselves disappointed in the constraints their role places on them.[45] So what is going on?

What do new mothers need from health professionals?

A number of studies have explored the impact of professional support on breastfeeding. By health professional I am generally referring to midwives and health visitors, or nurses in the USA, who are paid professionals. Research has explored the issue both from the perspective of what women feel is supportive and damaging, and from the perspective of the professionals providing support. Some key points emerge.

A systematic review identified clear themes in what support is valuable for women.[46] One key positive element was the concept of continuity of care. Mothers particularly liked building a relationship with an individual who they saw several times, even if this was over a short period of time in the hospital. However, many new mothers reported that their care was fragmented, and that they saw many different staff, even during a short hospital stay. A consequence of this was that different members of staff presented conflicting information and styles of approach, leaving mothers confused about what to do.

A second important finding was that women really valued time taken by professionals to sit with them. This allowed them to move past basic latch discussions and to form a connection and relationship. Mothers felt supported by the professional just 'being there'. In a related study, Professor Fiona Dykes describes this as 'touching base' – professionals taking the time to regularly spend time with the mum, even if it is very brief.[47] However, as you can imagine, many professionals simply do not have the time to give this level of care, and women feel that they are being rushed and that staff are disconnected from them.

The content of interactions with health professionals was also important. Although women did value information about how to latch the baby on, what they really valued was emotional support. Empathy. Affirmation. Reassurance. All good things. They valued discussion, and being facilitated to try things themselves and make decisions for themselves. In reality, what they often got was someone physically touching them and latching the baby on for them, without explaining what was going on, or standardised information that didn't take into account their wider emotions and experiences. Rather than being facilitated, many felt that they were being dictated to, with little room for manoeuvre. Women often felt that they had differing goals, with the professional determined to latch the baby on over and above everything else.

Likewise, in another similar study, lots of women reported that they didn't feel prepared to breastfeed and weren't given sufficient information, other than being told why breastfeeding should be chosen and perhaps how to latch the baby on. Mothers who had a more positive experience really valued realistic and honest information about what feeding a baby was like.[48]

Lots of research in this area has emphasised the need for personal interactions and care of the mum. One study noted how mothers particularly valued it when midwives saw them as a real person with needs, rather than there simply in the context of the baby. This included things like acknowledging the pressures new mothers faced, or that breastfeeding could be challenging, rather than simply insisting it was best. In particular, midwives who encouraged women to look after themselves while they were breastfeeding, not just the baby, were valued. It can be a hard thing as a new mother to put yourself first, even when you're exhausted, so someone in 'authority' giving a mother permission was important.[49]

Does support matter?

Yes, of course. Women who feel supported by professionals are more likely to initiate and continue breastfeeding. One mother summed this up perfectly:

> 'I simply couldn't have done it without her. She was my absolute rock. I must have called her over 10, 20 times when I was in hospital and every time she took the time to sit with me and reassure me. One time there was a bit of a lull in activity and she just sat with me watching him feed, reassuring me and telling me what a brilliant job I was doing. We chatted about what I would do when I got home and she told me about a great peer support group and a community midwife who would be able to help me. She made sure I felt confident in what I was doing and we talked about my fears for a bit. She didn't have to do that. She could have had a well-deserved break but she chose to give me that time. I will be forever grateful.'

There are many fantastic midwives and health visitors out there who are truly valued by the communities they support. These individuals make a real difference to the lives of families and if we could bottle what they do and sell it on, we'd make a fortune. However, not all women are so lucky. Inconsistent and unhelpful support is a common reason for stopping breastfeeding. One issue, of course, could be that health professionals are 'blamed' when mothers are unable to breastfeed. Cognitive dissonance theory explores how psychologically it is often uncomfortable for us to take blame or responsibility for decisions ourselves, especially if our actions do not match our ideals or intentions. Instead we look to attribute our behaviour to others. Health professionals are an easy target.

However, from looking at the literature around breastfeeding and listening to thousands of new mothers, it seems a lack of professional support – or for most, a lack of the *type* of support they needed – does play a key role in stopping breastfeeding.

What support do professionals give?

In a fascinating review of the literature exploring midwives' views on supporting breastfeeding, the concept of different 'types' of midwife emerges.[50] Midwives tended to take one of two approaches: midwife as a skilled companion to the mother, or midwife as a technical expert. Sometimes they had to swap between these roles, but professionals typically had a preference.

Midwives who see their role as a skilled companion focus mainly on supporting the relationship between mother and baby. Midwives in this group tend to be mother-centred, seeing the woman as important in her own right, not just in relation to the baby. Those that fall into this category tend to be very hands-off and follow the woman's lead. They listen to the woman and put her needs at the centre. Just what women want, right? Yes. And there are some absolutely fabulous midwives and health visitors out there who do this. But in an analysis of what midwives actually did in relation to supporting breastfeeding, this approach only accounted for 10% of all feeding interactions. Some midwives feel frustrated and angry about not being able to fulfil this role due to time pressures.[50]

In the other approach, the midwife is a technical expert. Midwives in this group are 'breast-centred', seeing their role as getting breastmilk from the mother into the baby. Successful breastfeeding, in terms of transfer of milk, is their goal. In a paper exploring how midwives who adopt this approach feel, transfer of milk was the key theme. Midwives saw themselves as the breastfeeding expert who is there to teach the woman how to breastfeed and use her 'breastfeeding equipment'. Many see their ability to get the breastmilk into the baby as an achievement that brings a sense of status, with some taking a very hands-on approach, literally holding the woman's breast and baby and bringing them together (often without consent to touch the mother's breast). If women cannot get the baby to latch on, these midwives may be insistent that she expresses, as the milk must reach the baby.[1]

Do women like this approach? No. Does it work? No. One study, for which midwives were taught how to give 'hands-off' support, found that far more women were breastfeeding at six weeks.[51] Why doesn't the technical expert approach work? Well, it's intrusive for a start. There seems to be an assumption that just because a few hours ago you were completely naked and someone was staring inside you to try to spot the baby, that they can then go on to touch you how they like forever more. And if mother and baby are manhandled into latching, it doesn't help women learn how to do it themselves. Physically manhandling a sensitive part of a woman's body that she is unlikely to have had touched by many people into a baby's mouth is, well, a little off-putting. It also puts significant pressure on the woman to 'perform'. She must breastfeed and she must do it now. Quickly, preferably, as the midwife wants to move on. All this can negatively affect her ability to actually breastfeed – remember all the stuff on stress hormones we discussed earlier? Gabrielle Palmer, in her 1988 book *The Politics of Breastfeeding*,[52] makes a sobering comparison about how we can sometimes treat breastfeeding today:

> *'Imagine a young man making his first attempt at sexual penetration. Ask him to set about the project in a special sex centre where there are "experts" he has never met before, ready to supervise and tell him how it ought to be done. Presume that his partner is as inexperienced as himself, and that he is asked if he is going to "try and achieve an erection". When he starts, a busy "expert", who may never have personally experienced sexual relations, starts telling him how to do it and inspects his body with a critical expression, prodding him and his partner in an insensitive manner. By the bed is an artificial penis, put there, as the young man is told, "just in case you can't manage it; many men can't make it. It's not their fault, nature often fails". Everyone knows how vulnerable the male penis is to psychological stress, and how sensitive sexual partners must be in order to nurture the psyche, as well as the body, of the male. Yet such sensitivity has been conspicuously absent from the experience of most women giving birth in hospital.'*

Do midwives want to be this way? Yes, some do. Some midwives take the view that they are the expert and the woman a student, using a directive tone and insistence that new mothers do things a certain way.[53] Some see mothers as milk-making machines and have been observed using condescending language such as 'sweetie' and 'girlie' when paternalistically telling the mother she needs to give her baby milk. Sometimes the midwives most likely to take this approach and stick to the 'rules' about infant feeding are the ones who do not have their own experience of feeding babies.[54] This dogmatic 'breast is best under all circumstances' approach, as it is perceived by some women, does little to help anyone to feed and can drive a wedge between mother and professional. Women talk about hiding bottles of formula, and not telling midwives and health visitors about their decision to formula-feed.[55] When introducing formula, a higher proportion of mothers raised concerns about telling their health professional, than were concerned about the health impact for their baby. That's just not right.[56]

However, other midwives desperately want to be the skilled companion type, but are so time-pressured that they are unable to do so. Many describe how they have so many women to care for that they need to get the minimum done and move on to the next. The main focus becomes latching the baby on and checking whether the baby is getting milk, rather than taking the time to sit and talk about how the mother feels. Some are so time-pressured that they resort to physically latching the baby on themselves, rather than guiding the mother to do it. Many feel a sense of relief once baby is latched on, as they can move on to their next task.[57] Others end up offering formula as a solution, even though deep down they know that with enough time they might be able to solve the problem.[58]

New mothers are often offered formula as a solution, which leaves them bemused after a pregnancy in which all they heard was that 'breast is best'. Many feel that huge effort goes into telling them to breastfeed, but as soon as there is a problem, formula is suggested, with the subtext that it will simply save time. One mother explained to me, exasperated:

> 'Sometimes it seems like they spend the whole pregnancy telling you that you must breastfeed, and then after birth try and persuade you to give a bottle whenever a problem arises. I was lucky in some respects that I had a community midwife that I saw both during pregnancy and after I had my baby. But on the other hand it was very surreal to hear the professional who had just spent nine months telling you breast is best suggesting that you top up with formula when you express concern about how much your baby is feeding!'

Unsurprisingly, wider issues such as short-staffing and midwives not having the time to sit and be with women after the birth are preventing midwives from being able to take the time to support new mothers.

Others think that everyone else must be providing the support, while everyone else thinks that someone else is – no one takes responsibility.[59] This creates a situation in which new mothers are uncertain and unconfident about how to feed their baby themselves. Women who aren't shown how to do something and supported to do it themselves are the ones who end up with the lowest confidence. Many feel that they cannot disturb their midwife, or feel guilty about taking up too much time. Others simply feel that their midwife doesn't want to help them.[60]

Midwives' own experiences

'One midwife actually told me that although she would never say it in front of anyone else she didn't believe in promoting breastfeeding and thought it made no difference, but she had to tell new mothers about it anyway. She told me her babies had been formula-fed and they were fine so not to worry about it. I was about to stop breastfeeding anyway at this point, but even I was open-mouthed at that one!'

Whether a midwife has breastfed her own baby, and her experience of doing that, can influence how she goes on to care for new mothers.[61] Some evidence suggests that those who have never had a baby of their own can be the most dogmatic, trying to get mothers to follow the 'rules' with little leeway for wider experience. This makes sense – on the surface breastfeeding can seem so straightforward when you haven't had the experience of doing it yourself. Surely women should breastfeed, right?

The most supportive midwives tend to be the ones who have had positive experiences of breastfeeding their own babies, or who have been affected by negative experiences and want to help other mothers. These midwives know how tough it can be and the emotions that go alongside it. They want others to have an easier time, or know what helps and what doesn't. They can empathise as well as give practical support, and it's easier to support someone through something if you've done it yourself.

This leads neatly on to the negative influence a midwife can have if she had a negative breastfeeding experience herself or chose not to breastfeed. As shown in the quote above, her beliefs can cloud the support she gives. Of course this doesn't apply to all midwives, but many struggle to encourage women to do something they didn't do themselves. They can feel hypocritical, or experience the cognitive dissonance discussed earlier, feeling 'I did the best for my baby and they're fine, so why am I bothering with this breastfeeding advice?' It is a complicated area, and midwives should be able to debrief their own experiences of breastfeeding during training, with emotional support.

What else gets in the way of providing mother-centred support?

Aside from time or personal experience, some midwives don't feel that they have the knowledge, training or skills to be able to support new mothers with breastfeeding. For those who trained some time ago when breastfeeding was not such a big part of the curriculum, many feel that they are unable to support women through anything other than a basic latch. Many from this generation note that breastfeeding was seen as a special interest, with only those who were really intrigued getting additional training on the subject. Sometimes, once midwives have lots of experience, they are called to work in more specialist areas, particularly the birth suite, rather than supporting women on the postnatal ward. Their experience of breastfeeding essentially becomes 'lost' – lost from the ward, and then lost over time as they don't keep up to date with their skills.[50]

However, some professionals don't see a need for training in breastfeeding, particularly when it comes to the concept of evidence based practice. Midwives in this group tend to question new research, especially if it contradicts older research. A good example of this would be the recommendation for the duration of exclusive breastfeeding, which has changed from 12 to 26 weeks during many older professionals' careers. Many in this group state that they ignore research findings and carry on as before. One midwife in a study referred to research as a 'bandwagon', and many were sceptical or even scornful, particularly when research is used to create policy that they feel is incorrect. Many doubt the need for a research base, preferring to rely on their own experience. One midwife noted that she didn't believe that breastfeeding reduced the risk of breast cancer in women, as she has seen women who breastfed go on to develop breast cancer.[50]

Others are wary about promoting breastfeeding, as they see their role as being protective of the mother above all else. Midwives want to encourage the mother to rest and recover from the birth and worry about breastfeeding causing her stress. These midwives report wanting to give supplements to the baby rather than waking the mother up if she is sleeping. Others are reluctant to talk about breastfeeding in case it makes women feel guilty or like a failure. You can really see where these midwives are coming from, but also how their approach could seriously damage breastfeeding in the early days.[62]

Research that aimed to promote knowledge and the importance of approach among health professionals in breastfeeding support has worked well. One study aimed to increase health visitors' knowledge of how breastfeeding works and the type of support new mothers need. At the end of the training health visitors felt more confident, and over time women in their care felt more supported.[63] Another study worked on challenging the negative approaches some professionals have to breastfeeding support by exploring attitudes and approaches to breastfeeding. Professionals were less disempowering and more facilitating after the course.[64]

What about other health professionals, particularly medical staff?

Women may approach different health professionals for advice while they are breastfeeding including medical staff and dieticians. Although there are some very passionate and skilled professionals working in these fields to support families, unfortunately a lack of breastfeeding content during training and other time constraints can sometimes lead to poor medical or nutritional advice damaging women's ability to continue breastfeeding.

Everything we've discussed about the pressures on midwives applies to doctors too: the lack of time, personal beliefs and their own experiences. Not all doctors are the same, but it can be a significant issue. My personal experience includes meeting a doctor who was amazed that I was still breastfeeding (he checked three times... *still?* Are you sure?). My son was just coming up to six weeks old. Another, in possibly the strangest interaction I have ever had with a health professional, on hearing I was still (*still!*) breastfeeding my four-month-old, asked me if I knew I could 'milk myself' (yes, exact words) and add it to my cornflakes in the morning. 'I prefer toast', I said.

Breakfast choices aside, doctors' knowledge of breastfeeding is particularly relevant when women need medication. Although many medications are suitable for use during breastfeeding, some doctors may focus on any potential risk of the medication to the baby, rather than the risk to the baby of not being breastfed. If a doctor thinks that a certain medication carries risk (even if there is no evidence for this), they are likely to consider this in isolation, rather than weighing up the risks against the benefits of a baby continuing to be breastfed. Many feel cautious, concerned about any potential risks, and sometimes confounded by fears or the threat of litigation.[65] Others do not value breastfeeding, feeling there is little real benefit over formula milk. This can obviously leave women feeling unsupported and that they are not getting enough information.[66] They may also feel societal pressure to reduce any perceived risk to the baby from taking a medication (of course, society does not simultaneously see any risk to not breastfeeding).[67]

We saw this in a recent evaluation we conducted for the Breastfeeding Network in the UK, exploring the impact of their Drugs in Breastmilk service.[68] We found that when women were prescribed a medication or medical procedure they faced two common issues: either being told they could not take the medication and carry on breastfeeding, or not receiving any information at all, leaving them uncertain. This led to them contacting the service and in almost all cases the medication or procedure prescribed was compatible with breastfeeding, or a suitable alternative could be prescribed instead. In the majority of cases the medications prescribed were common, with plenty of evidence that they were compatible with breastfeeding, for example antihistamines, antidepressants and antibiotics.

Without the service providing them with up-to-date evidence, many women in our research would have faced a dilemma between taking the medication and stopping breastfeeding, or continuing to breastfeed and risking their own health. We were surprised at just how many women indicated that they would choose the second, which highlights just how significant a risk this issue is. Breastfeeding meant so much to women that they were prepared to put their own health at risk to continue to protect their baby or their own mental wellbeing.

One core issue underlying misguided medical information when it comes to supporting breastfeeding women is a lack of depth of inclusion in the medical curriculum in the UK and many other countries. For example, in one study in Australia, 90% of general practitioners reported no formal training in breastfeeding, relying on informal experience and knowledge they had built over the years. Although all believed it was important to support breastfeeding, many lacked the skills or confidence to practically do so. Others believed it was more important to support maternal mental health and a good relationship with the mother than to encourage breastfeeding.[69]

Similar patterns can be seen in more recent research with medical students. Although attitudes towards breastfeeding are positive, students generally feel that they are lacking sufficient knowledge and skill. For example, a recent paper in the UK explored the education, knowledge and perceptions of medical students towards breastfeeding. Although almost all medical schools reported teaching some aspects of breastfeeding, this tended to focus on the physiology of lactation, whereas just 19% offered formal clinical teaching. Overall students did not feel confident in practical support skills for breastfeeding. Just 3% felt confident assisting with latching, 16% in recognising and managing mastitis and nipple thrush and 13% reasons for formula supplementation. Almost all wanted more breastfeeding education.[70]

Another study with medical students in Lebanon identified a core barrier as the curriculum focusing on pathophysiology and treatment as opposed to public health and disease prevention.[71] Students also reported relatively little opportunity to gain experience in obstetrics and gynaecology full stop, let alone in relation to feeding babies. Notably some students highlighted that they did receive pressures from infant formula companies to promote their products – something that will be considered in more depth in chapter 16. Other research has highlighted the pressures of an already full medical curriculum.[72]

Research that has tried to change doctors' attitudes to breastfeeding has worked well. One intervention in France sent doctors on a five-hour education programme and found that breastfeeding rates at their surgeries increased.[73] Another found that an interactive training session on how to manage breastfeeding problems effectively (e.g. not to just say 'stop breastfeeding') found that doctors emerged far more knowledgeable, particularly if they had their own children.[74] Finally, another study found that if medical students gained practical experience of seeing how breastfeeding worked in practice, their attitudes towards breastfeeding and subsequent breastfeeding advice were far better.[75]

Indeed, hands-on training and real-world clinical experience appear to be an important part of enhancing skills, rather than simple lecture-based delivery.[76] It's almost as if women and babies are real people and not data in textbooks! On a serious note, one fascinating study in the US developed a simulation model of a lactating mother. The students could practise showing 'her' how to hand express and have literal hands-on experience in examining the breast. Students very much valued having a realistic model to practise on before supporting actual women in real life.[77]

Another group of health professionals whose knowledge and skill can affect breastfeeding is dieticians. Research exploring breastfeeding knowledge among this group is relatively sparse, however. There are also no formal guidelines or standards in terms of supporting breastfeeding mothers, although breastfeeding is recommended by the British Dietetic Association. One recent study in Ireland exploring the experience of dieticians found that 59% had undertaken further training on breastfeeding since qualifying, however for half this did not include clinical skills. Overall 64% felt they would benefit from additional training with around half feeling that they lacked the skill, confidence or knowledge to fully support breastfeeding women.[78]

In terms of knowledge, although almost all felt that breastmilk was all that was needed for the first six months, over two-thirds believed a mother's diet needed to be well balanced for adequate quality milk, while over a third believed that formula milk is nutritionally similar to breastmilk. In qualitative responses, barriers included fear of upsetting mothers by being seen as too pro-breastfeeding, too many more common and complex issues to deal with such as allergies or malnutrition, and the often common ties between dieticians and formula companies. Indeed, 20% of participants gained information on breastfeeding from formula company-sponsored events.

The close ties between (some) dieticians and the formula industry, perhaps particularly in Ireland, remain an issue. In another study of 162 dieticians in Ireland, up to 50% received information on breastfeeding from infant formula manufacturers.[79] Again, more on this pressing issue in chapter 16.

What actually works best in increasing breastfeeding in terms of professional support?

Supporting women in the way they say they want has been shown by research studies to work best when it comes to increasing breastfeeding rates. One study found that the best outcomes for breastfeeding came when women had lots of positive support in hospital, in terms of praise and reassurance, and felt that they could ask questions and have them answered. Supporting a woman to latch her baby on, rather than doing it for her, and explaining why, also helped. Basically the gift of time. And understanding. And respect. The same study also showed that simply telling women during pregnancy that breastfeeding was a really good idea and they should do it, didn't work.[80] Strange, that.

One systematic review found that the things new mothers say work best to support them actually do. These included: home visits, telephone calls, peer support, hands-off teaching, support and encouragement, continuity of care across pregnancy and the newborn period and well-trained professionals.[81] Do most new mothers get all of these after they've had their baby? No.

Other research has shown that breastfeeding support works best when all professionals in an area are giving the same messages. In one trial, a coaching intervention aimed at new mothers worked better in some areas than others and the researchers were intrigued about why. It turned out that women in those areas where there were good working relationships between professionals who supported breastfeeding benefited most from the intervention. Essentially, they were supported best by all the professionals around them. Are most areas supported and encouraged to work like this? No.[82]

Timing of support is really important. Interventions in the antenatal period to try and increase intention to breastfeed don't work very well in isolation. Approaches that offer continuity, working with women antenatally, and supporting them postnatally, result in the biggest increases in breastfeeding rates. Typically these approaches offer information in the antenatal period and emotional support in the postnatal period. The support bit is critical. Education followed by education doesn't work well. And postnatal support needs to be ongoing – a one-off 'you're doing great' visit isn't enough. It has to be more regular – at least two to three contacts. An intervention with one of the best outcomes for breastfeeding at six months came from a study that started working practically with mothers in the hospital, followed up by a supportive telephone conversation when they got home, followed up again by visits from a community midwife and finally having peer support in the community. Breastfeeding is too complex to be 'fixed' just by getting the baby latched on.[83]

The role of specialised lactation consultant support

International Board-Certified Lactation Consultants (IBCLCs) are infant feeding specialists who have undertaken significant training and examination to qualify. This includes extensive clinical hours and formal learning with regular maintenance and recertification once qualified. The impact of receiving support from a highly qualified, experienced and motivated lactation specialist strangely enough tends to be positive. Who knew that providing women with the expertise and time they needed helped them to breastfeed and make them feel valued?[84]

Unsurprisingly, new mothers who have support from a lactation consultant breastfeed for longer. Research that has examined outcomes for early lactation support found that double the number of women supported by a lactation consultant left hospital exclusively breastfeeding compared to those supported by a nurse without lactation specialist training.[85] Another study found that breastfeeding duration and exclusivity rates rose up to six months after specialist lactation support was integrated onto the hospital ward.[86]

Other studies have looked at support within the community, after hospital discharge. One study found that discharging new mothers from hospital earlier, with a follow-up appointment with a lactation consultant at home, had better outcomes for breastfeeding than staying in hospital. It also didn't cost any more money.[87] Another found that even telephone conversations with a lactation consultant, one at 48 hours and then every week for four weeks, had a positive impact on breastfeeding duration. This really goes to show that it's also about what is said, rather than just physically latching a baby on.[88]

One of the most important skills that has been identified through research into IBCLCs is the format of support. Lactation consultants tend to adopt a counselling style that is more encouraging and woman-centred than the approach of health professionals. They tend to take into account the bigger picture and work with a woman and her concerns. They guide mothers rather than physically latch a baby on for them. What they offer is pretty much what new mothers want.[89]

Other interventions have focused on broader roles. One study used a small randomised controlled trial to evaluate the impact of IBCLC antenatal education and postnatal support groups. Those who received this over usual care had higher breastfeeding self-efficacy and longer exclusive breastfeeding rates.[90] Indeed, in a systematic review of 16 studies including 5,084 mothers, when breastfeeding education and support was delivered by lactation specialists, breastfeeding initiation, duration and exclusivity increased.[91]

So we have lots of lactation consultants in our hospitals, right? Er, no. The government is actually cutting funding for many of them.

Action 3
✓ Invest in expert support for all breastfeeding women right from the start.

8. A LACK OF UNDERSTANDING OF NORMAL BREASTFED BABY BEHAVIOUR LEADS TO PEOPLE THINKING SOMETHING IS WRONG

'It was all he did. Feed, sleep, cry. Feed, sleep, cry. Feed, sleep, cry. I knew something must have been wrong. This couldn't be right. Other people wanted to see him and I wanted to show my beautiful baby off but he was either attached to me, wanting to be attached to me or might as well have been attached to me as he only wanted to sleep on me. It was like he knew when I wasn't there or perhaps he just sensed his milk wasn't there and that was all I was to him. I was so worried I was doing something wrong. It was just nothing like I expected...'

This quote is taken from a research project I conducted exploring whether new mothers felt prepared for breastfeeding, or indeed felt prepared for caring for their baby at all. The general consensus was 'No'. This mother certainly wasn't alone. From the pages and pages of responses I had, the idea that babies weren't supposed to act this way came across very strongly. Babies were feeding seemingly all the time, not wanting to be put down and refusing to sleep at night. Nobody had told the mothers this would happen; they hadn't expected it and they worried it was wrong. You can see the emotion and anxiety in this mother's words: for many of you it will take you back to those early days when 'eat, sleep, cry' was on repeat. Those times can certainly seem overwhelming, and many feel unprepared, but is anything actually wrong? How often do new babies feed? How often do they wake up? How much do they cry? What is normal behaviour for a breastfeeding baby? And is it different from those who are formula-fed?

Throughout my research the same theme has cropped up time and time again. Women do not feel prepared for the realities of breastfeeding and end up worrying that their perfectly normal breastfed baby is broken. Knowledge of what breastfeeding and caring for a breastfed baby is really like is critical to preparing new mothers to breastfeed, yet we rarely do it properly. If women have any antenatal education at all they are often taught about latch, but the realities of breastfeeding? Rarely. Yet anxiety about whether they are doing it 'right', and whether their baby is 'normal', are key reasons given for starting to use formula milk, which is often seen as reassuringly measurable and predictable. One mother summed it up brilliantly:

> *'Saying breast is best to a woman who is desperate to feed but struggling to do so is like telling someone how great this bus is, how fabulous and cheap the journey, how much better it is all-round… but not telling them where the bus stop is…'*

Is breastfeeding difficult because we don't understand how it works?

Knowledge and confidence are intrinsically linked. Going back to the concept of a formula-feeding culture, do many new mothers really know what breastfeeding is going to be like? I don't think so. However, they do have some knowledge of what formula-feeding is like, whether from direct experience of feeding someone else's baby, comments from others or absorption of ideas from adverts and magazines.

The problem is that breastmilk and formula milk and breastfeeding and formula-feeding are intrinsically different. As we will see, breastfed babies feed more frequently than formula-fed babies, and when they need feeding, they need to be fed. And that is OK. In fact, it's more than OK: it's normal. But this one small fact is at the heart of a lot of breastfeeding problems. And many people don't realise it.

Some of the most common reasons for stopping breastfeeding are: 'he fed too much', 'I didn't have enough milk', 'he was never satisfied' and 'he wasn't sleeping properly'. Can these be true? Are there really so many babies out there who are dissatisfied with breastfeeding? Or is something happening to make breastfeeding go wrong so that women end up feeling like this? If we looked at how often those babies woke and asked to be fed, would it be abnormal? Or would it only seem abnormal compared to a formula-fed baby?

These 'problems' aren't just in mothers' heads. No one lives in a bubble. If mothers are doubting their babies, it is quite possible that their doubts are coming from others.

> *'Are you sure he needs feeding again?'*
> *'When you were little we just fed you every four hours.'*

'You really need to see how much he's getting.'
'Is your milk really enough for him?'
'I couldn't breastfeed, women in our family can't.'
'Are you sure he doesn't need a bottle?'

In what other situation would we behave like this? Last New Year I reflected on this behaviour. A quick glance at Facebook told me many friends had resolved to be more active, lose weight, drink less… the usual. Great. But what was notable was the comments underneath those resolutions. Most expressed support, awe or simply said it was a lovely idea. Maybe some people read the declarations and thought 'Ha! You said that last year and we all know you'll be eating cake before lunch on day one' – *but they didn't say it.* And that's what is important.

Imagine you declare (possibly after a glass or three of champagne) that this year you will get fit and run a half marathon. Instead of a handful of 'likes' and a supportive friend or two offering to come along, you get a stream of comments:

'I wanted to run but I just couldn't do it.'
'I tried that and I was in so much pain.'
'Women in our family can't do that.'
'But how will you know if you've gone far enough?'
'Why don't I drive along behind you and pick you up if it's too hard?'
'I'd really be happier if you didn't.'

Feeling demoralised yet? And yet these are the messages many pregnant and new mothers receive about breastfeeding. And it's likely to stop them breastfeeding. If you type 'is breastfeeding difficult' into Google, you get nearly 13 million hits. So here we have problem number one that needs to be tackled. Knowledge of what is normal behaviour for a breastfed baby, and why respecting that is important.

How often do breastfed babies really feed?

As we saw earlier, the first stages of milk production are pretty automatic, but what happens next is really important. Once that first milk has been triggered, it needs to be removed if more is to be made. Typically, the more a baby feeds (or a mother expresses) the more milk is made and vice versa. If feeds are replaced with formula, or delayed (perhaps by giving a dummy), then the body starts to produce less milk. The female body is pretty efficient and doesn't want to expend energy producing milk that the baby doesn't need.[1]

Numerous research studies demonstrate this. For example, trying to reduce feeds or feeding to a set schedule rather than when the baby asks for it can lead to a drop in milk supply.[2] When babies are breastfed on demand from birth, mature milk comes in earlier,[3] and babies are more likely to get back to their birth weight more quickly.[4] In fact, one study asked mothers to either feed to a set 3–4 hour schedule, or to feed their baby on demand, and then measured how much milk women were producing. Women who fed on demand had a far better milk supply than those who breastfed to a schedule, and their babies were taking almost a third more milk.[5] Not surprisingly, women who follow their babies' cues and breastfeed on demand are far more likely to be exclusively breastfeeding at six weeks.[6]

Frequent feeding is also really important from a hormonal perspective to keep feeding going. The more frequently a baby feeds, the higher the levels of prolactin (the hormone that supports milk production) in the mother. Suckling appears to send a signal for more prolactin to be produced, with a rise at the start of each feed.[7] Feeding lots at night increases prolactin levels even more than feeding during the day. More frequent feeds also help to flush any jaundice from the baby. In one hospital study, babies who were breastfed at least eight times in 24 hours had lower serum bilirubin levels than those who fed less frequently.[8]

Interfering with the baby's natural feeding cues by offering a dummy in the early days can reduce the frequency of feeds. One study explored how dummies were used and how babies were fed. Babies who used a dummy had on average one feed less and spent around half an hour less time feeding each day compared to those who did not. Babies who used a dummy also went around half an hour longer in between feeds. There also appeared to be a frequency effect; babies who used a dummy frequently fed less than those who only sometimes used it.

However, those 'sometimes' babies still fed less than the 'never used it' babies. What was really interesting about this study was that babies who thumb-sucked fed to the same pattern as the non-dummy babies.[9] This could work in a number of ways. Dummies might be used to deliberately delay feeds, or sucking on a dummy for a bit might delay the baby asking to be fed. Either way, feeds are delayed and the risk of milk supply dropping increases. Why doesn't finger or thumb-sucking have the same effect? Well, it's the baby's choice – the baby can put them in there and take them out. No one else is trying to distract them with their fingers. And fingers are finger-shaped, not nipple-shaped, so the baby doesn't think that if they suck hard enough milk will eventually come out.

What does feeding 'responsively' really mean?

Okay, so breastfed babies need to be fed lots and whenever they want it. But what does that mean in reality? Tins of formula and books suggest that formula-fed babies should be on a 3 or 4-hour schedule – so that's okay for breastfed babies too, isn't it?

In a word, no.

Newborn babies have tiny stomachs, around the size of a cherry or a walnut in the first few days, increasing to the size of an egg by around two weeks. Think about how much milk would fit in an egg. Not a lot. A four-week-old baby needs about 750ml of milk a day. Hmmm. That's a lot of eggs. At least eight, because the average intake of a month-old breastfed baby is about 90ml per feed.[10]

Breastfed babies therefore naturally feed a lot. If you look at the NHS website it suggests 8–12 times per 24 hours at least, but many women will laugh wryly at this. Babies can feed far more frequently and this is completely normal. In fact, looking at how often babies naturally feed, from a biological perspective, using anthropological studies, is fascinating. These studies typically report data from observational studies conducted in rural developing cultures where staying alive, rather than building a career or worrying about your baby's sleep, is the major task. Mothers in these cultures tend to sleep together as a family and have their children close to them during the day. They do not have the influences of Western culture suggesting they should stop their baby feeding at night, return to work or lose weight, so their feeding and sleeping patterns can give us an insight into what normal evolutionary baby behaviour is like. This is not to say this behaviour should automatically be picked up and followed in Westernised cultures, but it does show how breastfeeding and sleeping are biologically programmed, and where some of our issues may arise.

One good example is an observational study in Botswana looking at a very rural hunter-gatherer tribe known as the !Kung, where mother and baby are pretty much permanently together until the child is two years of age, and even then separations are pretty rare, at least until a younger sibling comes along. Researchers found that it was normal for babies to breastfeed very frequently, for just a few minutes at a time, for most of the day. Indeed, the average frequency was four times an hour, with the average feed lasting less than two minutes and an interval of around 13 minutes between each feed. It was rare for a baby not to feed during an observed 15-minute period, and although the baby who fed the least frequently who was something of an outlier, he still went only around 55 minutes between feeds.[11] And you thought your breastfed baby fed a lot…!

These babies are not alone. In two other observational studies measuring how often babies fed in rural Bangladesh, feeds averaged around once per hour.[12,13] Both studies observed feeds over an eight-hour period during the day among mothers who were often working in the fields but carried their babies while they did so. This frequency dropped as babies got a little older but was still 4–5 times over that eight-hour period when they were over six months old. Feeds at all ages tended to be fairly short – less than ten minutes at a time.

Studies conducted in Western cultures suggest that babies still feed very frequently, but not as often as the !Kung babies. An average of around 11–12 feeds per day during the first six months seems normal in studies that record feeds, although there is lots of variation, with studies often showing the top of the range to be around 18 feeds per day. One study in Sweden showed a remarkable variation. At two weeks the mean duration of all feeds was 4.5 hours, but the range was wide (from 2.5 to 10 hours).[14] Another Swedish study of babies aged 0–6 months found that the most common number of feeds started to drop from about 4–12 weeks, but increased again by 20 weeks. At 20 weeks babies were feeding almost at newborn frequency, particularly at night.[15] Women often notice this pattern and worry about it. Babies appear to have settled down a bit, then at about four months old they start feeding lots again. Of course, some then suggest that this is because breastmilk isn't enough for babies and they need solids, but actually there is a huge growth and developmental leap at about 4–5 months and babies need lots of fuel for this.

In an attempt to show just how often breastfed babies can feed I recently conducted a big study asking breastfeeding women how often their baby fed. I asked them to think about how many times their baby fed during the day and night and totted this up to give an overall figure. Looking at babies exclusively breastfed aged up to 6 months, most fed 6–10 times during the day (about 70% of babies), with the most common number of feeds being eight. The average number of feeds was also eight. However, the number of feeds ranged from four all the way up to 20. Less than 1% of babies fed four times a day and only 5% five times a day. However, 15% of babies fed more than 10 times a day (although only 3% over 13 times).

For night feeds only 6% didn't breastfeed at night and most fed 2–5 times (75%). The average number of times was three and the most common number was also three. The number of feeds ranged from none to 12. More babies fed six times a night or more than never. Overall, the most common number of feeds was 9–13 times per 24 hours (60%), but there was a range from five to 25. The average number of feeds was 11, which was also the most common. Over a quarter of babies fed 12 times a day or more. It was more common to feed 16 times or more than it was to feed five times a day. To sum up: lots of feeds, and wide variation between babies.

My data fits well with the other studies that suggest 11–12 times a day, although 20 women beat the top scorer in the Swedish study mentioned above. I did also have to exclude one mother for simply writing 'all the bloody time' as her response (although in hindsight I was surprised it was only one). What this shows is that the NHS suggestion of 8–12 feeds per 24 hours is a bit too low, as many babies fed more than this. It would be better to say that babies usually feed every two hours or so. And however you look at it, these results don't suggest a three-hourly schedule is normal, and they certainly don't fit with the old four-hourly schedules and the suggestion that babies should not be having night feeds from an early age. If we applied the old advice to feed every four hours (so six feeds per day), just 10% of breastfeeding women would be doing it. That's a whole 90% of women breastfeeding 'too much'.

Of course, defining a 'feed' is fairly difficult with breastfed babies. Some may start a feed, drift off to sleep and then resume. Is this one feed or two? So duration matters too. One of the Swedish studies mentioned above[14] looked at how long feeds lasted and found that at two weeks old the average feed time was 17 minutes during the day and 16 minutes at night, but with a range from 5 minutes to 98 minutes. So there's also a lot of variation in feed duration.

Why don't babies feed in a set pattern?

Do you? Do you eat and drink at set hours, around the clock? And eat and drink the same things at that time? No? Then why do we expect babies to?

Breastmilk isn't a uniform product. It changes over the course of a day and from one feed to the next, particularly in terms of fat and calorie content, which affects when a baby will next be hungry. Some studies show that in hotter weather breastmilk becomes less energy dense, encouraging babies to drink more. One study asked women to express milk before and after a feed and at different times of the day. They found that fat content was lower before a feed than it was at the end of a feed and that during the day fat content was higher than at night. Energy content in terms of calories was also higher during the day than it is at night.[16]

Babies will also feed more if going through a growth spurt, or if generally unsettled. Feeding more before and during a growth spurt makes sense, as more feeds will stimulate more milk production to support increased growth. Cluster feeding, when babies feed on and off for long periods of time (often in the evening) is also normal and is believed be an aid to increasing milk supply.[17]

Breastfed babies also seem to regulate their feeds according to their hunger. They don't take the same amount at each feed – just like as adults we don't eat the same amount at each meal. Formula-fed babies, in contrast, do tend to drink the set amount they are given, meaning their feeding may be more predictable.[10]

Why do babies feed so much?

Human breastmilk is notably different in content to the milk of many other mammals and has evolved to fit our lives (or perhaps we have evolved to fit the profile of breastmilk). As a species humans keep their babies very close, for a long time. Newborn humans are really quite helpless when you start comparing them to a foal or baby giraffe. They can't get up and walk about. We don't leave them on their own down a burrow while we go and find food (even if this idea sometimes seems appealing). Their brains develop an awful lot in the first year or so. In terms of brain development, ideally humans would be born at about 18 months old. Yeah, maybe not. So our milk is very different to other mammals.

Human milk is relatively low in fat and protein compared to the milk of some other mammals, but high in carbohydrates. It is digested quickly. This means that babies need feeding frequently, and certainly more frequently than mammals that typically leave their babies alone for longer. Lactose levels are also very high compared to other mammals. Fascinatingly, the more vulnerable a mammal is, the higher in lactose their milk is. The higher in lactose the milk is, the more frequently the baby needs feeding. Could this be an adaptation to make sure that mothers don't leave their vulnerable young alone, because they need feeding? Human babies need to be kept close and fed often, from a both a nutritional and a nurturing perspective. Indeed, if you look at the closest primates to humans, baby chimpanzees and gorillas spend their first years feeding very frequently and in very close contact with their mothers.[18]

Even between humans milk can vary. One study asked women to express milk and then measured its energy content. Fat content varied from 28–57 grams per litre. The researchers also found that women who produced higher energy milk reported reduced breast fullness, suggesting that women who made lower energy milk just made more of it.[19]

Is frequent feeding good for babies?

Aside from being what babies expect biologically, and building the mother's milk supply and keeping it going, frequent feeding has other long-term benefits, particularly around how a baby learns to control their intake of milk and, subsequently, their intake of food in later life. Feeding little and lots means that the baby never gets overly full and is always aware that they are able to have milk whenever they want. However, if feeds are less frequent, and particularly if they are not given when a baby is hungry, then they might be tempted to overfeed when milk does come along. It's a bit like being on a diet, but allowing yourself a day off. Suddenly you eat enough for five people on that day, just because you can and because you don't know when you're going to eat that stuff again. Taking big feeds can also stretch the stomach: remember how tiny a newborn baby's tummy is, and then think about the size of the feed going into it.

Every time a baby feeds, signals are sent to the breast to produce more milk. So the more the baby feeds, in terms of volume, the more the body makes, but if they also feed more frequently, the body gets this message more often. This helps to build milk supply. And in the early days this means that more milk is produced more quickly, helping to reduce the amount of weight babies lose and reducing those concerns women have about whether they have any milk.

Feeding little and often may also help build really positive eating behaviours for later life. For example, one study showed that babies who had larger but less frequent feeds were more likely to be overweight, as they drank more milk than those who fed little and often.[20] Another study looked at whether older babies were more likely to drain a bottle or cup of milk, or whether they left a bit when they were full. They found that only 27% of babies who had been exclusively breastfed in the early months drained the cup, compared to 68% of those only fed by bottle.[21] I also did some research following up babies when they were toddlers, and found that they were seen as better able to control their appetite and not overeat if they had been breastfed for at least six weeks.[22] Basically, if children learn to feed in response to hunger when they're babies, they're more likely to have this skill when they're older. This is a good thing.

Oh, and babies who are breastfed responsively cry less. Argument over.[23]

How does this differ from formula-feeding?

The feeding patterns I've described are different from how a formula-fed baby will feed. And this is where a lot of our problems come from. In general, breastfed babies will feed more frequently, irregularly and for longer than formula-fed babies from the first week of life.[24] Feeding every two hours or more is normal for a breastfed baby, while a formula-fed baby tends to be fed to a three (or more)-hour schedule.[25] In my study, formula-fed babies fed on average eight times a day rather than 11.

Studies that measure the time in between feeds show that formula-fed babies typically have longer gaps between feeds and more defined feeds from the first month of life.[26] Breastfed babies also continue, on average, to have night feeds for longer than formula-fed babies, although formula-fed infants do wake up just as frequently as breastfed babies. Furthermore, women who formula-feed report less variation in their infants' hunger across the course of the day than mothers who breastfeed.

As noted above, breastmilk content also changes across the course of a day. Formula is made up from the same tin for every feed and doesn't change in the same way. This means that formula-fed babies are more likely to feed predictably, whereas breastfed babies are more irregular, which is a good thing and normal for humans.

Finally, some studies show that formula-fed babies feed more quickly. One study that timed babies feeding (I'm imagining a giant stop watch and 'ready, steady, go') found that at two weeks of age breastfed infants drank on average 8ml per minute compared to 28.5ml in the formula-fed group.[27] Breastfed babies also spend more time in sucking pauses than formula-fed babies, drinking the milk at a slower rate.[28]

So if breastfeeding women start comparing feeding schedules

with their friends who are formula-feeding, it can make them really anxious. And this can be exacerbated when they see their friends making up set amounts of milk, and their babies draining their bottles.

Why do babies feed so differently?

Firstly, breastmilk is digested more quickly than formula milk as it is matched so closely to the human digestive system.[29] Breastfed babies will reach a 'fasting state' (where all milk has been digested and absorbed) more quickly than formula-fed babies. In one study examining how long it takes babies to reach a fasting state at 5–36 days, 75% of breastfed babies reached a fasting state within three hours of the last feed, compared to 17% of formula-fed babies.[30]

Breastfed babies also generally take less milk per feed than formula-fed babies (and often less overall over the course of a day). Studies have shown that this difference starts to develop as early as two days old and gets bigger as babies get older. At six weeks old one study showed that the maximum intake per feed in formula-fed infants was 450g, compared to 300g in breastfed infants.[31] In one study looking at intake from birth, the average intake of breastmilk on day 1 was 9.6ml/kg/day compared to 18.5ml/kg/day for formula-fed infants. On day 2, the average intake for breastfed infants was 13.0ml/kg/day compared to 42.2ml/kg/day for the formula-fed infant. And the difference kept increasing.[32]

One reason for this is that in the early days of feeding, only small drops of colostrum are available to the breastfed infant, whereas formula-fed infants essentially have access to an unlimited supply. Babies are designed to only need the small amount of colostrum, so large amounts of formula milk can lead to the baby being overfed. Parents are often surprised at the very small size of a newborn infant's stomach (about the size of a walnut) and may not realise that their newborn may be being overfed with formula. Many bottles designed for newborn feeds contain far more milk than a baby receiving colostrum would get.

Also, it is easier to persuade a bottle-fed baby to take a little more feed than is needed than it is a breastfed baby. When a breastfed baby has had enough, they can naturally slow down on the suckling and get less milk. When they've really had enough they can spit the nipple out, or fall asleep while gently suckling, as they won't be getting any additional milk. However, the same is not true when babies are fed from a bottle. Bottle-feeding, through holes in the teat and with the aid of gravity, requires minimal sucking effort. Babies still get full in the same way, but they are more likely to take more per feed.

Maybe it is because they have less control over the milk flow, and decide they might as well have a little bit more (A bit like when we decide we're full, but someone offers us a cake and we think… oh, go on then). A very tiny baby without good head control might find it quite difficult to stop the milk coming. Even if parents are very alert to the signs that a baby has had enough, the baby may still get slightly more than they need. Sometimes parents decide this is a good thing and try to persuade the baby to take more milk, hoping that they will feed less often or sleep better (more on this later).[33] This is fairly easy to do, and research has shown that even very young babies will take on average 10% more if you try to persuade them to do so.[34]

Overall, formula-fed babies take bigger feeds – or can be persuaded to take bigger feeds – and go for longer periods between feeds. This might seem like a bonus, but as we've seen, numerous studies show that formula-fed babies are more likely to be overweight than breastfed babies. Increased intake and the differences in milk content are likely to be the reason. Overfeeding is not good.

How does this affect breastfeeding?

Taking all of this into consideration, it's easy to see how a lack of understanding of how breastfeeding works, how often breastfed babies feed and how this differs from formula-feeding and why, can lead women to stop breastfeeding. In one study I looked at how mothers' concerns about intake, and their attempts to get their baby to feed less frequently, often led to them swapping to formula as breastfeeding was too difficult. 'My baby was breastfeeding too much' and 'I didn't have enough milk' were very common concerns before switching to bottle-feeding.[33] What probably happened was that they believed their baby was feeding too much and tried to stretch this out, which reduced their milk supply.

I spoke to Emma Pickett, IBCLC, Chair of the Association of Breastfeeding Mothers and author of *You've Got It In You: A Positive Guide to Breastfeeding* about the anxiety new mothers experience about feeding times and she agreed:

'A significant group of breastfeeding women perceive themselves to have low milk supply or are anxious they might develop low milk supply. But in the vast majority of cases, there is no reason to be concerned. A small

group of women can develop genuine supply issues, but this is a small percentage of women. For the vast majority, the crisis is perceptions of low milk supply. More often than not, this is what leads to unnecessary supplementation and then the creation of a real supply problem.

We are a society that likes to measure. From the minute the baby is born, we think in terms of grams and kilograms. In the first few days, it's about percentage of weight lost, centiles on a graph and weekly gains. Yet we expect mothers not to measure the element that contributes to this weight gain, their milk. When the calibrated bottle sits nearby and their mother and mother-in-law are not likely to have breastfed, the temptation to start measuring and controlling quantities is great.

There has been an explosion in the use of electric breast pumps and a consideration that this is a normal and expected part of breastfeeding. Yet there is very little understanding that pumping output does not indicate milk supply, and that some women may not even be able to trigger the milk ejection reflex with a pump or may only achieve one 'letdown'. Women also don't understand that milk volume may vary throughout the day and this is perfectly normal.

There is also a misunderstanding of what is normal newborn behaviour. Books and 20th century parenting messages emphasise the desirability of long intervals between feeds, and if your baby doesn't achieve the magic 2/3/4 hours, doubts about supply creep in. Antenatal education is nervous about 'putting people off' so information about frequent feeding patterns during growth spurts or evening cluster feeding doesn't always get through. When a newborn baby is overstimulated or overtired or simply doing their job of developing a new mum's milk supply with frequent stimulation, a mother imagines her supply is insufficient. Unfortunately healthcare professional training can also miss aspects of normal newborn behaviour.

When we live in a culture that perceives bottle-feeding as the norm, a lack of confidence in our own bodies and a lack of knowledge of what is normal leads to an epidemic of low supply fears.'

You can see how easily women can become anxious about their milk supply. All this information is critical to understanding and trusting in your body. But are new mothers taught this? No. Instead many become highly anxious about how frequently their baby is feeding or just feel completely overwhelmed by it. Given that they know little about normal feeding, it is highly likely that those around them know little either, and their anxiety is exacerbated by the concerns of others. As a society we are convinced that the feeding pattern and schedule of a formula-fed baby is normal and something to aspire to, when in fact the baby-led frequent feeding of breastfed babies encourages healthier eating patterns and weight gain. And is, well, just normal.

And what about sleep?

'People who say they slept like a baby clearly never had one.'

'Slept like a baby last night. Woke up every two hours and cried.'

'I don't want to sleep like a baby, I just want to sleep like my husband.'* (*not all husbands)

Baby sleep, or lack of it, is a popular inspiration for memes and social media humour in general. Many a Facebook status has mentioned sleep. Some are humorous, some despairing. Some brag and are smug about a full night's sleep (most of them are lying, I promise). But, like much good humour, underneath it all is something more serious: new parents worry about sleep. How much their baby is getting, whether this is normal and the hallowed notion of sleeping through the night.

As a culture we have strange views about babies and sleep, in that we expect them to do it and we expect them to do it alone. Even though at least one in three adults considers themselves to be at least a mild insomniac, and many sleep with a partner. But this isn't a book about sleep, so why is it important? Because many new parents believe the myth that formula milk will help babies sleep. And it won't, at least not in the long term. To consider this more fully, let's start at the beginning.

How much do babies really sleep?

Some older research described how babies slept through the night from an early age. However, when you look at what the researchers meant, 'sleeping through the night' actually meant 'not waking between 12 and 5am'. That's very different from 7pm–7am.

It is normal for babies to wake up at night, throughout the first year and beyond. We expect this for newborns who wake very frequently, around every two hours. But we quickly seem to lose our patience and from around six weeks, some start suggesting that babies should no longer be waking. However, it is still completely normal for babies to wake at this age, and most babies do at least once, if not more (and take it from me, it's usually 'more').

Night-waking remains normal for older babies aged 6–12 months, with 30–60% of babies this age waking at night depending on the study. Another study looked at how often babies this age woke at night and found the average number of wakings was 1.77.[35] Interestingly, the study found that almost half the mothers in its sample described their babies' sleep as problematic. Was it really a problem for the baby? Or simply a problem because it didn't fit with societal expectations of what a baby should be doing?

In one study we found that of babies aged 0–6 months, less than 10% didn't wake in the night, with most waking 2–4 times (60%). Three times was the average. For babies aged 6–12 months, 85% still woke up at least once, although it was a little less common, with most babies waking 1–3 times. Average number of times to wake up was around twice (yes, I know, if that's your baby that isn't really *less*). This was pretty much what we had found in an earlier study showing that most babies aged 6–12 months still woke at least once (80%) and most woke up once or twice.

There is data – often cited by the media and critics of baby-led parenting – showing that sleep problems in later childhood are linked to numerous problems for children in terms of behaviour, emotional development and academic achievement. However, there is a big difference between a sleep *problem* and just being a normal baby waking up. There is no evidence to show that the baby who wakes frequently at six months old will still be doing the same at six years (and highly unlikely by sixteen). Also, a great study has shown that sleep problems – no matter how big or small, transient or long-lasting, defined by the medical profession or self-reported – have no impact on sleep at six years old.[36]

So waking up lots at night? Just what babies do.

Where do babies sleep?

After how much sleep babies are getting, the next big worry is where they should be sleeping. Babies must be taught to sleep in their cot and transfer to their own room quickly, mustn't they? Or you risk the sin of 'making a rod for your own back'. But is this really true? Is it best for babies? What do they expect?

One eminent study exploring infant sleep across the world examined 127 different cultural groups and how and where babies slept (sounds like a fabulous research trip). The majority of cultures (79%) shared their bedroom with their baby, with 44% sleeping in the same bed (or surface, given that not all cultures use beds).[37] Some sleep close to their baby until the child is at least two or three, if not older.

Another stark study in 1992 compared differences in sleeping arrangements for a middle-class US sample of 18 mothers and 14 Mayan mothers living in a rural Guatemalan community. At 0–3 months and after six months, all babies in the Mayan group slept in the mother's bed. In the US group, no baby slept in the mother's bed at 0–3 months, with two doing so at six months. Conversely, three babies in the US sample slept in a separate room at 0–3 months and eight at six months. Notably the Mayan sample all felt that their way of sleeping was the only reasonable way, reacting with 'shock, disapproval and pity' when told of typical separate sleeping arrangements in Western cultures.[38]

Babies sleeping close to their mothers is not only natural, but may well be protective. In Western cultures, the baby sleeping in the same room as the parent reduces the risk of SIDS (Sudden Infant Death Syndrome) by 50%. This isn't simply a by-product of being close to anyone – the protection is not offered if sleeping with a sibling.[39] This may be because mothers become more vigilant about their baby's waking when they are close by, and may keep the room at an optimal temperature.

It is also possible that the mother wakes the baby more frequently by just being around – a factor that might seem very annoying at 2am, but may actually be protective for the baby. Sleeping too deeply, which is more likely when alone, is thought to be a risk factor for SIDS, and babies who have died of SIDS were shown to have longer periods of uninterrupted sleep and move about less in their sleep.[40] There is also a suggestion that babies mimic the breathing of those around them in the room, therefore 'remembering' to keep breathing (although I am not sure of the scientific evidence for this one).

Sleeping close to the mother may also help the baby feel more secure, which might make them a more restful sleeper. After all, it's pretty scary being a small, vulnerable baby, so sleeping close to your caregiver at night is going to make you happier than being in a room on your own. One study looking at hospital practices for rooming-in of babies confirmed this, showing that those sleeping next to their mother were far more relaxed in their sleep than those in a nursery.[41]

Western culture seems to have a particular problem with *where* babies sleep. Bringing a baby into an adult bed is labelled by many as dangerous, or perceived as the parenting sin of 'making a rod for your own back'. There is even a series of health promotion posters warning against it, with sensationalist images of a baby sleeping next to a large knife to suggest that co-sleeping is similarly risky. One has a fairy story that reads: 'Once upon a time, I was with my mummy. She fed me and we both fell asleep together. I didn't wake up. The end'. We are scared of bedsharing, as if it is somehow inherently unusual, non-instinctual and dangerous.

However, in the rest of the world, normal sleep is co-sleep. In the 1970s, while most parents in Western culture were putting their baby to sleep in a crib and trying desperately to avoid making that mythical rod, two researchers were busy studying sleep patterns in over 186 non-industrialised countries. What they found was that in 100% of tribes categorised as hunter-gatherer groups and 76% of the remaining non-industrialised groups, it was the norm to share the sleeping surface with babies and children.[42] This behaviour appears to survive transition to Western culture. One study found that over 80% of Thai mothers living in Australia shared their bed with their baby,[43] and another showed that Appalachian families who were now living in Kentucky in the USA also frequently shared their bed.[44]

When I wrote the first edition of this book in 2016, bedsharing was not recommended by the American Academy of Pediatrics (AAP). However, in 2019 the AAP revised their bed sharing and breastfeeding protocol,[45] stating *Bedsharing may only be a risk in hazardous circumstances… We aim to clarify the currently available evidence regarding the benefits and risks of bedsharing, and offer evidence-based recommendations that promote infant and maternal health through increased breastfeeding duration.* The updated protocol recognised how bedsharing protected breastfeeding and stated clearly that 'all families should be counseled about safe sleep', including the following:

'Discussion with open-ended questions from health care providers concerning bedsharing safety should happen with all parents, as bedsharing is likely to happen whether intended or not. These discussions should take place early in the perinatal course and continuously throughout infancy, and include as many caregivers as possible.'

Likewise NICE guidance[46] in the UK highlights the fact that professionals should discuss safer co-sleeping, and any risks, with parents-to-be during pregnancy and the postnatal period. They also note that:

'Evidence was reviewed relating to co-sleeping (parents or carers sleeping

on a bed or sofa or chair with an infant) in the first year of an infant's life. Some of the reviewed evidence showed that there is a statistical relationship between SIDS and co-sleeping. This means that, where co-sleeping occurs, there may be an increase in the number of cases of SIDS. However, the evidence does not allow us to say that co-sleeping causes SIDS. Therefore the term 'association' has been used in the recommendations to describe the relationship between co-sleeping and SIDS.'

So what do mothers in the UK do with their babies at night? Currently around one fifth of mothers report bedsharing with their baby, although this could be an underestimate, as many mothers still feel they cannot share this information with anyone for risk of being criticised.[47] However, many parents are unaware of the safe co-sleeping guidelines and end up doing it for the first time when they are exhausted, their baby is ill or even accidentally, which then increases the risk of harm – hence the AAP and NICE recognising the importance of open conversations with all parents.

Critics argue that bedsharing is unnecessary and unsafe. But is it really? No, it isn't – particularly if certain precautions are taken. The baby should sleep on a safe, flat surface, away from heavy duvets and pillows. They should sleep on one side of the mother rather than between mother and father. The mother should not have consumed large amounts of alcohol or drugs, and certain medications can make the mother very sleepy and should be avoided. One suggestion is that mothers should not bedshare when very tired… which always seems a bit nonsensical given that new mothers are perpetually tired, but in reality this means extreme exhaustion. Mothers who smoke or are very obese should also avoid bedsharing. Sadly, when co-sleeping deaths are reported these precautions have usually not been taken, or the mother (or someone else) has taken the baby to a chair or sofa and slept or fallen asleep with them on that surface. This sofa-sharing is not the same as co-sleeping, but unfortunately often gets mixed in with the data.

In fact, if you look at the actual statistics on co-sleeping, it is safe when done correctly. One study looked at SIDS deaths and found that 16% of babies died while co-sleeping with their mother. However, 36% died in a separate room.[48] Indeed, most incidences of SIDS do not happen in bedsharing groups. Most happen in areas of poverty, where bottle-feeding is typical. Most babies who die of SIDS are alone.[49]

Fascinating sleep footage of mothers and babies also shows that mothers often adopt a specific position when co-sleeping. Mothers tend to lie on their side, facing the baby, often with their legs curled up to the baby. They naturally, without prompting, put the baby on their back and the baby spends the night either in this position or curled slightly to face the mother. One study of 12 mother and baby pairs at night found that 7 out of 12 of them spent the whole night facing the mother. For the majority of the night mother and baby were less than 30cm apart.[50] McKenna and colleagues also looked at mother and baby sleeping patterns and how they varied according to where the baby was sleeping. When mother and baby were together, their sleep patterns overlapped far more than when they were apart.[51]

Indeed, cultures that have very high levels of bedsharing have far lower levels of SIDS, even though these countries often have far higher levels of poverty and overcrowding compared to Western cultures. One study in Hong Kong in the 1980s showed that SIDS rates in Western cultures were 10–15 times higher than in Hong Kong.[52] This can be protective when individuals move to Western cultures. One study in England and Wales found that babies of Asian origin were far less likely to die from SIDS, even though they were more likely to live in poverty. One explanation was the higher rate of co-sleeping.[53] However, this can decrease over time. One interesting study tracked SIDS rates among Asian immigrants in the USA. The study showed that the longer this group lived in the USA, the higher their SIDS rates. This was thought to be due to them starting to adopt Western sleep practices and reducing co-sleeping.[54]

Is it normal to be close at night?

If you think about it, of course it is. In the wild past we wouldn't have put a baby in another cave. And our babies still expect closeness. One study placed a mechanical breathing teddy bear next to babies and found that babies physically tried to get close to it if sleeping alone, although babies do not have the same reaction to normal stuffed toys.[55] Closeness at night may also be protective. Dependency between baby and mother is common among mammals, particularly primates who are born helpless and are relatively slow to develop. It has been suggested that the physiological influences of the breathing, heart rate and body temperature of a nearby mother are designed to support vulnerable babies.

Older monkey experiments show the physiological impact of separation. Temperature can drop, heart rate changes and babies sleep less deeply.[56] Some studies show a drop in immunity, which is likely tied to increased adrenaline and cortisol release – the stress hormones.[57] One study showed that growth hormone levels fell, alongside proteins needed for optimal brain functioning.[58]

In research with human babies, one study found that babies sleeping next to their mother matched her temperature closely and were less likely to get cold than those sleeping apart.[55] Another found that heart rate was more stable,[59] and still another that babies' breathing was steadier. Sleep apnoea, when babies appear to stop breathing temporarily in their sleep, is rare but of concern in babies. However, it is less likely in babies sleeping next to their mothers. In one study researchers asked mothers and babies to come into a sleep lab where they watched them sleep in different set-ups. On nights when babies slept alone they had far more sleep apnoea than when sleeping next to their mum, particularly when they were in deep sleep.[60]

Babies also stir in their sleep and wake up more frequently when co-sleeping. Again, this may be beneficial in stopping them sleeping too deeply, particularly in the deep sleep parts of their cycles. Another study measured the amount of CO_2 around the mother and baby when they were co-sleeping. They found that when co-sleeping, mother and baby spent around two-thirds of the night facing each other and therefore breathing in the same area. This led to a very slight increase in CO_2 around the baby; this increase was not detrimental, and may stimulate the baby to breathe.[61]

Co-sleeping might also be protective in other ways. Babies who were co-sleepers released less cortisol at bath time at 5 weeks compared to those who were not.[62] The benefits may even be long term. A number of studies have explored outcomes for children who shared a parental bed compared to those who did not. Many show improved social and emotional outcomes. For example, one study found that those who co-slept as babies were more adjusted as adults, with higher self-esteem, lower anxiety and less discomfort with physical contact and affection.[63] Another study found that toddlers who co-slept as babies were more independent than those who did not. They were more likely to be able to dress themselves and make friends by themselves.[64]

So how does this link to feeding?

Sleep concerns and feeding concerns go hand-in-hand for two reasons. Firstly there is a myth that how you feed a baby will impact on their sleep, and secondly there are concerns about where and when a baby should sleep, whether based on perceived risk or the belief it will make the baby too dependent, which lead to parents sleeping separately to their baby, which may have an impact on breastfeeding success.

Let's tackle the myth that how babies are fed affects their sleep, with more feeding leading to longer sleep. In early infancy (before three months), this is to some extent true. Formula-fed babies do tend to start sleeping for longer periods and have fewer night feeds at an earlier age.[65] They are also likely to have longer periods of deep sleep and be less likely to wake up between sleep cycles at this age.[66] This is likely to be because breastmilk is digested easily and quickly, meaning more frequent feeds are needed. Also, as we've seen, experiments have shown that bottle-fed babies can be encouraged to consume larger amounts in a way that breastfed infants cannot be. It is likely that some parents encourage this before sleep, in the hope that the baby will sleep for longer. However, this longer, deeper sleep may be one of the reasons why formula-fed babies are at a higher risk of SIDS.

Fewer feeds and less frequent waking don't necessarily mean more sleep for parents. One study explored what happened during night feeds and wakings and found that once you took into account things like where the baby was fed and for how long, and how long it took to prepare a feed and settle the baby back to sleep, mothers who were breastfeeding got more sleep overall, despite feeding the baby more often.[67]

A study in Australia looked at several different elements of sleep and found that feeding had no impact on difficulties getting the baby to sleep, or on whether the baby was restless during sleep. Breastfed babies were less likely to snore, wheeze, cough or have breathing problems during their sleep.[68] So breastfed babies had a much less restless night. Which meant their parents more likely did too.

However, one of the cruelest parts of being a new parent is that just when you think you've got it sussed, your baby changes the game. Some babies sleep very well in the early months, only to become more 'social' at night from around four months old. This can mean that a sleeping baby becomes one who doesn't sleep so well (if you post about your sleeping baby online, karma will ensure this happens instantly). And although formula-fed babies may sleep for longer in the early weeks, this doesn't hold true when babies get past six months. Recently we explored whether what milk a baby was given, or how much solid food they had affected sleep at 6–12 months and found it didn't matter how babies were fed. Most babies still woke up, and they didn't wake up more because of what they were fed.[69] Babies woke up… just because.

Recent research has also suggested there may be a genetic component in how much babies wake up. Other studies have suggested that infant sleep is affected by wider variables. For example, babies who had a difficult birth were less likely to be considered good sleepers at six months old.[70] So it's more about the individual baby than what you feed them.

What we did find interesting, though, was that breastfed babies were more likely to feed at night, *but formula-fed babies woke just as much*. We think this is because women are probably using breastfeeding to get their babies back to sleep and not really keeping track of how much their baby feeds. Women who are formula-feeding might think 'well he's had his set amount during the day' and not give a feed. Babies are far easier to get back to sleep if you feed them and this might be why breastfeeding women actually get more sleep overall.

Another interesting study from Professor Helen Ball and colleagues at Durham University's Baby Sleep Information Service (BASIS) highlighted just how important it was to measure sleep accurately when it came to looking at differences between breast and formula-fed babies.[71] This research involved asking mother-baby pairs to wear actigraphs to measure how much sleep they really got. Participants were also given a sleep log to record when their baby was awake or asleep. They collected data for one night every two weeks from 4–18 weeks of age, giving eight samples per mother and baby.

Overall measurements of total sleep time and longest sleep period duration as measured by the actigraph did not differ between babies who were exclusively formula-fed, or exclusively breastfed at any time point from 4–16 weeks. However, at 10, 12, 14 and 16 weeks, mothers who were exclusively formula-feeding reported that their baby slept 41–58 minutes longer per night than the exclusively breastfed mothers did. They also reported a significantly greater longest sleep duration at each of these time points, estimating it to be between 1.64 and 2.29 hours longer than mothers who were exclusively breastfeeding. Data from the actigraph actually showed the longest sleep duration was for breastfed babies (although it was not significantly different).

So for some reason mothers who were formula-feeding reported more sleep. Now if we relied just on this measure, the research could have concluded that formula-fed babies slept more, but the actigraph data showed otherwise. Why might mothers think they were getting more sleep than they were (or vice versa?). One reason could be that breastfeeding mothers are more likely to co-sleep, so might be more aware of every waking, but when the researchers controlled for sleep location this didn't explain the results. Maybe someone else was more likely to be involved in night-time care if the baby was bottle-fed? Or perhaps there is a placebo effect from everyone telling mothers that their formula-fed baby will sleep better.

Why wouldn't milk help sleep at this age? Well babies are past the point of not being able to get all their calories in the day – they're not only waking up because they are hungry. It's just as likely that they're waking up for all sorts of reasons. If you think about it, as an adult you likely wake because you are too hot or cold, to nip to the toilet, or because you're thirsty or had a nightmare. But as an adult you are able to sort out your own needs and get yourself back to sleep. Babies can't, so they wake up and call for someone to help them. Sometimes adults need a little help too. Ever woken up from a particularly bad dream and sought comfort from your partner? Imagine now that they refused to make eye contact with you and told you that you were old enough to be sleeping through, so you should just go back to sleep...

It makes little sense to think that introducing solids will help either. You often hear 'he needs more than milk to sleep', but this logic is skewed. Solids generally replace milk. And milk is far more energy-dense than most weaning foods. Carrots are great, but they don't help you sleep. And anyway, back to adults waking up... it's not (always) because they're hungry.

But this isn't what most parents hear every day. There are so many myths around sleeping and food. Not sleeping? He needs solids. Not sleeping? He never will while you're still breastfeeding him. He's too old to be waking up now. You're making a rod for your own back by going to him. Leave him to cry, he needs to learn. And so on. Sleep myth bingo at its finest. But many new parents don't know that all this is nonsense, so they think they are either doing something wrong, or need to stop breastfeeding to help their baby to sleep. We got so enraged about this that we made a public service video, cute animated baby style. You can watch it here (apologies if the music gets stuck in your head): www.youtu.be/KIoS897cp-c

How much do breastfed babies really feed at night?

It is important to remember that when we think about differences in behaviour between breast and formula-fed babies, the breastfed baby is the norm. Even if there are differences, we need to think about our language. We shouldn't be comparing breastfed babies negatively – by saying that they are doing anything 'too much' – compared to formula-fed babies. So what is normal for breastfeeding at night?

In cultures where co-sleeping is the norm, babies feed lots at night.[72] A study in rural Tanzania found that co-sleeping babies fed on average four times a night.[73] This was echoed in a Bangladeshi sample showing that babies took around half their milk between 6pm and 6am.[74] Another study of rural Thai babies and mothers found that as children got older, they actually took more of their feeds at night. Children over one year old consumed about half of their intake at night, compared to around a quarter for younger babies. This makes sense; toddlers like to run around during the day, but if they are sleeping next to their mother at night and are allowed free access to the breast, they will fill their tummies. This reflects the ideas of McKenna and Lee Gettler, who recently proposed the concept of 'breastsleeping' in one of the best-titled papers I have ever read 'There is no such thing as infant sleep, there is no such thing as breastfeeding, there is only breastsleeping'. Babies don't sleep *or* feed. They do both, moving between both states throughout the night, usually not waking properly at all, and drifting back to sleep while still feeding.[75]

However, babies in Western cultures often consume more milk during the day. One study in the USA found that far more milk was consumed between 6am and 6pm than in the remaining 12 hours.[76] Another study of exclusively breastfed infants aged 0–6 months in Sweden found that for all ages the average number of night-time feeds was 2.2 feeds a night at two weeks, dropping to 1.3 at 12 weeks. Incidentally, feeds then increased to an average of 1.8 at 20 weeks. At four months 48% fed once at night, 37% twice, 11% three times and 3% four times. One mum, however, was up five times a night breastfeeding. Doing the maths, what is notable is that only 2% of infants at any age from birth to six months never breastfed in the night.[77]

Incidentally, when mothers in the !Kung tribe were asked how often their baby fed at night, common responses included 'many times' and 'all night'.[78] Only Western nations perceive babies feeding at night as something unusual that needs to be measured and reduced.

Does where a baby sleeps affect feeding?

Babies in cultures where co-sleeping is normal feed far more at night than in Western cultures where babies often sleep separately. This pattern is reflected in co-sleeping pairs in Western cultures. But does co-sleeping help with feeding?

The answer is yes, or at least bedsharing and breastfeeding are closely linked. One study found that twice as many co-sleeping babies were breastfeeding at 3–4 months than those who slept alone.[79] But is it just because mothers who are more determined to breastfeed are more likely to bedshare?

It's probably a bit of both. Durham University Professor Helen Ball and colleagues, who are behind the Infant Sleep Information Source, recently showed that mothers who decide during pregnancy that they are going to breastfeed are more likely to go on to do so. However, certain aspects of bedsharing definitely promote breastfeeding. Babies who bedshare breastfeed far more frequently – twice as much in fact – as babies who are sleeping separately.[80]

Just keeping baby close appears to enhance breastfeeding. Another interesting study looked at sleeping arrangements in hospital and patterns of feeding. Babies who were in bed with their mothers, or in a sidecar crib, fed more often than those in a standalone cot. What was so interesting about this study was that no differences were seen in the sleep of either mother or baby, which detracts from the argument that keeping baby close will stop everyone from sleeping.[81] Indeed, one study found that compared to bottle-feeding mothers, mothers who were breastfeeding and co-sleeping actually got more sleep.[82]

Another rooming-in study at a hospital measured milk intake in rooming-in and nursery babies. Those who roomed-in fed far more frequently. As a consequence women produced more milk by day three, with babies losing less weight. These babies were also less likely to have any formula milk.[83]

From a practical perspective, once mother and baby get used to being in bed together, dealing with night feeds becomes far easier. There is no getting up out of bed or trying to resettle the baby after a feed; in fact they hardly change position. Mother and baby typically sleep close to each other, facing each other and older babies can even latch themselves on.[84] After a while the mother may not even notice she is feeding. In their study comparing Mayan and American families, Morelli and colleagues found that Mayan mothers who bedshared with their baby, when asked how often their baby fed at night, simply responded that they didn't notice.[85] If they did realise, it wasn't perceived as a problem; mothers simply turned over to allow the baby to access the breast and fell asleep again. In contrast, American mothers were very aware that they had to stay awake at night in order to feed their baby, often taking the baby to a separate room to feed. Only one mother in the American group slept with her baby and fed the baby in bed. She responded that night feeding did not bother her.

Mothers who breastfeed also tend to bedshare differently from those who formula-feed, suggesting that there is a natural link between breastfeeding, night-time feeding and bedsharing. Breastfeeding mothers very closely follow the safe sleep advice in terms of who bedshares, where and how they bedshare. Professor Helen Ball explains:

> 'Bedsharing mothers appear to avoid the presumed hazards of sleeping in adult beds (for example, suffocation, overlaying and entrapment) due to the presence and behaviour of their mothers. But this may not be the case for babies who are not breastfed. When we have compared families videoed sleeping at home, formula-fed infants were generally placed high in the bed, level with their parents' faces and positioned between or on top of their parents' pillows. In contrast, breastfed babies were always positioned flat on the mattress, below pillow height. Mothers who did not breastfeed spend significantly less time facing their baby than did breastfeeding mother-baby pairs, they did not adopt the protective sleep position with the same consistency, and they experienced less sleep synchrony.
>
> The hormonal feedback cycle experienced by breastfeeding mothers promotes close contact with, heightened responsiveness toward and bonding with infants in a way that is absent or diminished among mothers who do not breastfeed. The implication for bedsharing – that breastfeeding mothers and babies sleep together in significantly different ways than do non-breastfeeding mothers and babies – suggests that future case-control studies of bedsharing must take feeding type into account.'

So what's the problem?

Aside from critics who continue to ignore the frequency of bedsharing and its importance in enabling easier breastfeeding at night, myths about breastfeeding causing sleep problems and formula or solids helping a baby to sleep are everywhere in our society. Most people do not realise how normal – and even protective – it is for a baby to wake at night. They feel under pressure from smug social media posts or grandparents who insist that babies should be sleeping by now. If their baby wakes often, they feel they're doing something wrong. If they are breastfeeding they may be accused of making the famous rod for their own back – in other words, it's all their fault their baby wakes. Some anxious parents are willing to try anything to get their baby to sleep as they feel so isolated and exhausted. They may stop breastfeeding, or try and overfeed their baby, both of which have negative health consequences. Or they may fall prey to the self-proclaimed 'baby sleep experts' and try to train their baby to sleep.

Encouraging sleep can have negative consequences for breastfeeding. One intervention study that aimed to reduce night waking in babies aged 6–12 months found that breastfeeding rates fell more rapidly than would be expected. Breastfeeding rates fell from 81.8% at the start of the study (so mothers were highly motivated to breastfeed) to 53.6% at the end. Co-sleeping also fell from 70.1% to 26.1%, suggesting that mothers were being encouraged to be separate from their babies, which in turn made breastfeeding more difficult.[86] There is a concern that mothers' worries about sleep have the same effect.

No one will deny that it is extremely tough being a parent of a waking baby. It's exhausting and parents worry that it will never end. But perpetuating a myth that babies *should* sleep, and if they are not you should do something about it, only causes harm to all concerned. Rather than looking at ways to persuade babies to sleep, we should be recognising normal baby behaviour and looking for ways to support new parents through this time.

Action 4

✓ Tell all new parents and those around them about normal feeding and sleep, and support them in other ways to get more rest.

9. OUR OBSESSION WITH BIG BABIES AND RAPID WEIGHT GAIN LEADS TO UNNECESSARY SUPPLEMENTATION

'I hated it when everyone started talking about weight. Oh he's put on 9oz and she's put on 12oz and I'd be keeping quiet as Oliver had never put on as much and they used to give me these really sympathetic looks like there was something wrong with him and I should feel upset.'

Along with how many feeds, and how much sleep, a baby is or is not getting, how much weight they are putting on is another one of *those* questions. People seem obsessed with how much babies weigh. At no other time in our lives will anyone take so much interest in our weight, or indeed so openly comment on it. It appears to be socially acceptable to wander up to a mother and baby and ask 'How much did he weigh at birth?', or say 'Isn't he a big boy' or 'Oooh, look at the legs on that.' Try it with an adult stranger in the supermarket and see where that gets you.

We have a particular love for a big chubby baby, don't we? There is a certain pride in growing a baby and making them bigger. And culturally food is equated to love and care. Rolls of fat are idolised while babies are young, but demonised once they are over the age of two. But what if your baby doesn't have Buddha rolls? What if they're happy and hydrated and healthy… but, you know, just not stacking it on. Is there something wrong?

The issue of infant weight is *so* tied to our concepts of normal feeding. We live in a society where formula-feeding is the norm and therefore have a natural tendency to judge the minority group (breastfed babies) against the majority group (formula-fed babies). And on average (but not always) the breastfed babies gain weight a bit more slowly. And this is perfectly normal, and actually a good thing. Just because a breastfed baby is smaller than a formula-fed baby, doesn't mean the breastfed baby has a problem. Rapid weight gain is not necessarily good in terms of long-term health, even though it can be reassuring in those early days and weeks. Very rapid weight gain in the first week of life is associated with an increased risk of overweight in adults and subsequent cardiovascular illness, compared to growth in any other time period.[1]

Anxiety over weight gain

Anxiety about weight is a common reason for women to stop breastfeeding. Doubts about growth often trigger a belief that the baby isn't getting enough milk. Women who are worried about their babies' growth are more likely to stop breastfeeding.[2] One study found that mothers who were told their babies were losing weight during their hospital stay suffered more anxiety at two weeks and were less likely to be breastfeeding at six months than mothers of babies that were gaining weight.[3]

Growth charts can play a big part in this anxiety. The WHO promoted the use of growth charts as a way of combating malnutrition. The idea was to track whether babies were losing too much weight, and the charts can be a useful tool for measuring weight trajectories. However, they can also be a significant source of anxiety, particularly when misinterpreted by parents and professionals. A growth chart looks at the normal distribution of baby weight over a population. What that means is that it splits every weight into a percentage and plots the spread. A baby on the 80th percentile weighs more than a baby on the 20th percentile. On the 80th percentile, only 20% of babies are bigger. On the 20th percentile, 80% are.

But babies come in all shapes and sizes, and there is no 'right' figure unless they are towards the extreme ends. Babies below the 3rd percentile are considered underweight, but again that is only an indication that something might be wrong. Some babies are just naturally very small. At the other end of the scale, babies might be considered at risk of overweight if they are above the 95th percentile. And weight is only half the issue: length matters too. A baby on the 30th percentile for weight and the 30th for length is well proportioned. A baby on the 90th percentile for length and the 30th for weight might have something going on that needs investigating. We know that adults are all different heights and weights and the same applies to babies.

Where a baby lies in relation to other babies doesn't matter unless they are beneath the 3rd percentile (and maybe not even then). What matters is how a baby tracks the percentile line. If a baby is at the 70th and then drops to the 30th, this may be a sign of something to worry about, but not always. Sometimes, particularly in the early weeks, babies jump about the growth charts a bit. Sometimes babies are born smaller than their genetics suggest because the father is taller and the mother is smaller. The human body generally only grows babies to a size they can be born at, so in this case the baby might be born slightly smaller. What they then do in the early weeks is 'catch up' this growth and go up the charts.

The opposite can also happen in that if the baby got lots of calories in the womb and grew to be a bit bigger than their genes suggest, they can 'catch down' and appear to fall down the charts. This is why weight on its own is not a sign of health. If a baby is smaller or weight gain appears to slow then this needs to be considered alongside other factors. Is feeding going well? Is the baby feeding often? Are they having lots of wet nappies (and lots of dirty ones if under six weeks old?) Do they look alert and happy?

Many think the 50th percentile is the 'target weight' and become anxious if their baby is not on it. This can be a considerable worry for women who are breastfeeding as they come to see weight gain as a sign they are producing enough milk.[4] One study looking at who attended a baby weighing clinic found that those who went most frequently were more likely to have a smaller baby, even if growth was steady.[5] Getting a baby weighed becomes a central part of motherhood. A study in London asked parents why they took their baby to baby clinic, with 93% stating that it was to get their baby weighed.[6] Data from another study showed that 45% of parents take their baby to be weighed at least once a fortnight.[7] The costs of this frequent weighing to the NHS are substantial – one economic analysis suggested that it cost 64p for a child to be weighed and for the parents to have a discussion about growth, which seems a tiny amount per baby, but for every baby, repeated many times, it adds up.[8]

How is weight linked to feeding?

On average, breast and formula-fed babies grow in different ways. Again, the pattern of growth of the breastfed baby is normal. Formula-fed babies tend to lose less weight after birth, and grow more rapidly in the first year, but this doesn't mean breastfed babies lose 'too much' weight, or don't put on 'enough'. They are growing in a way that is biologically normal, and the increased growth of formula-fed babies is a risk factor for later obesity. However, if you spend time in a baby weighing clinic or in a parenting forum online, you will soon see increased anxiety among women of 'smaller' breastfed babies. The difference often isn't communicated, let alone explained, to these mothers.

A few years ago the WHO formally recognised this difference by issuing growth charts based on the normal patterns of breastfed babies. The WHO had originally adopted the US National Center for Health Statistics (NCHS) growth reference charts, which were based on data collected in the USA in 1929. However, most of the babies in this initial data set were formula-fed and had an early introduction to solid foods – two factors we know are associated with greater weight gain. Further research into the differences in growth of breastfed and formula-fed infants led to a realisation that weight was being overestimated, particularly for breastfed babies.

The WHO undertook the Multicentre Growth Reference Study from 1997–2003, to create new growth charts that better reflected breastfed babies' weight. They made sure that data was collected from babies from a range of backgrounds, but that babies were from families with good nutrition and no socio-economic or environmental factors that might affect weight. Importantly, all babies in the data set had to be exclusively breastfed for at least four months, and support was given for women to do this.[9] The result was a brand new set of charts that took into account how breastfed babies initially gained weight quite quickly, but then started to slow down from around 2–3 months. But why might the pattern of weight gain be so different in breast and formula-fed babies?

Weight loss after birth

Firstly, from the very start of feeding formula-fed babies have access to a large supply of milk, and the amounts given are often bigger than their tummies naturally hold. Compare this to breastfeeding, where babies receive very tiny amounts of colostrum until the mature milk comes in, and you can see where differences might arise. Colostrum is the biological norm. Remember those studies looking at intake of milk in the early days? How formula-fed babies quickly start taking in more milk, and this difference gets bigger every day? Well this is what can lead to differences in weight (or weight loss) in those first few days. There is simply more formula milk potentially available than babies would naturally expect to have.

Some weight loss after birth is actually normal. In fact, up to around 7% is considered fine and expected, although this isn't often communicated to women. One study weighed newborn babies every 12 hours to chart their weight loss. The average weight loss after

12 hours was 2.8%, after 24 hours 4.5%, after 36 hours 5.5%, after 48 hours 5.7% and then climbing back up to 5% after 72 hours. By discharge, 30% had lost more than 7% of weight, 12% more than 8% and 4% more than 9%. No baby had lost more than 10%.[10] So babies naturally lose a bit of weight early on.

However, one issue that can exacerbate concerns is that growth charts only show an upward trajectory. The physiologically normal weight loss is not reflected in the charts. Researchers in Scotland followed babies from birth to six weeks, weighing them at birth, five and 12 days and at six weeks. They found that 20% of babies had not regained their birthweight by 12 days, with the biggest babies at birth showing the biggest losses, but only 3% were 10% or more below their birth weight at five days. They found that weights in the first fortnight were about half to one centile space lower than the charts suggested, but that the babies had no health issues.[11] If a baby is weighed during this weight loss period, and then a mother reflects on the growth chart, she may presume that there is something wrong with her baby (or her breastfeeding).

So breastfed babies naturally lose more weight in the early days, taking longer to regain their birth weight, which makes complete sense given that they are having small amounts of colostrum compared to their peers having larger feeds. However, colostrum is jam packed with immunity-boosting properties, which is Mother Nature's priority for the baby in those early days: get that concentrated immunity in, and we'll worry about weight gain later. But Mother Nature didn't count on the invention of weight charts, scales and formula-feeding to make mothers doubt her ingenuity.

Breastfed babies do of course regain their birth weight, just a little more slowly than formula-fed babies. One study showed that the majority had regained their birth weight by around eight and a half days, whereas formula-fed babies took about six days. Mixed feeding didn't have much impact, with mixed-fed babies regaining at about eight days. Researchers have also looked at when babies have their lowest weight point after birth. This typically happens on about day three, around 60 hours old, and babies start climbing again after this point. One study showed that at this 60-hour dip the average weight loss for a breastfed baby was 6.6%, compared to 3.5% for formula-fed babies, and 5.9% for mixed-fed babies.[12]

There are additional factors that influence this weight loss. How frequently a baby feeds, rather than what they are fed, can affect how much weight they lose. If they are fed lots, on demand, their weight loss is less than those fed less frequently. Women who feed more frequently also have more milk on day three, suggesting that these babies are getting more milk.[13] Conversely, women who report that their milk doesn't come in until after three days are more likely to have babies with a bigger weight loss at 72 hours.

Weight loss isn't just affected by feeding, and this needs to be recognised. There is growing evidence that if women have a lot of fluid during labour, either by drinking it or through an IV, their babies might weigh more than they should at birth due to taking in some of this fluid – and these babies might then have a bigger weight loss as they lose it. One study showed that if a mother had more than 1.2 litres of fluid during labour, an average weight loss at three days was 6.9% compared to 5.5% for those with a lower intake,[14] and IV fluid babies typically lose 50% more weight than those whose mothers had only oral fluids.[15] Another study showed that if women had a lot of swelling, particularly after the birth, their babies were more likely to have greater weight loss. Presumably this water retention got passed on, to some extent, to the baby![16]

Birth itself can also affect how much weight babies lose after birth. Babies who are born by caesarean section are more likely to end up with greater than 10% weight loss, and are more likely to experience dehydration.[17] Another study found that over a quarter of babies born by caesarean lost more than 10% of their birth weight by 72 hours, compared to 5% of babies born vaginally. Notably, weight started to rise for vaginal birth babies after 48 hours, but took until 72 hours for c-section babies. At 24 hours weight loss for both was similar (4.2% for vaginal and 4.9% for c-section), but at 72 hours it was 6.4% for vaginal and 8.6% for c-section. By 96 hours, mean weight loss for c-section babies was 5.8%.[18] Linked to this, babies who are separated from their mother after birth, even if only for two hours, are more likely to have greater early weight loss.[19] Epidural use is also associated with increased weight loss at 48 hours old.[20]

Finally, weight loss can be seasonal too! In cold weather, fewer babies lose more than 8% of their birth weight in the first three days than in hot weather (23% versus 32%). Babies who have more wet nappies also have more weight loss![21] Small things like these might seem obvious when you start thinking about them, but are they always considered and communicated to new mothers in practice?

There has been some debate about whether a greater than 7% weight loss by day three is too small a loss to raise concern. Some researchers looked at a lot of different studies examining weight loss patterns in breastfed babies and found that although the average weight loss was 6% at three days, there was a pretty consistent range between babies of about 3–7%, suggesting that 8% or more might be a better cut-off. When they looked at what happened to babies in this cut-off, 89% had regained their weight by day ten and 92% by day 14.[22]

Finally, one useful study looked at how much weight breastfed babies lost after birth and created 'nomograms' – charts that looked at normal and expected weight loss after birth. This means that professionals can look at a baby in relation to where they fit with normal weight loss expectations, so rather than saying 'Your baby has lost 7% of their birth weight at two days old', they can say 'Your baby has lost a normal amount of weight for this time point. They are on the 50th percentile for weight loss'. What these charts show is that the normal low point for weight is at 60 hours of age, or the third day of life. And that's, well, normal.[23]

Neonatal hypernatraemic dehydration

Neonatal hypernatraemic dehydration (NHD) is rare, and happens when babies become very dehydrated after birth. This is a serious issue because it can mean that their sodium levels rise dangerously. A level of around ≥150 mmol/L is considered to be dangerous and needing treatment. When this happens due to a low intake of breastmilk it is called breastfeeding hypernatraemia. One of the biggest signs that a baby may be developing hypernatraemia is if they lose a lot of weight after birth, usually more than 10%.[24]

NHD usually occurs in breastfed babies, although formula-fed babies can experience it too. NHD can be very serious. In extreme cases untreated babies can suffer brain damage, have fits and amputation is a risk. However, despite scary headlines, the number of babies who experience this level of dehydration and have any type of lasting consequence is very small. In fact, one study showed that it affected two in 10,000 babies, and only a minority of those had any kind of lasting damage.[25] Most babies who suffer NHD lose at least 15% of their birth weight, rather than the 10% which is considered a risk.

So what causes NHD? One study in Italy, which didn't look directly at NHD but at babies that lost more than 10% of their birth weight, found that around a quarter of these cases were linked to milk insufficiency and the rest were due to poor breastfeeding technique. Of course these are interlinked. Another study looked specifically at the causes of milk insufficiency in NHD babies and found a number of factors, including no breast growth during pregnancy, breast surgery, hypoplastic breasts, fertility difficulties, retained placenta, no engorgement and the absence of colostrum.[26]

Milk insufficiency can simply be delayed rather than absent milk. Indeed, one study suggested it may increase the risk of NHD seven times.[27] In a study in California, delayed onset of milk was linked to many interventions during the birth, but also maternal weight and diabetes.[28] Other studies have shown that infants who experience birth complications (long labour, assisted delivery and pain medications) are more likely to experience excessive weight loss.[29] This may be because these babies find it more difficult to latch on to the breast after birth, and we will look at this later.

What is particularly interesting is that the number of babies who experience NHD appears to differ significantly between countries, which suggests that something more complex is going on than simply breastfeeding not working out. It is likely that factors around the birth, healthcare system and health of pregnant women are affecting this. For example:

- Italy: in a study with 686 healthy breastfed babies, 7.7% lost more than 10% of birth weight but only 2.8% of those babies had a sodium level ≥ 150 mmol/L.[30]
- UK: the risk of a sodium level level ≥160 was 71 per 100,000 breastfed infants (1 in 1,400).[31]
- Netherlands: 58 in 100,000 breastfed babies were readmitted for dehydration. Out of these 20 in 100,000 were at serious risk of hypernatraemia but only two in 100,000 had documented cases of hypernatraemia.[32]
- USA: in a study of 3,718 breastfed babies, 71 were readmitted with hypernatraemic dehydration – a much higher rate of 1.9%.[33]

From that data it appears that NHD risk is much higher in the USA than in other countries. We also know that the USA has higher levels of numerous risk factors that are associated with a more challenging breastfeeding experience. These include higher levels of intervention in labour, higher levels of maternal obesity, and critically, a lack of universal healthcare. It is likely that these factors exacerbate breastfeeding complications and in turn increase dehydration risk.

However, dehydration and normal weight loss must not be confused. Greater than 10% weight loss may be an *indicator* of NHD, and it is vital that mother and baby receive feeding support. It is however important to make sure that the right type of support is received. Caution should be exercised about multiple daily weighings from birth because of the anxiety it can cause. Weighing a baby on day 3–5 is recognised as being optimal. If a baby is identified as having lost 10% or more weight (or in some hospitals 8%) a plan should be triggered. The NICE Clinical Guidelines on faltering growth recommend that this should begin with a detailed breastfeeding assessment which includes observing feeds and checking the health of the baby. If feeding is not going well NICE recommend that a woman should be supported to increase her milk supply.[34] This may involve:

1. Expressing between feeds to stimulate milk supply
2. Feeding that expressed milk to the baby after a feed
3. If these do not work, using small amounts of formula while continuing breastfeeding support to increase supply if possible.

At this stage a baby should be weighed once per day and a referral made to a pediatrician if weight loss continues. It may be that the mother will struggle to produce sufficient breastmilk due to an existing condition, or it may be that with a plan in place, she will be able to increase her milk supply if she wants. It is also important to remember that in some cases this will be nothing to do with her milk supply at all – a health problem in the baby may mean they are not absorbing milk or nutrients. NHD can occur, although it is rarer, in formula-fed babies clearly being fed sufficient milk. All in all, the message is to be aware of risk factors and act promptly if an issue occurs.

Growth during the first few months

Aside from early weight loss, babies who are breastfed also typically put on weight more slowly than formula-fed babies in the first year. A number of studies have shown that although breastfed babies don't put on as much *weight* during the first year as formula-fed babies, there is no difference in *length* or head circumference (pretty important given the brain is in there). So babies are growing perfectly well, just not gaining weight so quickly.[35]

Once babies have regained their birth weight, most studies find that breast and formula-fed babies put on weight similarly in the early weeks, but by about three months differences start to emerge. In the randomised controlled trial in Belarus, for example, they found that formula-fed infants gained weight more rapidly than breastfed infants during the first year, and this difference was strongest at 3–6 months.[36] Another study in Holland compared the growth of exclusively breastfeeding or mixed feeding babies, finding that no difference was seen in these groups up to three months of age, but from 3–6 months of age the babies who received formula milk gained more weight.[37] Finally, in the NOURISH trial, an intervention designed to promote healthy early feeding practices, babies who put on weight rapidly (defined as crossing a centile line) were more likely to be formula-fed.[38]

Some studies don't show differences in weight between breast and formula-fed babies, but look closely at what they are comparing. Data from the Millennium cohort study found that the biggest difference in weight comes when babies who are exclusively breastfed for at least four months are compared to those who have only ever had formula.[39] A similar pattern was found in the Gemini birth cohort study, which is a fascinating study exploring the development of twins in the UK. One of the benefits of the study is that it has regularly weighed babies – 10 times between birth and around six months – and looked at their feeding. Data from this study has looked at how quickly babies grow and found that babies who were breastfed for at least four months weighed less at three and six months.[40]

It may not just be the milk that contributes to this difference, but also the way in which it is given. A study in the US compared bottle-feeding of either formula or expressed breastmilk to feeding directly from the breast. They found that babies who were bottle-fed either formula or expressed breastmilk gained weight more rapidly during the first year of life than those breastfed. When babies were fed from the breast they gained an average of 729g per month, compared to 780g when they were fed breastmilk in a bottle.[41] As we have seen, it is likely that babies take more milk from a bottle than they do at the breast, and this small difference adds up over time.

How do differences in growth affect breastfeeding?

Weight loss after the birth is normal and expected, but mothers who are breastfeeding may be concerned, especially if they are not expecting weight loss or they start to compare notes with their peers who are bottle-feeding. It is natural, when you can't see how much milk your baby is getting and people start comparing weight gains, to put two and two together and assume that the breastfed baby is not getting enough milk.

Our love of a big baby, and the association of weight with health and feeding a baby well, makes this anxiety worse. You can see why some women might start to use formula top-ups in the early days. Ironically this increases their risk of not producing enough milk. All new mothers should be told about normal baby weight loss after the birth, and the signs that show baby is getting enough milk.

At around four months other people often start putting pressure on mothers to give solids to encourage sleep, suggesting that the smaller breastfed baby is not getting enough milk and must be hungry. Babies are often unsettled around this time due to a big growth spurt and developmental leap, meaning that they start feeding lots and not sleeping. However, this is perfectly normal. The problem comes from considering the formula-fed baby as normal and the breastfed baby as underweight, despite the knowledge that overfeeding can contribute to longer-term obesity.

Action 5

✓ Tell parents and those around them about normal patterns of weight loss and weight gain in breastfed babies, and why this doesn't mean that they are underweight.

10. OUR OBSESSION WITH ROUTINES AND GOOD BABIES CAUSES UNNECESSARY PROBLEMS

'Is she good?'

Three little words that cause me to pause and stare slowly at the stranger who has just stopped me in the street, wondering if today will be the day that I launch into my speech regarding our cultural loss of understanding of normal baby behaviour and the damage that this causes.

'Is she good for you…?'

I realise the stranger is staring quite intently at me now, clearly expecting an answer. It's probably my own fault for having reeled off the answers to the first two questions on the script for stopping a new mother in the street. ('Is it a boy or a girl?' and 'How much did they weigh?', if you are wondering. Responding 'yes' to the first question causes too many awkward stares).

That day I chose humour. 'Oh yes, well so far this week no banks robbed – just don't ask me about last week'. Depending on how much I had been awake the night before, and therefore how high-pitched my voice was, this response would either elicit a laugh or the stranger would back slowly away. Apparently it wasn't the socially acceptable reply.

On a serious note – what is a good baby? And why do we stop new mothers in the street and ask them if they have one? Why does it matter and what answer are we expecting? Some will say it's just polite conversation, showing interest, no harm done… you're over-reacting… it's just what we say in the UK, once we've exhausted talking about the weather.

The conversation I recall happened often when my children were babies. I gave various answers (although rarely the full-blown semantic critique). It also happened often to people I know. When I repeat the question in a lecture or talk, it always gets a chuckle as so many have experience of it. It is clearly one of The Questions To Ask New Mothers. But is it really a benign enquiry?

In case you are not aware of the job description for a 'good' baby, it is usually taken to mean a baby that is silent and still, but wakes at appropriate times to smile and coo happily. Good babies sleep long periods at night, nap when you fancy a coffee and are happily passed to anyone who wants a cuddle. A 'good' baby doesn't interfere with your life at all, it simply adds value through occasional cute smiles. And what's more? If you have a 'good' baby, you have the holy grail and are a 'good' mother. Which of course is what we are all aiming for. Or at least, we're all typing it into Google. Seriously, go to Google and try it. My searches brought up:

- How to be a good mother... 721 million hits
- How to be a good mom... 316 million hits
- How to be a good mum... 158 million hits

This is clearly a topic that is of concern to new mothers. Incidentally, my searches only bring up 16 million for being a good father, and to put it into context 668 thousand on how to solve world hunger. But the real issue is that we're searching for the impossible – no matter how 'good' we are as mothers, the 'good' baby doesn't exist (or at least is very rare). But this doesn't stop parents from trying to achieve 'good' baby status.

The 'normal' baby

The problem is that we are so far removed from understanding what normal baby behaviour is like, that we see normal behaviour as problematic. Normal babies are not like the ones on the front cover of baby magazines or in nappy adverts. Normal babies wake up lots, like to be held and want to feed very frequently. And, as the name suggests, that's normal. However, this doesn't prevent others from suggesting that a baby should be 'good'. And 'good' babies do three things; they don't feed very often, they sleep well and they are predictable. Does it sound as if this is going to fit well with breastfeeding?

It is perfectly normal for babies to want to be held close and to stay near to their immediate caregivers. Being born is a shock to the system. One minute you're all cuddled up warm and snug, with food whenever you want it, being swayed gently to sleep, and the next you're out in the big, bright, noisy world all on your own. It is the most natural thing in the world for a baby to seek to stay close – if they were left alone they'd be rather screwed, wouldn't they? Baby giraffes might be able to get up and walk within moments... but humans? Kind of helpless. Working out strategies to stay close to mother and keep her attention is crucial to survival and backed up by a lot of psychology and attachment theory. Babies generally do best when they have a primary caregiver who is responsive to their needs and keeps them close. It makes them feel all loved and happy and they go out into the world with positive vibes about it being a lovely place. Peace.

Research has shown that being cared for while in close contact with mother is important across animal species. In rats this equates to how much licking and grooming goes on – the more attention paid to the baby rat, the less stress activity it has in its body.[1] In humans, babies who have parents who are responsive and interactive respond better to a stressor than those who do not (responsive generally means responding quickly to babies needs, rather than the licking – but feel free to give it a try). In particular, when parents are responsive the baby's cortisol (stress hormone) levels drop back to normal far more quickly after a stressful event.[2] A typical stressor in this type of test is the 'still face' – mother and baby play together and interact, then mother puts on a 'non-responsive' face. How stressed the baby gets is measured.

Much of this research contributes towards a model that considers the impact of whether babies experience many of these early stressors and how it might affect them. The 'Early Life Stress' model by Loman and Gunnar suggests that lots of stress in early infancy and childhood can programme the nervous system to respond in a certain way.[3] If a baby gets stressed a lot, their stress system becomes over-stimulated, so that they react more strongly in future – or in other words, get stressed and anxious more easily. This over-activity can also damage other areas of the developing brain, particularly around emotion regulation. This is one of the reasons why early stressful experiences can increase the risk of mental health difficulties in children and adults. For babies who spend most of their time sleeping, feeding and being held, how responsively this is done is really important. Babies do best when they are fed on demand, sleep close to their mother and have their needs met promptly. This doesn't fit very well with the concept of a 'good' baby, does it?

Self-styled parenting experts

Hot on the heels of mothers who are finding the transition to motherhood difficult are the self-styled parenting experts. Remember the bit about maternal identity formation, where you look for other experts to see if you can identify with them? The authors of baby care books have taken advantage of a gap in the market for maternal role models. They know new mothers feel overwhelmed during their transition, and they know all about the importance of good babies... and they make money out of telling you how to ensure your baby is one of the 'good' ones. Unfortunately, in Western culture we have the perfect environment for such experts to thrive; a lack of family around to support and guide us, no knowledge about what babies are really like and serious pressure to get this mothering thing right. Oh, and a 'one click order' function on Amazon. Lethal.

The baby parenting book market has taken full advantage of parental anxiety and the need for advice and a guru to follow, so Western popular culture is now awash with books by self-styled 'experts' (who often *do not* have their own children) about how to care for babies. Although books that advise a more responsive approach to caring for young babies exist, many parenting books are based around the idea of routines for feeding and sleep for young babies, with structured guides explaining how to get your baby to fit into the structure. Or in other words, how to get a 'good' baby. The ideas go completely against the concept of responsive feeding and care for young babies.

Although books about infant care have been available for many years, this most recent style of parenting publication first arose in the 1940s, with the publication of Dr Spock's *Commonsense Book of Baby and Child Care*.[4] This book became a bestseller, outsold in its time only by the Bible, and was available when today's mothers were babies (their mothers and mothers-in-law probably read it, and they are now telling today's mothers what to do). Spock was to some extent supportive of responsive parenting, declaring:

> 'Every time you pick your baby up – let's assume it's a girl – even if you do it a little awkwardly at first, every time you change her, bathe her, feed her, smile at her, she's getting a feeling that she belongs to you and that you belong to her. Nobody else in the world, no matter how skilful can give that to her... Don't be afraid to love her and enjoy her. Every baby needs to be smiled at, talked to, played with, fondled – gently and lovingly – just as much as she needs vitamins and calories. That will make her a person who loves people and enjoys life. The baby who doesn't get any loving will grow up cold and unresponsive'. (p2–3)

However, Spock also had some very clear ideas about infant sleep and the precedents for how, when and where babies should sleep can be seen in his writing:

> 'A 5 or 6 pounder needs to be fed every 3 hours. Most 8 and 9 pounders are happy to average 4 hours between feeds… somewhere between the fourth and fifth month, a majority of babies show a preference for a 5 hour interval' (p95)

On night feedings he has this to say:

> 'They come to realise that they don't need the late night feeding and most of them give it up at 1, 2 or 3 months of age.' (p95)

> 'If babies reach the age of 1 month and weigh 9 pounds and still wake for a 2am feeding, I think it's sensible for the parents to try to influence them to give it up' (p98)

Consider this in relation to what we know about normal baby feeding and waking. There is also no evidence that babies need fewer feeds as they weigh more – at least not within the weight and age range he is talking about. Yes, they can take in bigger feeds as their tummy gets bigger… but then they are also bigger so need more milk. These statements, however, are very specific and issued by a doctor – a person of authority. Many would have followed his advice, and many would be trying to pass his advice on to their children as mothers.

However, Spock pales into insignificance when you look at some of the ideas of the more modern parenting authors. Take Tizzie Hall, who runs a business called 'Save our Sleep' and has written a parenting book of the same name with the subtitle 'helping your baby sleep through the night from birth to two years'.[5] She has no children of her own. In her book she describes her beliefs about how and when babies should be sleeping and feeding, and these are based heavily on routine.

> 'By week two it is important to be developing some sort of sleeping and feeding routine.' (p3)

> 'I advise my clients whose babies are born full term and weight to offer breastfeeds of six minutes on each side every three hours in the first 24 hours. On the second day, offer him 9 minutes on each breast every 3

hours, and on the third day (if your milk has not come in yet) offer him 12 minutes on each side every three hours. On the fourth day, if your milk is still not in, give him sixteen minutes on each breast.' (p26)

This advice goes completely against what we know about boosting milk supply in those early days (frequent feeds, on demand). However, she does not stop there, going on to link sleep to a baby's weight:

'In my experience, babies don't start to surface between sleep cycles until they reach 6kg, usually around 8 to 16 weeks. This means you can help a newborn baby to go to sleep and she will stay asleep for a long time.' (p5)

She goes against safe sleep advice, actively suggesting that babies should sleep where the mother gets most sleep (e.g. needs to feed them the least).

'I feel your baby should sleep in the place that enables you to get the most rest… if every noise wakes you up and you feel you would get more sleep with her in a separate room, put her in her own room… but wherever she sleeps first, I do recommend moving her by 5 months to where you would like her to sleep for most of her babyhood.' (p8–9)

However, her views on routine and milk quality are the most perplexing, as she likens breastfeeding women to dairy cows:

'One aspect I considered is whether the quality of the mother's milk changes when she puts her baby on a routine. Because cows' milk is close to human milk, which is why we drink it and feed it to our children – I decided to discuss it with various dairy farmers.

Dairy farmers stick to strict routines in relation to their milking. Most will milk their cows at 5 am and 3pm every day. When I enquired why it was explained to me that milking the cows at a set time every day meant their metabolism knew exactly when and how much milk to produce.

The farmers said that if they milked their cows earlier or later than scheduled, the milk would not be of the highest quality or quantity. It's not such a leap to come to the conclusion that this might be the same for a breastfeeding mother's milk supply.' (p19)

Not such a leap? Say what? This is more a giant expedition across the galaxy than a leap! Newsflash – human babies and cow babies are not the same thing in any form. They are not physically the same, cognitively the same or have the same care needs. They are different. They need different milk. If we're going to be making leaps across species, perhaps we should be looking at those closest to us: chimpanzees and gorillas (who in fact feed their babies far more often than we do). As noted in previous chapters, the content of cows' milk and breastmilk is very different, based on the different physiological needs of babies and calves (babies – cognitive growth, cows – physical growth) and the care needs (human babies need closer care than calves do). So of course they will feed differently.

Secondly, dairy farming is not the same environment as naturally caring for a calf. Information from farming websites suggests that most cows would naturally feed their calves around 4–6 times a day if able to do so. Dairy cows don't have their calves. The set-up is completely artificial. Tizzie also fails to account for the fact that many cows consume huge amounts of antibiotics to prevent mastitis, levels of which would rocket if human women fed just twice a day.

The messages in Tizzie's book work to subtly undermine maternal confidence. Consider what we've already discussed about new mothers feeling unsure of themselves and looking to experts to tell them what to do. Tizzie's approach manipulates that uncertainty perfectly. She suggests that parents are unskilled in recognising their own baby's needs and need an expert to tell them what to do (so they need to buy her book).

'I feel that in today's society with less family support, it is too hard for most new parents to learn the skill of interpreting their baby's cries early enough to demand feed.' (p22)

'The good thing about my routines is that when your baby starts to cry, you can look at the routine and see what is due to happen next, a real help when learning to distinguish tired and hungry cries.' (p21)

However, there is lots of evidence that women learn to tell what their baby needs from the sound of their cry from an early age. (And more than one need is served by whipping out a boob – tired, hungry, thirsty, grumpy... so does it really matter if a mother isn't sure what a cry means?) A further theme is that she suggests you should not respond to your baby's dependency – babies must be prevented from being manipulative and taught 'correct' behaviour. This flies in the face of what we know about the importance of loving relationships and attachment for development.

> 'Be conscious that some babies think your sole purpose in life is to help him fall asleep.' (p20)

> 'During night feeds try not to talk to your baby.' (p84)

Finally, let's look at her dreamfeed advice. Parents are advised to feed their baby while they sleep, in the hope that this will stop them waking up. A bit like putting petrol in a car. Dreamfeeding to increase sleep duration is a strange concept, and the parallel with the evidence showing sugary drinks can increase obesity risk is stark. People who drink too many sugary drinks are more likely to be overweight because they don't consider the calories in the drinks to be food. And this is essentially what dreamfeeding encourages; you're trying to feed the baby without them realising it.

> 'How to dreamfeed: To do the dreamfeed gently pick up your sleeping baby, place the bottle or breast on her lower lip and allow her to drink taking care not to wake her.'[84]

Save our Sleep is not the only baby care book that is based on routines. The Contented Little Baby Book[6] by Gina Ford advises parents along the same lines: feed to a routine to teach your baby to sleep and make your baby as independent as possible. 'Routine' is a real buzz-word, it keeps popping up:

> 'I personally believe that the majority of babies thrive and are happier in a routine.' (p27)

So routines, according to the 'experts', will help your baby grow and thrive and become a happier baby overall! (I wonder how you measure baby happiness?) And routines must begin from the start, as this will mean the baby will be sleeping for long periods by around two months.

> 'If you want your baby to sleep through the night from an early age and ensure a long-term healthy sleep pattern, the golden rules are to establish the right associations and to structure your baby's feeds from the day you arrive home from the hospital.' (p76)

'The majority of babies I helped care for personally usually started to sleep to 6–7 am somewhere between 8–12 weeks.' (p75)

Gina thinks that a baby's weight somehow determines how much a baby needs feeding, with the inverse logic that bigger babies need less feeding:

'Once your baby has regained his birth weight and is regularly putting on at least 6–8oz each week you can look at establishing a regular bedtime of 6.30–7pm.' (p80)

'I believe by the end of the second week a baby who weighed 7 pounds or more at birth should really only need one feed in the night.' (p205)

Aside from the lack of evidence (or indeed logic) that such small weight changes in the early weeks would magically remove the need to feed at night, this advice is particularly baffling in the context of mothers who stop breastfeeding a 'big' baby, because they perceive, or have been told, that they can't 'fill them up'. Gina also perpetuates the myth that formula milk will make babies sleep, giving advice that contradicts the Department of Health's recommendation to breastfeed exclusively for six months:

'By three to four months: If your baby is totally breastfed and is still waking up early in the night… it may be worthwhile talking to your health visitor about replacing the late breastfeeds with formula-feeds.' (p102)

And finally, the theme of 'creating dependence' rears its head once more, with Gina's belief that interactions should not be responsive, but should be used to train your baby's behaviour:

'I suggest avoiding eye contact at 10.30pm and during night feeds to help you show your baby it is not play time.' (p44)

'Feeding him to sleep … in the long term can create sleep problems.'

So there we have it: three popular books that ignore what we know is normal behaviour for breastfed babies and encourage parents to use routines rather than responsive interactions. Apart from being harmful, the idea that you can simply train your baby to sleep may be irrelevant. Some babies are just born to be more sociable at night. One study of infant temperament and sleep found that babies who were rated as having an 'easy' temperament generally slept a lot more at night than those rated 'difficult'.[7]

Notably, in the Mayan–American study discussed earlier, the concept of a night-time routine, or the need to 'encourage' a baby to fall asleep, was alien to the Mayan mothers. None had set routines to encourage the baby to fall asleep. Babies just fell asleep when they were ready to sleep – whether that was in a parent's arms, before the parents went to bed or at the same time as everyone else. Most fell asleep while being held, with 70% being fed to sleep. No parent reported a routine such as a bath, bedtime story or comfort object… babies simply went to sleep. Conversely, the majority of American parents reported a routine. The authors quote one mother in the paper jokingly noting that when she tells her friends it's time to put her baby to bed, they say 'See you in an hour'.[8]

Do baby care books work?

I first came across baby care books when I had my own first baby in 2006. As an academic mother, I read them and had questions about their approach, so I turned to Google Scholar to get a sense of the evidence that *must* be underpinning them. Given their readership, and the strength of the authors' opinions and recommendations, *surely* these books must have a substantial evidence base? Not so much. Although my search brought up over 11 million hits, and told me that hundreds of millions of copies of these books had been sold worldwide, the academic literature was sparse. And by sparse, I mean non-existent.

In terms of broader evidence, research had looked at the importance of responsive parenting for older children. Generally speaking, when parents were responsive to their child's needs during infancy and childhood, children had the best outcomes educationally, socially and emotionally.[9] In particular there is evidence that suggests that mothers who responded sensitively and promptly to their baby's signals have the most positive attachment bonds with their baby.[10] How could this fit with routines and not looking at your baby during the night?

The evidence exploring the idea of trying to manipulate and shape a baby's behaviour was mixed. On the one hand, allowing babies to cry for long periods of time, rather than responding to their cues, caused high levels of cortisol to be released in babies as they were so stressed.[11] Among other things this may have an impact on the infant's developing brain.[12] However, a mother's risk of postnatal depression also increases with sleep deprivation,[13] infant crying[14] and maternal feelings of loss of control or identity.[15] In turn, postnatal depression can negatively affect infant attachment[16] and infant development.[17] When you read this it's easy to think that perhaps using routines to help shape a baby's behaviour could be a good idea.

Unfortunately, when you look more closely at research examining whether it's even possible to get a baby into a routine or to sleep longer at night, then the evidence is very weak. Although some studies might claim an impact, when you start looking at the detail of the studies, there are often a lot of issues with the methodology used. Take for example one study conducted in Australia.[18] Researchers asked mothers who were experiencing sleep difficulties with their baby to sign up to a study that would look at the impact of controlled crying on baby sleep and maternal mental health. They assigned one group to learn all about controlled crying and left the other as a control group. They reported that mothers in the controlled crying group had improved wellbeing and their baby slept better at the end of the study.

That sounds promising, right? Well not really, when you look at what they actually did. First of all, we know from other research that if you simply offer one group support and not the other, the support group will have an improvement in wellbeing just because someone is doing something. Mothers who were at the end of their tether with a baby who wouldn't sleep were probably relieved that someone was helping. Of course their mental health would improve. And in fact, mothers in the intervention group received one-to-one support from a research nurse, including ideas for how to protect and support their own wellbeing. Is it any wonder their mental health improved compared to those who received no support? Also, when asked what they found most useful about the study, mothers rated having someone to talk to as the best thing.

Second, sleep problems were identified by the mother. Mothers were asked whether they felt their baby's sleep was problematic. But as part of the intervention mothers were taught what normal baby sleep looked like. It's likely mothers in this group reduced their perceptions of a sleep problem compared to those who had no education. So did the intervention actually improve sleep? It wasn't measured, so no one knows.

Eight years after my initial ponderings, my MSc student Victoria Harries and I conducted some research exploring what impact these books actually had for babies and parents. Did they work?[19] And how did they make them feel? We found that mothers were split. One group followed the books closely and found them useful. These mothers had fewer depressive symptoms, experienced less parenting stress and had higher confidence. All good, yes? But only around one in six mothers experienced positive effects.

The rest of our mothers found the advice in the books less useful. They were more likely to have exhibited symptoms of depression and lower confidence. Of course it could be that mothers who were already miserable found the books difficult to follow, but when we asked them directly about the impact of the books on their emotions, many talked about feeling more anxious, more confused and even like failures. It's unsurprising really. These books sold them a hope, a dream. And when that didn't work either, they felt worse than ever, blaming themselves and feeling like nothing would ever work.

How do baby care books impact on breastfeeding?

There is also growing evidence to suggest baby care books and promotion of strict routines can impact negatively on breastfeeding. Around nine years ago fellow psychologist Dr Bronia Arnott and I decided to explore how the concepts outlined in baby care books affected infant feeding experiences. We designed a questionnaire based on the concepts in these books, asking how much mothers used a routine for sleep and feeding and the types of interaction they had with their baby. We tested the questionnaire on mothers with babies aged 0–12 months and found that five different types of behaviour emerged that echoed the behaviours in the books.[20] These included use of routine (for sleep, feeding and day-to-day activity), nurturance (how quickly a mother responded to her baby), discipline (belief that a baby's behaviour needed changing), anxiety (over infant health, wellbeing and her role as a mother) and finally concern for development (a concern that she must enhance her infant's development through different activities).

Overall, we found mothers who breastfed longest had higher levels of nurturance, lower levels of anxiety and low levels of routine.[21] These findings could be interpreted in two ways. Firstly, it is possible that mothers who want to follow a parenting approach that is high in routine and encouraging of independence may not choose to breastfeed at all, as it does not 'fit' with their preferred approach. Alternatively, given the literature we have already looked at about the importance of baby-led feeding, it is possible that those mothers who try to implement the messages of the books only manage to breastfeed for a short period of time. If they try to restrict feeds, have a strict activity routine for their baby or are encouraging their baby to sleep to a set timetable, it is likely that this will negatively affect their milk supply. Alternatively, they may experience anxiety that their baby is feeding 'too much' or 'too irregularly' based on what the books suggest, and believe that they are not producing enough milk. Or they may respond to rumours from friends and family that formula-fed infants sleep for longer, and decide to stop breastfeeding. It was clear that following the ideas in the books was linked to stopping breastfeeding. Given what we know about how breastfeeding works, it's not difficult to see why.

Then a few years later, in the second part of our study into the impact of specific books on parenting, wellbeing and behaviours, Victoria and I found that mothers who followed the advice to use routines and found it to be useful were less likely to breastfeed at birth, less likely to continue breastfeeding if they did start and more likely to feed to a routine. Notably this was embedded within a wider parenting style in which babies were more likely to sleep in their own rooms and mothers were more likely to encourage sleep routines and wait longer to respond when a baby cried. Given that these behaviours were also indicative of formula use, it illustrates a wider, less responsive parenting style.

Overall, our cultural beliefs about how babies should behave have the potential to damage breastfeeding. In the absence of close-knit family and a general knowledge of babies, self-styled experts have jumped on the 'good' baby bandwagon, teaching parents how to train their babies to be 'good' while setting up breastfeeding to fail. Breastfeeding is not compatible with routines. How breastfed babies feed is normal, and we should be thinking about wider ways in which we can make life easier for new parents, not training their babies out of normal and healthy behaviour.

Action 6

✓ Bin all the rubbish baby care books.

11. OUR LACK OF VALUE FOR NEW MOTHERS MAKES EVERYTHING FEEL MORE DIFFICULT

Motherhood is tough. Whichever way you look at it, life changes. We have what we know about breastfeeding… and then we have modern life. Modern mothering. Modern expectations. And the two can be a challenge to merge.

It's all very well to know that breastfeeding works best if you feed on demand. And that babies feed frequently. And wake up a lot. And don't much like being apart from you. And this is all natural, and if you look at other cultures, just what babies are designed to do. But how does this all fit into modern everyday life? Does knowing this help when you are challenged from every angle? As a society we are not baby friendly. Mothers have so many expectations placed on them, at a time when they are getting to grips with an enormous change in their life. On the one hand we tell them breast is best and urge them to do it, yet on the other hand we demand that they get back to participating in life as it was before baby. Is that baby sleeping yet? Come out for the evening! When are you going back to work? Must lose that baby weight!

Feminism has made enormous strides for women. We have far more opportunity to work, be educated and have equal power in relationships than our mothers and grandmothers did. But it also means that there are more demands on us. Education means many become highly sensitised to the 'right' or 'scientific' way to do things (although babies typically don't read the books). Our careers mean we need or want to get back to work. Around a third of women with children are now the main wage earners, with many more in families that need two incomes to make ends meet. Becoming a mother is even more of a shock to the system when babies weren't part of your former life and you had a powerful job and an organised social life. Social media screams at us that we need to get our figures back and get out there socialising and Having Lots Of Fun All The Time.

Some of this will mean that women make the informed decision that breastfeeding will not fit with their family. More will want to breastfeed and struggle to fit it all in as they attempt to do everything society insists they do, with little support from others. Society continues to demand that they breastfeed, while simultaneously refusing to realise just how challenging it can be to 'have it all' in this situation. Women's home and work lives are all different. Their expectations and experience of mothering, their concern over getting it just right and personal feelings about their body and the constraints of their employment can combine to mean that breastfeeding itself is the straw that breaks the camel's back. Until we start to realise this, and work with new mothers to support them, we won't solve the problem.

Transition to motherhood

'I'm not sure what I thought would happen. I guess I hadn't really thought about life much with the baby. The birth, yes. But the baby? I thought we'd take him home, bursting with pride in what we had made and I would sit on the sofa and watch him peacefully sleep. I had great plans of coffee with friends, trips to the hairdresser after not getting it coloured during pregnancy and lots of walks in the park laughing and playing with my beautiful son. I'd even planned my new mum wardrobe like the magazines showed. And breastfeeding would be beautiful right? Then reality hit. I had stitches that stopped me walking for a while. Then it rained. A lot. He cried, a lot. I cried a lot. He had colic. I sometimes didn't get changed out of my pyjamas. My hair lived tied back on top of my head. I didn't drink a cup of coffee whilst it was still hot for a long time. My friends all had jobs and lives. And most of all I felt very alone, both physically and in terms of how I felt. I didn't think anyone else could feel this way.'

I often talk about the concept of 'supermum' in my teaching, and explain to students how in Western society we praise or even idolise new mothers who appear to 'get their life back' – to how it was before baby – as soon as possible after the birth. Usually my international students, who have come from cultures where family, mothering and babies are celebrated and accepted, look at me in horror. I regale them with stories of mothers stopping in to do a full shop on their way home from the hospital, while they tell me stories of new mothers being cared for, fed and massaged daily after birth for six weeks. It's usually at this point that I make a mental note to move to their home country if I ever have another baby.

We don't idolise and protect motherhood in the same way, do

we? It's a very weird concept, this 'getting life back to normal'. Let's have a baby! A whole new dependent person! But let's not change our lives! Instead of adapting to this humungous change we expect women to simply do it all. And look happy about it. The wonderful Sheila Kitzinger talked about this in her book *Ourselves as Mothers*,[1] describing how the media bombards mothers from every angle, insisting that they must care for their baby perfectly while keeping up their former lives. To quote, a mother is instructed to 'keep the romance in her relationship good, cook gourmet food and produce candlelit dinners and at the same time be a perfect mother'. This was back in 1992. Nearly 25 years ago. Have we made progress? No, we've gone backwards and now put even more pressure on new mothers to live up to impossible standards. Today the headlines might scream 'Celebrity gets back into skinny jeans half an hour after giving birth', but the message is still the same, and just as unrealistic to live up to. Kitzinger had it spot on: 'A woman who catches sight of herself in the mirror sees a very different picture. And the message is clear: she is a failure'.

Although we have made huge strides in women's rights, inequality still exists. Women still do more housework and childcare than men (on average; of course, there are some great men out there who do more than their fair share). Bizarrely, the more money a woman earns, the more housework and childcare she does. Women who work full-time and have a child who is primary school age have higher stress levels than everyone else in our society. And the least time to themselves. Strange, that link, isn't it? In one study of how new mothers' lives had changed, over half of all mothers reported that they had no time for their own interests, had no social life and desperately needed a break from their child. Over a quarter admitted they did not like their new lives.[2]

But this is only half the picture; this is what mothers become. When women have a baby for the first time, they have to go through the transition to motherhood: from independent woman to putting the needs of someone else above hers, 24/7. Plus they have to get to grips with feeding a whole new person to keep them alive. One who seems to want to feed frequently, just to remind them of the freedom that they're now missing out on, and makes them wonder whether life will ever be the same again.

Becoming a mother

'But nobody told me I was having a baby! Where on earth did that come from?!'

That's my own quote. One I shared with so many new mothers, and they all nodded in agreement. 'My first thought was to put him back,' responded one. 'There were more checks and processes involved in getting my rescue cat,' said another. Humour, or truth? The best humour is often based on the truth. We are woefully underprepared to become mothers. And yet somehow we don't speak out about it.

Parents-to-be rarely consider what caring for the actual baby will be like. No one really thinks about how life is going to change. Few ever dare to think that it might not change for the better. And certainly no one says that out loud. Few really know what they are letting themselves in for. In one study into non-mothers' experiences of babies, three quarters of women surveyed had never held a newborn. Only around 20% had ever babysat a very young baby, bottle-fed or changed a nappy. Their vague experience of babies was playing with dolls as a young child. Anne Oakley, who led the research, concluded 'Adoptive mothers may be carefully scrutinised for their mothering abilities... and nannies and children's nurses are professionally trained, yet women who give birth to babies may not know one end from the other.'[3]

Susan Maushart sums this up perfectly in her book *The Mask of Motherhood: How becoming a mother changes our lives and how we never talk about it*. It's a great book, go and read it (after this one).[4] She talks about an exchange she had with her sister, who had a baby, about the realities of motherhood:

'I recalled asking later in a playful sort of way, "Well, tell me about motherhood. What's it really like, anyway?" I was taken aback by the intensity of her response. She looked away from the baby (and that itself was a rare occurrence) and stared straight into my eyes. "I'm going to tell you this now, and I want you to remember it," she began. "Everyone lies. Do you hear me? Everyone lies about what it's like to have a baby. Don't listen to them. Just watch me, and remember".'

We don't tell the truth about motherhood, do we? We don't say the negative things. They're not socially acceptable. But in what other job would we be entirely happy? And this is a job that wakes us up every hour through the night and prevents us from showering! A recent study explored the impact of having a first baby on happiness. They followed people from adolescence until older age and asked them regularly how happy they were with life, then looked at whether anything that happened to them made them more happy or less so. They found that a partner dying young had less of an impact on overall happiness than having a first baby. Death is less disturbing than a first baby! Of course, not all mothers feel like this and as always there is a continuum of feeling. Some feel totally overwhelmed, others just a bit and some are never happier. But many new mothers do struggle to some extent in the early months. And when you think about it, it is a kind of loss, a grieving for a former life. Yet few can voice these feelings.

What does it feel like to become a mother?

Aside from positive emotions, when mothers were asked how they felt about motherhood, common responses included 'shocked', 'unprepared', 'panicked', 'out of control' and 'anxious'.[5] Other common thoughts included feeling overwhelmed, burdened and an awful realisation of responsibility.[6] Others are simply shocked by how much they needed to do... and how different it was from what they expected. It feels unfair, when you think you are so prepared and ready, that you end up totally overwhelmed by the reality.[7] Further distress can be caused by work issues and simply having to say goodbye to your work identity. And on top of all of that, marriage satisfaction rapidly declines in the first year of parenthood as stereotypical roles become embedded and jealousy mounts, as typically a father is able to continue his old life to a greater extent.[8] Maushart sums it up: 'Mothering is the most powerful of all biological capacities and among the most disempowering of social experiences.'

I recently did some work with academics Dr Rebecca Clifford and Dr Kate North exploring this concept of the transition to motherhood. Rebecca is a historian interested in people's life stories and Kate is a creative writer. Together we designed a creative writing project designed to get mothers talking about the hidden emotions of motherhood; the emotions we found you couldn't really share. As part of the project we asked over 1,000 mothers to describe the emotions they experienced on becoming a mother. The usual suspects jumped out – the ones you would expect: love, proud, rewarding, lucky, euphoric. But actually the most common words were things like overwhelming, exhausting, terrifying, unprepared and lonely.

You can see our work in progress at www.creativemotherhoodproject.com.

Maushart (I really like this book) goes on to describe how it felt to have her first child:

'Anna was born at a civilised 7.30pm. By midnight I was not only ready for sleep but I desperately needed it... Every time I tried to put her in that damned crib she screamed as if scalded... my weariness had turned to exhaustion... I found myself wondering guiltily when a midwife would pop in and take Anna to the nursery. But surely this would defeat the whole point of rooming-in... And yet I was so tired. So tired. I had never been more tired in my life.'

And there we sum up motherhood. Who comes first? When do I sleep? Who have I become? When do I get to be me? Can I have a break yet? Hang on, should I feel this way? Am I allowed to say anything to anyone else? Where's my support?! Some describe motherhood as transitioning to an entirely new reality. Mothers may need to change their goals, behaviours and responsibilities and basically construct a whole new self. Many realise there is no going back to their old self, or at least not for a long time, and start to build their new reality and new definition of self. This can include seeking out new role models who represent their new normal, seeking lots of information about what to make the new self into, and then testing out their new role. Things around the woman can influence this, including how much money she has, the community she lives in and her culture. It is a time of rapid change.[9]

There are lots of theories about what happens during this time but one is the concept of maternal role attainment – or the process that leads to a mother emerging at the other end. During this she watches those around her, trying to decide who she might follow or who she will not be like. She will note how people act, what they believe and what they say and think about adopting these behaviours. Being like other people is comforting (and this may in part explain why we end up with breast and formula-feeding 'camps'). Grief is part of the process as she says goodbye to her old life and forms a new one. A woman's own mother is the potential strongest role model in all of this, and conflict and distress can arise as a woman decides whether she will adopt those same behaviours or not, or starts to question how her mother could act so differently.[10]

Most studies suggest that the first three months of motherhood are the hardest in terms of this transition. Most have made a transition by three months, although 4% have not done so by a year.[11] This can be disrupted at about eight months when babies become more wilful and independent (and at the same time more clingy), just at the time that mothers are seeking even more independence and trying to regain aspects of their pre-baby identity, such as weight, appearance and work.[12] Another study suggested that as the baby gets older, mothers feel more and more confident, but not necessarily more satisfied.[13]

Those who cope with the transition well tend to rapidly shift their goals in life to become more family-centric. Mothers who have more family-orientated goals have lower rates of depression than those who are aiming for more personal achievements. Others fully transform into a 'mummy' and adopt a very traditional family set-up.[14] For some this will mean a whole new friendship circle as they look to role models on whom to base their behaviour, and in turn on who can validate the new them. Old friends may be forgotten as they may remind the woman of what she has lost.[15]

Professional, educated, high earning mothers often experience the shift most harshly, feeling particularly out of control and as though their identity has been stolen. The skills they worked so hard to achieve no longer matter. They rapidly move from a world in which they knew what they were doing and their qualifications, experience and reputation put them in control, to a world where the stuff they don't have, like close family support and a network of mothers with babies, is what matters. Many women in this group admit to fiercely loving their children, but not loving the task of caring for them. Frustration, tedium and chaos were words they used to describe their lives and although they wouldn't change their children, they didn't enjoy being with them. For others it was not the baby that they resented, but the loss of their former identity and life. If they could just combine both… but there was no going back.[16] And on top of this? A big dose of guilt for feeling that way.

The ecstatically happy new mother image doesn't however fit with what the research actually tells us about new motherhood. Research suggests that for first-time mothers, happiness increases during pregnancy and can peak just after birth. Then things start to decline, levelling at a point worse than before you got pregnant. It's not so much you don't love your baby, but that you don't necessarily love everything that goes alongside it. The lack of freedom, sleep and money. Increased tension or arguments with your partner. The relentlessness of it all. The feelings of loss or grief for your own life.

They all mean that this idyllic image is, well, a myth.[17]

The main problem is that for some reason we don't talk about any of this. We keep it hidden, maybe out of fear that we are the only ones who feel this way. Or that what we are feeling is wrong. So then the next mother feels like this too, and so on. We need to be more honest and open. Motherhood was never meant to be a time of total joy, all the time. Struggling with your new life is not the same as not loving or not wanting your baby.

Becoming a mother and feeding your baby

So how does this all fit with how babies are fed? Looking at the bare facts of breast and formula-feeding, we can see why formula milk might appeal to those who want a more convenient feeding method. Breastfed babies feed very frequently, whereas formula-fed babies feed less often. People believe that formula-fed babies will get more sleep. Formula-fed babies gain more weight, and weight is an outward badge of 'good' mothering. On the surface breastfeeding looks like it will be a lot more intensive, at a time when intensive is really overwhelming and society is putting pressure on you to get back to normal. In that pressure to get your ordered life back, how does breastfeeding fit with that? It doesn't.

However, some women find that during this overwhelming transition breastfeeding actually really helps. It helps them feel closer to their baby. They identify with breastfeeding being a huge part of mothering. Although they might find it challenging overall, they feel it is worthwhile, and it makes them feel like they're doing something right. For some it can heal the trauma of a difficult birth, making them feel like their body has achieved something. One mother explained to me:

> 'I was absolutely exhausted and overwhelmed with it all and a few people suggested I give up breastfeeding to get a break. I felt like a useless mother in so many other ways but the breastfeeding was the part I really loved and felt like I was doing a good job at. It helped me stop, escape and just be whilst I was feeding. It was all the other things I wanted to escape from and stopping breastfeeding wouldn't solve that.'

Others find breastfeeding exhausting. It's a step too far. Overwhelmed by how much their life has changed, and the little rest and free time they have, it is easy to see why breastfeeding gets the blame, especially if people think that formula-fed babies will feed more and sleep less. Breastfeeding is one aspect of mothering that can be a choice. You can't really just ignore your baby all night or leave them alone all day while you pop to the gym. But feeding? Other people want to do that.

All this is a *huge* issue for breastfeeding. People offer to help by feeding the baby, not by supporting the mother in other ways. Sometimes her only ray of light is someone with a bottle in hand. However, many new mothers are so isolated from any help that they really are doing it all on their own. As humans we aren't designed to look after babies in isolation. In other cultures mothers may be able to put the baby in a sling and life goes on, because they have wider support circles around them, but in Western culture we often just aren't set up to do that. Little fears about sleep, separation and independence creep into our thinking and we worry that this dependency will continue, along with the lack of support, forever.

'I just couldn't do it any more. I was suddenly on call for this tiny person all day and all night and it was such a shock. I love my sleep. LOVE my sleep and now I could barely get an hour at a time. She wanted holding all day too. She was glued to me. I grew so envious, and then angry, at my husband lying there sleeping. How dare he sleep? He should be helping me with feeds and caring for this baby he helped make, not sleeping and then escaping to work in the morning.'

Sometimes breastfeeding itself can be too overwhelming. If women are having problems every time they try to feed their baby, it can make motherhood seem so difficult. For these mothers, breastfeeding doesn't help them bond or adapt to mothering; it's a reminder in their minds that they're failing.

'He used to get so hungry and upset. He'd bang his little fists on my breasts and throw his head around, mouth wide open and screaming trying to latch on and failing. It was as if he hated me, and every time I watched that and couldn't console him I died a little bit further inside. I'd come to hate breastfeeding and everything it made me feel.'

For these mothers it's not so much that they want to formula-feed, but that they can't stand the experience of breastfeeding any more. And you can see how this links in with all her previous experiences. The woman quoted above had a really difficult birth. She'd been separated from her baby and was so exhausted she asked for him to be given a bottle of formula so she could sleep, without realising it might make breastfeeding more difficult long term. She hadn't been able to access any support and felt completely overwhelmed.

However, one of the main draws of formula-feeding is the concept of someone else being able to feed the baby with milk you haven't had to express. On the surface it's easy to see the appeal of this idea. Someone else being able to feed the baby does mean that someone else will be around to feed the baby! In a survey of women who had chosen to formula-feed, around a quarter did so because they believed it to be easier and more convenient. A further 15% stated that they wanted others to be able to share the feeding. And 12% stated that they were working or looking after another child. Three-quarters of these women were pleased to find a solution that made things easier, and 88% were pleased the baby was getting fed.[18]

One study explored how much time mothers spent feeding and caring for their six-month-old babies in relation to how they fed them. They found that mothers who were exclusively breastfeeding spent more time feeding their babies than those who were partially or fully formula-feeding. Overall, the exclusively breastfeeding mothers spent 18.2 hours a week feeding their babies, while the partial or full formula group spent 11.6 hours. But that wasn't the full picture. The partial or full group spent more time feeding solid foods and preparing feeds, meaning that the total feeding time for both groups was 18.7 versus 15.4 hours. So the exclusively breastfeeding group were still spending more time… but this still wasn't the full picture.[19]

The researchers then asked what help the mothers had in caring for their babies, both specifically in relation to feeding and more general care. Mothers who were exclusively breastfeeding had 9 minutes a week of help with feeding, compared to 35 minutes a week for the partial or full group, which counters the belief that if you formula-feed you will suddenly get lots of help with feeding the baby. Interestingly, the exclusively breastfeeding group had far more help with general care (324 minutes) than the formula-feeding group (235 minutes). I'm imagining a lot of 'I've been up all night feeding this baby, it's your turn now' conversations.[19]

I am not about to suggest that a woman who has looked at her life and made an informed decision to bottle-feed to fit in with her family's lifestyle shouldn't do so. Some may also argue that how a baby is fed is only one part of mothering, and choices have to be made that enable a family to be the happiest it can be. However, I do want to ask which factors mean that breastfeeding a small baby is seen as so inconvenient and overwhelming? Also, who decided that those factors are more important than feeding a baby? And how did we get to the point in our society that a mother's choice about how to feed her baby is based on pressure put on her by other people about what her life should look like? If a mother wants to make that decision herself, fair play. If someone else's pressure or rules make it impossible for her to exercise her right to breastfeed her baby, then we need to be taking action.

Furthermore, if we're abandoning mothers to 'do it all' alone, is it any wonder they 'give up' on one of the things they can give up on? We need to take a long look at how we treat mothers during the postnatal period. And we need to think about how we can help and support them *without* using a bottle. We need to care for our new mothers, to 'mother the mother': cook her a meal, hold the baby for a bit, do some housework or just sit and let her talk honestly. If we supported and cherished mothers in this way, rather than expecting them to snap back to their normal lives, breastfeeding would seem less overwhelming. We need to get to the point where breastfeeding is the easiest choice, rather than something perceived as inconvenient or overwhelming.

How does this fit with maternal mental health?

'The "breast is best" obsession and a mother driven to take her own life.'

'British mother fell to death after problems breastfeeding baby.'

'Tragic fall missing mother "stopped taking medication so she could breastfeed".'

These headlines are devastating. But does breastfeeding increase the risk of, or exacerbate, postnatal depression or other mental health difficulties? This is an increasingly important area of research and not one that is easy to disentangle. After all, it is not as if you can set up a trial to deliberately induce postnatal depression in new breastfeeding mothers and see what happens. Moreover, separating the experience of postnatal depression from the experience of feeding (and overall mothering) is extremely hard.

As we've seen, it's not surprising that new mothers are depressed, given the expectations placed on them combined with the shock of motherhood and a general lack of support. Breastfeeding difficulties can seem like the last straw. And for mothers who are feeling depressed, all aspects of caring for a baby can seem even more demanding than they would if they were not depressed. Conversely, as we discussed earlier, when breastfeeding is going well, it can be protective for maternal mental health from both a physiological and psychological perspective. I think it is safe to say that breastfeeding *itself* is unlikely to cause mental health difficulties, but the experience of breastfeeding not going well, or not being supported, can be destructive.

One nagging thought I always have in the back of my head when we discuss breastfeeding and mental health difficulties is not that the experience of breastfeeding itself is causing depression, but rather that our experiences of new motherhood are making everything seem challenging. When you're feeling low or anxious, you search for anything in desperation that could be blamed or changed to make it all go away. Breastfeeding is an easy fall guy, but rarely does stopping breastfeeding miraculously fix all the other issues.

Postnatal depression is thought to affect around one in five new mothers, although these estimates could be very conservative, as new mothers may be worried about the implications of telling other people how they feel. Concerns about being perceived as a 'bad' or 'unnatural' mother, or simply being seen as not being able to cope with motherhood, can stop women from telling others how they feel. This secrecy serves to prevent others from speaking out, as they believe they must feel differently from everyone else. Others worry about social services becoming involved, or their baby being taken away from them, which is highly unlikely based on a diagnosis of postnatal depression alone.

Postnatal depression can have a wide range of symptoms and does not necessarily reflect the stereotypes of depression we may be familiar with. Sadness can play a considerable role, but often this sadness is not connected with anything specific and is more of an overall feeling of loss and loneliness. Anxiety can play an important role in postnatal depression, with mothers feeling anxious about themselves, their baby or just in general. Behaviourally mothers may feel very lethargic and not want to leave the house (or even get out of bed), have sleeping problems (either too much or too little) and appetite problems (again, too much or too little). Stereotypical examples of how a mother with postnatal depression must feel: that she regrets becoming a mother, or even wants to harm her baby, are rare. Many mothers report feeling overwhelmed and anxious about life, but very much in love with their baby.

Considering the causes of postnatal depression is vital if we are to reflect on whether it could be caused by breastfeeding. Although there are some genetic components to postnatal depression, and women who have had previous episodes of depression are more likely to experience it, most causes of postnatal depression are thought to be psychological or social. Research suggesting that hormonal changes may lead to postnatal depression is inconclusive, as all new mothers go through significant hormonal changes. It is possible, however, that some mothers react differently to these hormonal changes than others. Likewise, sleep deprivation and exhaustion are believed to increase the risk, but this is difficult to research because well-rested new mothers are hard to find.

Unpicking the causes of postnatal depression often leads to consideration of a woman's wider experience. Western culture has changed the way we care for new mothers and their babies. Often women are in hospital for only a few hours, before being discharged home to return to their everyday lives. Many women now live far away from any family, and if they have a partner, once they return to work after a week or so, she is predominantly on her own day to day. We have babies later in life, and less experience of being close to our families, so often the first baby we hold is our own. Other cultures focus on 'mothering the mother' after childbirth, with family coming to support her while she focuses on her baby and recovering from the birth.

Our pre-baby lifestyles are now often so baby-unfriendly that the transition to motherhood can be a shock. With more mothers now working, and in senior roles, the significant changes to lifestyle that having a baby bring can be a major shock. Watching a partner's life continue as 'normal' as they leave for work in the morning can challenge even the strongest relationship. Rachel Cusk, in her book *A Life's Work*, records the following quote from a mother:

> *'The Doctor said "I think you are a bit depressed". I am exhausted, I have no job, I have no life, I am stuck at home with this crying baby and these pointless domestic tasks to do... You go nuts just walking around with these books, thinking can he have butternut squash... wouldn't you be depressed?'*

The two key factors of social isolation and birth shock combine to create a feeling that is very common among new mothers – that having a baby is nothing like they expected it to be. This is all made worse by the comments of strangers, who admonish the mother for feeling like this. 'You have a new baby. A gift. Why would you be depressed? You should be grateful'. What mothers hear is 'What an awful mother you are for feeling like this'. These comments fuel a mother's anxieties and guilt.

But how does this fit with breastfeeding?

Mothers who breastfeed longest have the lowest level of postnatal depression. However, women who stop breastfeeding in the early days, or who don't start in the first place, are more at risk. Experience can also play a role; breastfeeding difficulties are linked to postnatal depression.[20] Understanding postnatal depression is critical in unpicking the relationship between postnatal depression and breastfeeding. If there is a relationship between a short breastfeeding duration and postnatal depression then we need to understand why. There are three possible options at play here:

Option one: Postnatal depression makes breastfeeding more challenging

When a woman presents with both postnatal depression and a difficult breastfeeding experience, it is easy to jump to the conclusion that the difficult experience is leading to the postnatal depression. But that is not necessarily true. It is feasible that a mother who is experiencing the symptoms of postnatal depression will find breastfeeding, or mothering in general, more problematic. Indeed, mothers who have symptoms of postnatal depression are more likely to find caring for their infant more challenging than those who do not. This can work two ways. A baby who has a more difficult temperament or additional needs is associated with an increased risk of postnatal depression, but mothers with postnatal depression are also more likely to perceive their baby's behaviour as more challenging.[21] One study showed that mothers with postnatal depression are more likely to perceive that their baby cries excessively, and find it more difficult to regulate their behaviour, than those who do not have symptoms.[22]

It is likely, at least in part, that mothers who are feeling over-whelmed by their baby's needs want desperately to find something that they can 'fix'. Blaming breastfeeding for being challenging can be an obvious solution, as formula-feeding may be portrayed as offering hope. Given how often babies can feed, it is likely that breastfeeding is sometimes blamed 'accidentally': the fact that you have to do it often means that it is at the forefront of your mind.[23]

Postnatal depression may also make breastfeeding more difficult physiologically. Studies that have explored mothers' interactions with their babies have shown that depressed mothers often interact differently with their babies than non-depressed mothers. For example, one study found that mothers with depression had poorer interactions with their newborn, with reduced touching, less sensitivity and less skin-to-skin contact.[24] Another study found that mothers with depressive symptoms were less sensitive when touching and positioning the newborn on the breast, and also reported poorer latch, lower milk intake and lower weight gain.[25] Given what we know about the importance of interactions, frequent feeding and responsivity to cues for breastfeeding success, it is easy to see how poorer-quality interactions can affect breastfeeding success.

However, breastfeeding may protect depressed mothers' babies. Babies of depressed mothers are more likely to show patterns of brain activity that mimic those of depressed adults. One study found that the babies of mothers who were depressed displayed this brain pattern, but not if they were breastfed. Mothers who were breastfeeding tended to touch and stroke their babies more, which was thought to explain the difference.[26]

Option two: A negative breastfeeding experience leads to postnatal depression

We conducted some work a few years ago exploring the relationship between breastfeeding and postnatal depression in more detail, particularly considering women's individual experiences of breastfeeding and how this might explain the link. A number of studies had suggested that a short breastfeeding experience increased the risk of postnatal depression, and that 'breastfeeding difficulties' played a role in that. We wanted to be more specific, so we asked women who had started breastfeeding but stopped before six months why they had stopped, and then looked at their symptoms of postnatal depression. Overall we found that the reason they stopped breastfeeding was linked to their risk for postnatal depression, rather than the duration of breastfeeding alone. Stopping breastfeeding because of pain or physical difficulty was the biggest predictor of postnatal depression. And that makes a lot of sense.

As we've discussed, pain and physical difficulties are common reasons for stopping breastfeeding. Experiencing chronic pain in any situation is linked to an increased risk of depression,[27] and this includes breastfeeding pain.[28] We also know that the immune system may play a role in depression. Research has shown that mothers with higher levels of inflammatory immune response (cytokines) had more symptoms of depression and anxiety than those who did not.[29] Sleep disturbance, pain and stress can all increase inflammatory cytokines.[30] The stress hormones – cortisol and adrenaline – increase the immune response in an attempt to heal the body. However, high levels of cytokines increase levels of depression.

If a mother is having difficulty getting her baby to feed (perhaps a poor latch, a lethargic baby or a weak suck), this is likely to make her overall experience of feeding, and therefore caring for her baby, more difficult. A baby who has difficulty feeding often takes longer to feed, or feeds more frequently as they find it harder to get milk out of the breast.[31] This doesn't only have an impact on feeding experience; it can also mean that the mother is exhausted or feels she is unable to care for other children or do tasks. Alternatively, she may have high levels of anxiety that her baby isn't feeding or getting enough milk. Anxiety, exhaustion and lack of sleep are all key predictors of postnatal depression.

Stress also interferes with the oxytocin reflex that supports milk production, thus leading to a decrease in milk supply, further confounding the problem. It is also possible that stress inhibits prolactin, although studies on humans haven't been conclusive.[32] Some 'interesting' (they wouldn't get away with it now!) studies were conducted on breastfeeding mothers back in the 1940s to explore whether stress affected their milk supply. The first was conducted with a mother of an older baby (7 months) and involved immersing her feet in ice water for 10 seconds every 30 seconds, giving her verbal maths problems to solve, with electric shocks if she got the answer wrong or took too long to answer, and random pulling on her big toe to cause pain. They labelled these tests 'distractions' (I don't want to know what counted as stress to these researchers).

On days that 'distractions' were experienced they injected the mother with either saline solution (a placebo) or oxytocin (to stimulate milk supply) a couple of minutes before she fed her baby. Milk intake per feed was then measured on control and distraction days. Intake on the control days was on average 168g compared to an average of only 99g on the distraction and saline day (with particularly low readings with ice water). However, average milk intake on a distraction and oxytocin day was an average of 153g. The authors concluded that the distraction interfered with her milk ejection reflex.[33]

A less intrusive study (but still not great) randomised breastfeeding women a week after birth to one of three groups: control, mental stress (more maths problems) and noise stress (building construction noise). They then collected blood samples before and after a feed, as well as weighing infants before and after as a rough guide to intake. There wasn't any difference in how much milk the babies received in each group, but oxytocin was 43% lower in the mental stress group and 52% lower in the noise stress group compared to the controls. It seems to me like a good excuse for a holiday on a quiet beach post-birth. It's for my milk supply, darling.[34]

A far kinder study explored how milk production could be enhanced for mothers in a neonatal unit. Understandably, having a baby in neonatal care is a stressful experience, particularly when mothers also need to express milk for their infants. Mothers with a premature baby (average age 31 weeks) were split shortly after birth into control and relaxation groups. Those in the relaxation group listened to a relaxation tape daily, just before they expressed milk. The amount of milk mothers in this group could express after just one week was almost double that of those in the control group.[35] Note that this study is over 30 years old. Is relaxation current practice in all neonatal care units...?

In addition to these physical pathways we need to consider the role of expectations. Mothers who find breastfeeding painful and difficult will likely not have expected this when they thought – if they thought at all – about what their breastfeeding experience would be like. Mothers often report that they believed breastfeeding would be straightforward and when they encountered difficulties they felt guilty, let down and upset, and that they had failed. These feelings themselves may increase the risk of postnatal depression.[36]

Linked to this, if mothers decide that they need to stop breastfeeding due to pain or physical difficulties, it is more likely that they feel they are being made to stop, rather than stopping for reasons they feel will benefit them (such as for convenience or choice). Instead they feel that they need to stop breastfeeding because the experience is too distressing, rather than seeing stopping as benefiting themselves in some way (even if the pain and discomfort recede). Indeed, considering breastfeeding intentions and readiness to stop is a critical element of understanding the relationship between breastfeeding duration and stopping.

In another study we found that mothers' readiness to stop

breastfeeding was key in predicting her risk of depression, regardless of breastfeeding duration. If mothers were ready to stop, it didn't matter if their baby was six days or six months old. Likewise, if they weren't ready to stop, the age of the baby didn't matter either – they still felt the loss.

Option three: Other underlying factors

Behaviour is complicated and we do very little in isolation. It is likely that wider factors, at least in part, contribute towards both breastfeeding difficulties and postnatal depression. One of the key factors, as discussed earlier, is the impact of birth experience. As noted, birth complications can have a significant effect on breastfeeding success, both physiologically and due to reduced confidence in the body's abilities and anxiety over milk production.[37] However, birth experience can also affect maternal wellbeing, both physiologically and psychologically, with mothers who have a difficult birth, or perceive their experience to be difficult, having an increased risk of postnatal depression.[38] As we saw, mothers who have a caesarean section, interventions or pain relief may feel that they have not been able to birth 'naturally', and thus now feel unable to feed their baby 'naturally'.[38] Residual pain from the birth can also prevent a mother from sleeping properly, which further increases the risk of postnatal depression.[39] It is unsurprising that mothers who have a difficult birth may find breastfeeding more difficult and are at increased risk of postnatal depression. All these factors in her life add up, damaging her ability to breastfeed.

What is the solution?

Does all this mean that breastfeeding 'causes' postnatal depression, and that we should stop encouraging women to breastfeed as it makes them depressed? No. This idea often comes up in arguments about breastfeeding, when it is suggested that 'pressure' to breastfeed causes postnatal depression. But it's not that simple. Of course, if a woman feels so overwhelmed by breastfeeding that she wants to stop, then that is her decision and it should be respected. But stopping encouraging breastfeeding in this situation is simply putting a plaster over a broken bone. The real issue is why so many women find breastfeeding so difficult in the first place (and why so many experience postnatal depression) – and that is what we need to fix. More support services are needed, for both practical and emotional support. In fact, support should be more than breastfeeding support; we should be protecting and caring for new mothers in general. New mothers should not get to the point where they feel overwhelmed and alone in feeding and caring for their baby.

Action 7

✓ Give new mothers the emotional and practical support they need, every step of the way.

12. PRESSURE ON WOMEN TO DOUBT THEIR BODY OR GET THEIR 'PRE-BABY BODY' BACK

'I think women who have breastfed understand what I'm saying – that if you get a boob job it's more reconstructive surgery, actually, than cosmetic surgery.' Gwyneth Paltrow

Wow. Pretty influential stuff. But what is so wrong with this statement? Firstly, its definition. And secondly, its potential impact. Oh and thirdly, a small matter of the truth... If you look at the definition of reconstructive surgery, it is this:

'Reconstructive surgery is all about repairing people and restoring function. It is performed to repair and reshape bodily structures affected by birth defects, developmental abnormalities, trauma/injuries, infections, tumours and disease.'

Breastfeeding is not an injury or a disease. It is not a trauma. It is the primary function of breasts. A body part doing what a body part is designed to do, and able to perform that function multiple times, does not need 'reconstruction'.

Gwyneth is not the only celebrity quick to emphasise the importance of appearance soon after the birth. Amanda Holden, who experienced significant trauma after her birth, was naturally concerned about the impact of her being so ill on her young daughter. Her response was to try to appear to be a 'normal mummy' as soon as possible. Understandable, no? However, in Amanda Holden's world this happened:

'When Lexi came into hospital to see her baby sister, it freaked her out seeing me so ill. She said "Momma, what's that tube? Your hair looks horrible". So I had to be "normal Mummy" in her heels and hot pants and went back to work.'

Despite her traumatic delivery, Amanda went on to note 'I survived childbirth remarkably well. I didn't get any stretch marks, my boobs are the same shape and still up, but I didn't breastfeed.' So emergency surgery, losing significant amounts of blood and needing intensive care is actually *surviving childbirth well* because at least you don't have stretch marks? The pressure on new mothers to accept the trauma of childbirth and to fit into a certain image of success is overwhelming.

Finally, Jordan (Katie Price, the reality TV star). After the birth of her daughter in 2007, Jordan caused global furore with a magazine spread (complete with formula advertising on the opposite page) of her dressed scantily and feeding her baby with a labelled, pre-prepared bottle of formula. In the accompanying interview Jordan noted 'I don't want a baby drinking from me – the thought of it makes me feel really funny. I think only a certain person could handle my knockers!'.

Each of these women can of course do exactly what she wants to her body and make the choices right for her and her family. However, they all have a significant fan base and influence both women (who go on to be mothers) and men (who have expectations about what the women in their lives should look like). Comments like these plant seeds of doubt, make suggestions about what a woman's body should look like and do, and increase feelings of insecurity and body dissatisfaction in women. And in just these few comments there are so many 'seeds'. So many seeds.

Body dissatisfaction and pregnancy

Body dissatisfaction is rife during pregnancy and the early months postpartum. A quick search reveals over 29 million hits for 'how to lose weight after pregnancy', with articles promising the solution to 'getting your body back... fast'. Magazine covers feature svelte, immaculate models (thanks, Photoshop) holding strangely clean babies and posing as the pinnacle of motherhood. There are even magazines dedicated to having a 'fit pregnancy', with other pregnancy magazines increasingly having articles about body image and exercise, or models on the cover in gym gear.

Although changes to the body during pregnancy are inevitable, dissatisfaction relating to these changes is pretty high. Body image issues during pregnancy, and especially after pregnancy, are now so common that it is considered 'normal' for new mothers not to like how they look.[1] The issues are compounded by growing pressure on new mothers to maintain their figure throughout pregnancy and the postnatal period. Although some women report feeling liberated by the changes pregnancy brings, pregnancy can trigger or intensify negative feelings about the body or disordered eating.[2] Whereas women used to have more confidence to 'eat for two' during pregnancy, growing numbers of women now feel pressure to not gain a lot of weight and quickly return to their 'pre-baby' selves.[3]

All of this is compounded by public ownership of the pregnant body. People start commenting on the size of your bump or want to touch it (top tip – try commenting or touching back, this usually puts a quick stop to it). Then there are the public images of pregnant women. They either seem to be very slim, long haired and standing in a field in dappled sunshine, or are just a pregnant bump with no head alongside an article criticising or warning pregnant women about something. I don't literally mean no head – but rather the photo is cut off somewhere around the breasts placing all focus on the bump. The subtle and not so subtle messages are clear – this is about the baby, you are just a vessel and you as an individual don't matter.

Somewhat unsurprisingly, this can have a negative impact on maternal mental health. Body image dissatisfaction during pregnancy is associated with a higher risk of low self-esteem, anxiety and depression.[4] New research has even found a link between body image during pregnancy and attachment to the baby during pregnancy and beyond.[5] It can also further impact on eating behavior. We are seeing a rise in women controlling their diet or even trying to lose weight during pregnancy. One fascinating study exploring how women felt about their pregnancy and changing shape used the phrase 'unruly maternal body' to highlight how body image and eating behaviour are often tightly linked to feelings of control.[6] Women felt stressed not just by their changing shape, but also by their changing lives – losing weight or controlling food intake was a way of bringing feelings of control back. Unsurprisingly, these bodily changes contribute to women deciding not to breastfeed, particularly younger mothers who might be more concerned about their appearance.[7,8]

Breastfeeding and weight

Firstly, weight can affect the decision to breastfeed. Mothers who are obese are less likely to plan to start, or continue breastfeeding.[7] To some extent this is physiological. Women who are obese are more likely to report low milk supply. If a woman is obese it is more likely she will have a delay in her milk coming in, as she can have lower levels of prolactin and may have higher levels of hormones, such as progesterone, stored in her body, which can decrease initial milk supply.[9] Sometimes very large breasts can make latching a baby on more difficult, and she is more likely to experience pain. She is also more likely to have had complications at birth.[10]

These are statistical relationships and I know there will be readers shouting at me now that they, or someone they know, breastfed for years and were obese. And you know what? Although there are physiological reasons why weight would affect breastfeeding, overall I think the relationship is more about wider pressures on women. Interestingly, mothers who are overweight are less likely to seek support when they have breastfeeding difficulties and are generally less likely to feel confident about breastfeeding, experiencing more embarrassment and discomfort when breastfeeding in front of others. And when researchers consider how confident a woman feels when they look at the relationship between weight and breastfeeding, it turns out that confidence is a huge contributor.[11] And at the other end of the scale mothers with anorexia are also less likely to breastfeed.[12]

However, perhaps a bigger predictor of whether a woman breastfeeds or not is her body image. How she feels about her body, regardless of weight, seems to be important. Body image refers to the thoughts people have, and the behaviours they undertake, related to aspects of their body such as appearance, shape and weight. Non-weight-related aspects of body image are particularly relevant to pregnancy and the postnatal period and include stretchmarks and changes to breast shape and function. The body goes through changes at this time like no other.

Mothers who are concerned about changes to their body shape, how pregnancy and birth affect their body and weight gain are less likely to plan to breastfeed. If they do breastfeed at birth, they only do so for a short period of time. Interestingly, this isn't anything to do with weight; body image issues affect those with a healthy BMI and even those who are underweight.[13]

Why might body image affect breastfeeding?

Firstly, general body consciousness might make breastfeeding more difficult, particularly if women are feeling unsure about the changes in their body. Mothers who are less confident about their body, or who dislike the changes pregnancy has brought, can find the idea of breastfeeding in front of others embarrassing, and decide to use formula instead.[14] Negative or 'humorous' comments from others exacerbate this.[15] If a mother has serious body image concerns, it is likely she is more aware of herself in front of others. She may worry that others are paying her high levels of attention, which may exacerbate her anxiety over public feeding. This may mean she tries to stretch out feeds, or offer additional formula milk in front of others, reducing her milk supply and increasing the likelihood of her stopping breastfeeding. Feeling uncomfortable about feeding in front of others is very common. In the Infant Feeding Survey in 2010, half of mothers reported feeling uncomfortable feeding in front of others, with 13% feeling uncomfortable breastfeeding in their own home. Women were far more likely to cite feeding in front of men being uncomfortable than feeding in front of women, suggesting that society's view of the breast as sexual is affecting their behaviour.[16]

Dr Ruth Newby, lecturer at the University of the Sunshine Coast in Australia, explored this issue in research which showed that women who were obese were three times more likely to have stopped breastfeeding by six months, compared to those with the lowest BMI. She said:

'We asked women who were obese during their pregnancy how they anticipated feeling about breastfeeding in front of other people. Almost half of all the women said they expected to be embarrassed if there were strangers present. Of concern, though, was the finding that significantly more overweight women compared to smaller women expected to feel uncomfortable when breastfeeding their infant even in the presence of their close female friends. This seems to imply that poor body image may stop many larger women from continuing to breastfeed their babies. There may be value in equipping healthcare professionals to provide larger women with supportive interventions and strategies during pregnancy to address body image concerns and overcome personal, social and psychological obstacles in relation to breastfeeding.'

Secondly, women might not like the idea of using their breasts in a different way. Functional changes also play a large part in body image dissatisfaction after pregnancy. It's not all about shape, appearance and weight, but what the body suddenly starts doing. Breasts grow, can feel tender and produce and leak milk. It is a constant reminder right in front of your nose (well, 8 inches or so away) of your changing role. Breasts, which may once have been viewed as purely sexual, now have another function. These changes can require alterations to clothing, nursing bras and the use of breast pads. This 'new' function can sometimes interfere with the 'existing' function if breasts are too sore to touch, or mothers have concerns about milk leaking, or not fitting into nice underwear and so on. Although we all know that making milk is breasts' actual function, it can still be a huge mental hurdle, especially for those 'grieving' for their former lifestyle.

There is also the issue of control over bodily functions. Some women report that they simply wanted their body back to themselves after a long pregnancy and birth.[17] They want their body to go back to its pre-pregnancy self, when it just had to support the woman, rather than grow and sustain another life. When put that way it seems fair enough, but given that breastfeeding is our biological norm, why is this happening? Personally I think it goes back to the way in which we treat and support (or not) new mothers. Whereas once new mothers had family around them, and less pressure to think about work or being the 'perfect' mother, now new mothers are often alone. Discharged in hours from the hospital and isolated from family, they are pressured to 'get their life back': meaning, do all the cooking, shopping and running round after other children on their own as if nothing had happened! No wonder new mothers want a break. Many report that intense visceral emotion of feeling 'touched out' and just wanting to lock themselves away in a dark quiet room (or even the bathroom… but that's not necessarily peaceful when you have small children either).

Common myths also persist. One fear is that breastfeeding will 'ruin' the shape or volume of the breast and that these changes will be permanent. Although research in this area is sparse, all studies conducted, including those by plastic surgeons who you would expect to be more invested in outcomes, show that it is actually pregnancy that leads to changes in appearance of the breast and not breastfeeding itself.[18] Anecdotally, many women report a short period after stopping breastfeeding when breasts can seem a bit forlorn, but they soon perk back up again. However, this concern is real. Pregnant women who are concerned about the impact of pregnancy and breastfeeding on their breast shape are less likely to even think about breastfeeding at birth.[19]

Wanting to go on a diet

Women who are concerned about their weight, and want to lose excess pounds, are more likely to diet. Women who are actively dieting are less likely to breastfeed.[20] This extends to pregnancy. Women who are worried about their weight during pregnancy are less likely to plan to breastfeed. Wanting to diet is one of those reasons that often crops up when a mother stops breastfeeding. Sometimes this is related to a genuine need to lose weight, but often it is not, or at least there is no need to do so quickly.

Studies that look at what a new mother eats support this. Mothers who are breastfeeding tend to eat more, including eating lunch (as if this is something novel), snacking and having dessert.[21] (Or that flapjack for its milk-boosting properties… or the biscuit because I need to keep my strength up… or that chocolate bar… Not talking about my own personal experience here at all, obviously). To what extent this is causal I am not sure. Does hunger increase in breastfeeding mothers to make sure milk is produced? Anecdotally many breastfeeding mothers will recognise *the hunger* especially at that 3am feed. A few crumbs in the cleavage (or an escaped bit of spaghetti on the baby's head) never hurt anyone, after all. Especially if that's due to eating all meals with one hand over a cluster-feeding baby's head (again, nothing to do with me, honest).

Wanting to go on a diet may be a common reason women give for stopping breastfeeding, but it is completely unfounded. Sensible weight loss, at around two pounds per week, does not impact upon milk supply or how much weight a baby puts on.[22] In fact, breastfeeding can help with weight loss as it uses up to 500 calories a day,[23] with women who breastfeed losing on average more weight postnatally than those who formula-feed.[24] Most studies show no effect on the calorie or nutrient content of a woman's breastmilk despite her diet.[25] After all, we've evolved to be able to feed our children in times of hardship and plenty. It's not lack of breastmilk that is killing millions of children in developing countries, it's the introduction of formula milk.

There is some evidence that mothers who are restrictive in their eating are more likely to have difficulties breastfeeding and stop. Mothers with a history of eating disorders are more likely to report difficulties feeding their baby, even when they are consuming enough calories to produce milk.[26] One explanation for this could be the link between a mother's own eating and how she feeds her baby. Those who are very restrained are more likely to try and feed to a routine. Breastfeeding doesn't allow for the same tracking and monitoring of intake that formula does. Formula is very visible and measurable, with guidance for how much a baby needs. With breastfeeding, however, the 'power' over feeding times and amounts is taken away from the mother and given to the baby. Mothers who are high in restraint do report feeding their baby less responsively, as do mothers with a history of eating disorders who report becoming distressed if their infant wants to feed more frequently.[27]

A distrust in our bodies

Another issue underlying body image, weight and breastfeeding is how women are taught, particularly during pregnancy and breastfeeding, not to trust their bodies to work. Medicalisation and intervention during pregnancy and birth (although obviously sometimes lifesaving) sow the seed that bodies are dysfunctional. Messaging around breastfeeding and breasts extends this. Women are taught to expect that breastfeeding may not work out, far more often than it genuinely does not work out. How many times do you hear a woman say she'll give 'breastfeeding a go' or someone say that 'lots of women can't breastfeed'?

All this fits into what we discussed and will discuss in future chapters around a lack of understanding about milk supply, beliefs that babies can and should be in routines and how industry fuels all this anxiety. We want to measure milk and track intake and bring in external validation of whether our baby is getting 'enough' milk.

One increasingly common anxiety that I think stems from this distrust in our bodies is women worrying that their breastmilk is not good enough. I mean, this belief or anxiety has always been around, but it feels like more and more women are worrying specifically about breastmilk content. This is happening alongside a growth in websites and information suggesting to women that they very much need to eat a healthy and balanced diet if they want their milk to be sufficient and nutritious for their baby. Now how many new mothers genuinely have the time and energy to invest in a perfect diet? Actually, how many of us do full stop? But as soon as you plant that concern, women naturally start to worry.

We have survived for millennia on less than perfect diets and our babies have too (and thrived). Maternal diet has very little impact on breastmilk content in real terms – there isn't, for example, a point where it would be better for an infant to be formula-fed. However there appears to be a growing number of studies examining how maternal diet affects breastmilk. I am really uncomfortable about this type of research because much of it is so one-sided. Numerous studies seem to conclude that maternal diet affects breastmilk content – and that is the headline we see. But what it doesn't do is explain a) whether a significant relationship between diet and milk is actually significant in real life or is just a numerical difference, b) what the actual impact on babies is, and c) how this compares to them being formula-fed.

There is a major difference between there being a statistical relationship between diet and milk content and that actually meaning anything in real life. My major fear – and it is too early in relation to the growth in this research to really see the impact – is that no one is following this through to look at the consequences of sharing this type of research, without context, with women. My bet is that women are stopping breastfeeding because they are worrying that their diet is not perfect enough. Even though that diet in pregnancy grew a healthy baby. And even though breastmilk is more than just whatever slight variation in nutrient has been examined. Whether a woman's breastmilk is lower than average in a certain nutrient, possibly due to her diet, doesn't invalidate all the other components of breastmilk and their impact upon health – but focusing on a nutrient in this way can lead to thinking that her milk is 'deficient'.

The problem is that these comparisons to formula or the bigger picture are often not made. Take this study for example: researchers looked at maternal intake of long-chain polyunsaturated fatty acids [LCPUFAs] and the level in mothers' milk, finding maternal dietary intake was associated with levels in breastmilk.[28] LCPUFAs are important for infant growth and development and have been added to some infant formulas. However, those added to formula milk are often not as well absorbed as the type found in breastmilk, and have in some cases been seen to have a potentially detrimental impact on growth. You can see the train of thought women might experience on reading the study: my diet is not high enough… my milk is deficient… oh this formula has fatty acids added to it… I'll use that instead.

There is also a tendency for studies to highlight associations between maternal diet and breastmilk content, without actually going further and seeing it if impacts on infant growth or development. We do not know whether variation in the content of breastmilk really affects the infant, or how much variation needs to occur for a significant impact. Lots of studies only use small time points too – few look at variation over a significant duration.

When studies do look at the variation in breastmilk content and then infant growth or development, few find any knock on impact. For example, one study compared the diet of Swedish and Chinese women and the LCPUFA content of their milk (seems to be a popular area of study). The paper is called 'Long-chain polyunsaturated fatty acids in Chinese and Swedish mothers: Diet, breastmilk and infant growth' – you'd be right in expecting an impact upon growth, yes? Well actually, although they found significant differences in maternal diet… and significant associations between diet and LCPUFA content which are highlighted in the paper abstract… buried away in the paper was a paragraph saying there was no association with growth or differences between Swedish and Chinese babies.[29]

Another consequence is that women keep breastfeeding but worry about the content of their diet and milk and start taking supplements. Given the obsession with LCPUFAs, one area of research over the years has looked at whether it is a good idea for women to take fish oils during breastfeeding. Some research has suggested that supplementation can support preterm brain development, although intriguingly there doesn't seem to be an association between maternal intake and brain development in term babies.[30] However, worryingly, new research has shown an association between fish oil supplementation during breastfeeding and reduced immune protection for infants.[31] This just goes to show that adding 'more' is not necessarily better and that breastmilk is more complex than one component or nutrient. In my opinion we need to promote trust in our bodies to carry on nurturing our babies, unless perhaps women are severely malnourished.

There is also the big question of who is funding and sharing all of this research or information around breastfeeding and maternal diet.[32] A recent study is a classic example to support what I just said. They examined maternal diet in terms of sugar intake and found that breastfeeding mothers who consumed more sugar (specifically fructose) when their baby was one month old had babies with lower cognitive scores at 24 months. My main issues with it are:

1. Correlation is not causation. Just because two things are linked doesn't mean one causes the other. It could well be that factors that lead mothers to eat a high-sugar diet are affecting cognitive development.
2. They didn't measure breastmilk content.
3. They didn't give specific details of real-life differences in cognitive development and what that meant.
4. They didn't measure the same relationship in mothers who were formula-feeding. I would bet, if you did, the same relationship would occur. Instead the reader is left to assume this just happens in breastfed babies.

And then you get to the small print about funding. It was funded in part by Gerber. Gerber, who make formula milk and baby foods. Now why would a formula manufacturer be funding research trying to show that maternal diet during breastfeeding is really important?

I'll leave you to answer that, but it reminds me of the story of when Coca-Cola invested loads of money into researching the relationship between exercise, weight and heart disease.[33] They wanted to draw attention to factors other than diet i.e. away from their own products. Recent research is highlighting just how much sugar is in many baby foods.[34] Again I'll leave you to your thoughts there.

This isn't an isolated funding incident though. Some more examples include:

- *Maternal diet and nutrient requirements in pregnancy and breastfeeding* – funded by Danone.[35]
- *Associations between human breastmilk hormones and adipocytokines and infant growth and body composition in the first 6 months of life* – Mead Johnson.[36]
- *Effect of maternal diet and milk lipid composition on the infant gut and maternal milk microbiomes* – funded by Strauss Dairy Foundation.[37]
- *Importance of maternal diet in the training of the infant's immune system during gestation and lactation* – Nutricia Research Institute.[38]

The bigger picture

There are other factors associated with negative body image that can make breastfeeding more difficult. Mothers who have strong body image concerns are more likely to experience low self-esteem and low confidence, while experiencing high levels of self-criticism, which can affect breastfeeding.[39] These women are also at more risk of postnatal depression and anxiety, which we know can make breastfeeding seem more difficult.[40] Women who are anxious about breastfeeding are more likely to find it difficult, worry that their infant is not getting enough milk, or feel unable to solve problems if they arise.[41] Finally, wider personality traits such as introversion[42] and perfectionism[43] are associated with finding breastfeeding more challenging. These traits are both associated with poorer body image.[44]

Breastfeeding as sexual

Society continues to scream 'breasts are for sex' at us from all angles. Pushed-up breasts. Adorned breasts. Enhanced breasts. Breasts with tassles on. Images that glorify 'breasts for feeding babies' are like hens' teeth. Sometimes breastfeeding breasts do make the media, but only when they are attached to a styled celebrity.

Mothers therefore face pressure from 'society' as to how they should be using their bodies. The concept of the female body being sexualised and open to public comment is certainly nothing new. Unfortunately we expose women to it from birth. Baby girls are labelled 'pretty' or 'delicate' (and are more likely to be handled gently, as obviously they'll break due to those dainty X chromosomes), marketing companies target children and pre-teens with make-up sets and princess clothing and teenagers and older women are hammered with adverts suggesting their entire worth is based on plump skin and eradicating fine lines (or whatever they have decided to make women feel guilty about now... last time I checked I think it was wrinkly knees that voided a woman's entire existence on this planet).

These subtle and not-so-subtle messages affect women's perceptions of their bodies (and therefore breastfeeding) in two main ways. Firstly in terms of how they 'should' look, and secondly in terms of how they 'should' act. Objectification theory states that women are socialised to view and evaluate their own bodies from the perspective of others' views and desires, rather than their own needs. The view of others becomes internalised, so they strive to meet the desires of others. Typically these desires are focused on sexual appeal and beauty, but extend to the way in which women should use their bodies.[45]

Although female reproduction (which naturally includes breastfeeding) demonstrates a woman's success at another female function (motherhood), it is at odds with these desires as it implies that the woman is not focused on her purpose of being sexually attractive and available for others.[46] Alternatively, disgust can arise from seeing others break out of their role of being 'decorative'. If a woman has strongly internalised the desires of others, she may feel uncomfortable when some manage to choose another route – and this discomfort is reflected in disdain of or disgust at their behaviour.

I spoke to UK academic Dr Sally Dowling about this idea of society's view on how women should be using their bodies in a pre-prescribed way. She agreed with the main points above, but also felt that the breastfeeding body confused people, or made them uncomfortable in some way, because breastfeeding women do not fit neatly into a little box of 'pregnant' or 'available'. Sally explained:

'Breastfeeding – however long it lasts, but particularly when it goes on for extended periods – can be seen as a liminal activity. This means that breastfeeding women are neither one thing nor another (not pregnant, not breastfeeding); being in a liminal phase is sometimes described as being 'betwixt and between'. People in liminal states can be disturbing to others; this is sometimes reflected in comments about breastfeeding in public or about long-term breastfeeding. Women in this state refuse to conform to the norms of what we expect and that challenges others and makes them feel uncomfortable. It is not an expected state as such.'

Others have a child-like response to breastfeeding. Humour is frequently seen in tabloid reader comments. For example one *Daily Mail* reader noted on an article debating breastfeeding in public: 'I think it's rude... they should at least spike my tea with it'. Hilarious. But why do we find breastfeeding so funny? Is it because deep down we are so hung up about the female body that anything to do with it turns us into seven-year-olds laughing at the underwear models in our women's catalogues? Actually, that's insulting to seven-year-olds. But you get my drift.

These views can be subconscious. Those who perceive breasts as sexual and therefore feel uncomfortable if they witness breastfeeding may not be consciously aware of the views they hold, but their attitudes prove otherwise. A common finding is that fathers can be supportive of their partner breastfeeding, but dislike her doing so in public or in front of friends and family. If they were not attaching a sexual element to it, why would this discomfort occur? In one study of undergraduate students, those who felt uncomfortable with sexual stimuli held stronger negative views about breastfeeding, suggesting an inability to distinguish the sexual breast from the nurturing breast.[47] This actually says more about individuals than whether women should be allowed to breastfeed in public. Perhaps we could use it as a test of whether someone has deep-rooted issues... what do you think of this photo of a woman breastfeeding?

Action 8

✓ Stop this ridiculous body image pressure on new mothers and come to terms with our own illogical sensitivities and prejudices about human milk and the female body.

13. FAMILY AND FRIENDS: WHEN IT'S NOT YOU, IT'S THEM*

There's an old saying that it takes a village to raise a child, which highlights the importance of being surrounded by supportive family and friends during the transition to motherhood and throughout the parenting experience. We know that women who feel socially isolated are often at far higher risk of postnatal depression, and adjusting to motherhood can be a whole lot easier if your parents look after the baby from time to time. Countless models of human behaviour suggest that the likelihood of any given behaviour is predicted by how much social support someone has to undertake that behaviour. People who are supported by others generally feel happier and more confident in their decision and ability to do something and can seek support when they find that behaviour difficult. Those around them can also help practically, giving advice or support in other ways to make it easier to follow that behaviour.

But does this same notion apply to breastfeeding? Yes! If those people in the village are knowledgeable, skilled and supportive of breastfeeding, then it's a resounding yes. And I really want to go and live in that village. But what if your 'village' isn't that supportive of breastfeeding? Or really wants to be supportive but doesn't understand how breastfeeding works and inadvertently ends up damaging it instead? What happens then? The attitudes and experiences in relation to breastfeeding and feeding babies can really have an important influence on a woman's experience. This can be direct in terms of how they feel about breastfeeding, and more indirect in terms of their ability to support breastfeeding in reality. Often family and friends are theoretically supportive of breastfeeding, but all their knowledge is based on their own experience of bottle-feeding, meaning advice and support can end up being unhelpful.

A really useful paper was published a few years ago exploring how understanding and reflecting on the experiences of those around you in relation to breastfeeding can help a mother identify

---

* Disclaimer: There are lots of people who are very supportive of breastfeeding. It's not them either.

who may or may not be able to support her.[1] The paper produced an infant feeding 'genogram' – or diagram – as a tool for exploring how different individuals around the mother may be involved in or affect her experience of caring for a baby, and thinking about how they may end up influencing her breastfeeding experience, deliberately or otherwise. Emerging research suggests that it could be a useful tool in clinical practice for a woman to think about who she has around her who could help her with breastfeeding and whose advice she may want to avoid.[2]

Your mother's experience of breastfeeding

A big predictor of whether a woman breastfeeds is whether she was breastfed herself, and whether she knows that she was.[3] I'm sure Freud would have come up with some theory about the baby learning or something, but of course it's not physiological but all to do with relationships. And the reasoning is quite complex.

If your mother breastfed you, it's likely that your breastfeeding experience, at least with regard to your interactions with your mother, will be far more positive. Firstly, unless something drastic has happened in the meantime, she's probably supportive of breastfeeding. And that's a pretty good thing. No pursed lips or snide comments when you mention that is what you want to do. No persuasion to do what she chose. No 'you were bottle fed and you're perfectly fine'. This is a pretty big deal. In one study that explored what new mothers wanted from their mothers, two main things arose: valuing breastfeeding and loving encouragement.[4] Feeling that your decision is accepted and supported is very important, especially in a world that seems so anti-breastfeeding.

Secondly, depending on whether you are the oldest child or not, you may well have grown up seeing other babies being breastfed. This might have been your sibling, or a cousin or other relative, because once one person breastfeeds successfully in the family, others are more likely to do so too. It's more catching than chicken pox. You might have been a toddler at this point, but we all know that toddlers learn pretty quickly about what is going on around them (if you disagree with me, try swearing around a toddler and see what happens... Actually, don't do that – but you get the idea). What children see is what becomes 'normal' to them. They think that is just the way that babies are fed. It's just their baby sister eating (again... and again... and again). Nothing more. So, consciously or otherwise, you probably grew up thinking that breastfeeding was normal. You might not think that this is that remarkable, but many children never see a baby being breastfed. Actually, many adults have never seen a baby being breastfed, at least not up close. And let's face it, once you are an adult it becomes a lot less acceptable to stick your nose two inches from a woman's nipple and enquire 'What are you doing?'.

So, you know your mother thinks breastfeeding is OK and you may have grown up seeing a bit more of it. But what is really on your side is the fact that your mother knows what it is like to breastfeed. If she breastfed for a few months she knows that babies feed all the time. She knows that they wake lots in the night. She knows the practicalities of how to latch a baby on, how to recognise when they are hungry and maybe the different positions to hold them in. Perhaps a trick if there's too much milk or what to do if you feel sore. Importantly, she may be able to give you practical advice on how to breastfeed, and she hopefully won't be saying 'He can't be hungry again can he?'

She may also be able to remember what it was like to breastfeed and, depending on her experience around other people, know exactly what was helpful to her… or exactly what would have been helpful. She'll know to offer to cook you dinner rather than asking to give the baby a bottle. She'll know to offer to cuddle the baby after he's had a long feed, but give him back when he's hungry. And importantly she'll be able to say to you 'It's really tough when they feed lots, but it will pass. I promise'. If she didn't breastfeed, then even with the best will in the world she won't know what it's like or be able to support you in quite the same way.

If your mother breastfed you, and your dad was around, then he is far more likely to be supportive of breastfeeding too. If she breastfed he'll be more likely to think it's normal, and he'll have seen her breastfeeding. This is important because so many men have never seen a baby being breastfed.

What if she didn't breastfeed?

This is quite complicated, and it all depends on why she didn't. The mothers of the mothers of today quite likely gave birth when there was less encouragement to breastfeed. It is entirely possible that she didn't breastfeed because the messages she got at the time were that there was really no need. Formula was marketed as a scientifically-produced product that was equal or even superior to breastmilk. It's possible that since then she has come to realise that mothers are now encouraged to breastfeed, and the reasons for this, and she may fully support her daughter to breastfeed.

Women with mothers who didn't breastfeed, but are supportive of breastfeeding, are more likely to be able to breastfeed than those whose mothers are unsupportive of breastfeeding, but in some cases less likely than those whose mothers breastfed. Why? Aren't positive messages and encouragement enough? Sadly, no. This comes back to that 'simple' message about how breastfeeding works. New mothers naturally turn to their own mother for advice (assuming a good relationship, and sometimes even if not). If a woman has no experience of breastfeeding it is likely she does not understand fully how breastfeeding works (although of course there are exceptions). She may not realise that frequent feeding is normal, or that bottles of formula or formula top-ups can be damaging. And if problems arise she may not be able to offer practical support. She might not know how to solve problems such as low or high milk supply, or how to position the baby. Even with the best will in the world she will not have her own expertise of breastfeeding a baby.[5]

Others may not know how to deal with a breastfeeding woman, in terms of being unsure how much privacy to give her. One study explored how many new mothers felt that they were being sent away to another room by their non-breastfeeding families to breastfeed in private. They felt isolated and as though no one wanted breastfeeding to be part of family life. But when asked, families thought they were doing the best thing for the breastfeeding mother and that she would want some space. So little differences in approach can make a big difference.

What if she wanted to but couldn't?

On the one hand, mothers who really wanted to breastfeed but couldn't may be very supportive of their daughters. They have positive views of breastfeeding and may be very educated about it, but simply could not do it themselves for whatever reason. They are, however, more than happy to support their daughter to breastfeed and actually encourage her to do it. On the other hand, this all depends on that mother's experience of why she couldn't. Back in the 1970s, 80s and even some of the 90s, beliefs about 'how' you breastfed a baby were very different. Far less was known about the importance of demand and supply, frequent feeds and keeping mother and baby close. After birth babies were often routinely separated from the mother while she was in the hospital and brought to her for feeds (and she was likely to be in the hospital for several days). Ideas about when a baby was fed were often based on the clock. Feeding was often three or even four-hourly.

Those parenting books were also very popular and often had strict ideas about when a baby should be breastfed (including for how long and from which breast – thanks, Dr Spock). With hindsight, this had a negative effect on milk supply and the number of women who simply 'couldn't' breastfeed rose. Babies were 'topped-up' with formula (leading to an even bigger drop in milk supply), or breastfeeding was simply stopped and replaced with formula. Those formula-fed babies tended to fit the schedules and formula became the 'magic solution'.

Now that mother's daughter is breastfeeding her baby every two hours, for varying lengths of time. You can see why she says 'Is he feeding again? He can't be hungry'. Still holding the faulty belief that babies shouldn't feed so frequently, and wanting to give her support, the grandmother offers her experience: 'I couldn't breastfeed either, you fed too much as well'. The daughter gets the message that 'women in our family just can't breastfeed'. Her mother, believing her experience was the 'right' one, tells her daughter that she needs to give formula because babies 'must' be fed every three hours.

It may also be that the mother sees her daughter struggling and remembers how she felt during those struggles 30 years ago. All she wants to do is support her daughter, so she suggests that her daughter give formula so that the baby feeds less frequently and she can get on with other things. Or – still not understanding how breastfeeding works – she suggests that the daughter 'just give one bottle of formula' so she can have a break from the feeding, not realising the damaging effect this could be having on her daughter's milk supply.

It is also possible that mothers who did not breastfeed may try and sabotage, deliberately or not, their daughters' experience of breastfeeding. Cognitive dissonance theory explores how we like to think that we are doing the best possible thing in all situations, and if we are unable to do the perceived 'right' thing, we need to be able to explain why our way is best. People who do something different can challenge our thinking, especially if we are not confident in the choice that we made, or would have preferred to make a different choice.

You see this time and time again with parenting decisions, often because we are led to believe that the stakes are so high.

Although there is considerable evidence that early experiences are very important in life, a tendency to over-emphasise this can lead to feelings of immense guilt, anxiety and regret. This can lead to huge tensions – you only have to look at the lengthy arguments online about different parenting ideologies to see this for yourself. Of course, when you are doing things differently from your own mother, this can be very challenging for her.

...If she formula-fed and believed she was doing the best thing for her baby, then she may question why you are not doing the 'right' thing.

...If she wanted to breastfeed but couldn't she may feel that your ability to breastfeed is 'exposing' her perceived failure to breastfeed.

Your different choice can seem like an attack on her entire parenting ideology; a statement that you are doing things the 'right' way and they are different to hers, ergo, you believe that she is 'wrong'. Indeed, many studies suggest that mothers will actively try and dissuade their daughters from breastfeeding if they don't agree with her decision.[6]

Does this actually have an impact?

Yes. Mothers who have more contact with their own mother stop breastfeeding sooner if she didn't breastfeed.[7] This is for two reasons: first her inability to support breastfeeding and her formula-based advice, and second her active attempts to get her daughter to change her mind. Mothers who feel actively supported by their own mothers breastfeed for longer.[3]

One way in which breastfeeding can be damaged is that women's mothers often influence wider decisions around breastfeeding. They may pressure her to give a bottle, or to allow them to care for the baby, which can interfere with milk supply. Even when their reasoning is based on kindness and wanting to give their daughter a break, these wider decisions can affect successful breastfeeding. In theory women's mothers may be completely supportive of breastfeeding, but because they don't understand the physiology behind it, they inadvertently damage it.[8]

Younger mothers' own mothers are particularly influential. Firstly, younger mothers are more likely to feel inexperienced and turn to their mother for advice, often taking her advice over and above that of health professionals. They may also feel that they need to listen to the advice of their mother as they are less independent. Adolescent women may be dependent on their mothers financially, emotionally and practically. Going against the grain is therefore much more difficult.[9]

One study highlighted this. The researchers developed a counselling intervention to support younger mothers with breastfeeding. The intervention worked well to improve breastfeeding rates, but only if the mother was living away from her own mother. When mothers still lived in the family home, the intervention didn't work, because their mothers ultimately decided how things were done.[10]

You can see the importance of this for the cycle of breastfeeding. If a mother was formula-fed, she is more likely to formula-feed, and her baby is more likely to formula-feed. The cycle continues. Unfortunately, given the promotion of formula milk in the 1980s (more on that later), the majority of mothers giving birth today will have been formula-fed themselves. You can see how this affects both their choice and their ability to continue. However, if we want breastfeeding rates to rise, we need to consider wider interventions that improve the breastfeeding knowledge of the whole family, and not just mothers.

Partners and breastfeeding

I have written this chapter predominantly from the perspective of a couple within a relationship. The word father has been used, given a lack of literature exploring same-sex couples and breastfeeding, but many of the issues can be translated. There is generally a complete lack of research exploring how same-sex couples may have different experiences when it comes to breastfeeding – more on this in a bit.

'I went to all the antenatal classes with her, but when it came to the breastfeeding session, we were all sent down the pub, with a wink, for a male bonding session. I could really have done with staying.'

This quote comes from research I conducted a few years ago exploring men's experiences of supporting their partner to breastfeed. Sadly this father was not alone. Despite the important role fathers play in bringing babies into this world, we fail to equip them with the information and skills they need to properly support their partners. This study only looked at the experiences of dads whose wife had breastfed – so if even the most motivated fathers are not receiving the information, what hope do those who are less interested or even averse to breastfeeding have?

But do dads really matter? Should we be spending time giving them information during pregnancy, when there is the important issue of birth to get through first? Of course we should. Fathers can have a huge influence on how their baby is fed and can be critical in ensuring breastfeeding goes well, or play a large part in determining whether breastfeeding is stopped. So why are we not paying more attention?

Fathers are now expected to play a central role in their babies' lives. We've come a long way since they paced outside the delivery room or went to the pub to receive the news of the baby's birth, before having another pint and a celebratory cigar. Fathers are now involved in pregnancy and birth and are expected to be involved in the care of their newborn babies. There are now certain expectations that fathers will be involved in shared parenting and childcare, and there are more extreme movements that call for more power for men in their children's lives.[11] For good reason. Fathers who are involved in their children's lives tend to have children with better health, wellbeing, educational achievement and social development. And this is important right from the start. Mothers who feel well supported by their partner during pregnancy are more likely to give birth to a baby who is a healthy weight.[12]

After the birth, the relationship a mother has with her partner can also be predictive of her wellbeing. Marital problems or a lack of support from her partner during pregnancy or after the birth are predictive of postnatal depression.[13] And the support (both emotional and practical) of a partner can affect breastfeeding success. The good news is that most fathers, at least during pregnancy, want their baby to be breastfed (although unfortunately many have other ideas). The reasons why men are supportive of breastfeeding tend to be based on health benefits or simply believing that it is more convenient (and cheaper!).[14] But how do dads influence breastfeeding?

Fathers who are supportive

Fathers who want their partner to breastfeed, or at least support her decision to do so, are more likely to have a baby who is breastfed. Studies have shown that a father who is supportive of breastfeeding is predictive of a woman planning to breastfeed in pregnancy, to breastfeed at birth, to be breastfeeding on discharge from hospital and to breastfeed for a longer period of time.[15] But why is there such a strong link? The men are not actually feeding the baby themselves, and we no longer live in a culture in which men can tell their wives what to do. So what's going on?

One explanation may lie with the woman herself and how she has selected her partner. Looking at a lot of my friends who have breastfed for a longer period of time, I know they'd never have a baby with a man who was against breastfeeding – or he'd learn to change his opinion pretty quickly! Joking aside, there is an element of truth in this.

Increased maternal confidence is another factor. Lots of studies show that if a man supports his partner's decision to breastfeed, or supports her as a mother more generally, then she feels more capable, competent and empowered. She is also more likely to be able to overcome problems and he is more likely to be her advocate.[16] He is also more likely to act in ways that support her breastfeeding, whether that's reading up about breastfeeding, just being there at 3am or taking the baby out for a walk when she is exhausted. A father can really boost and protect his partners' chances of breastfeeding.[17]

The 'cycle of breastfeeding' also plays an important role. Fathers who grew up around family members who breastfed are much more supportive of their partner breastfeeding. They tend not to have any problems with embarrassment and know that babies feed whenever and wherever.[14] However, not all fathers are supportive, either because they dislike breastfeeding, or because of wider factors around baby care.

Fathers who are disinterested

Fathers do tend to respect the idea that the decision to breastfeed is down to their partner.[18] However, there is a big difference between enabling your partner to be the decision-maker, and having no opinion. A sub-group of men really have no opinion on how their baby is fed, with fathers of teenage mothers being the most dismissive. In one study two-thirds of fathers simply had no opinion.[19]

Why does this matter, if they genuinely don't care? Well it's difficult to get support from someone who doesn't care. It's far more likely that at 3am when you're feeding *again* and are wondering out loud if you'll ever get a full night's sleep again (you will, I promise) that you'll simply get a muffled 'well give him a bottle then'. Fathers who don't care are unlikely to stand up for breastfeeding or get involved with problem-solving. Formula is likely to be seen as the easiest solution to a problem. Any problem. And they'll likely see lots of problems.

When fathers feel overwhelmed

We talk about the transition to motherhood and how stressful it can be, sometimes forgetting that fathers are going through a time of huge change too. Admittedly they are not the ones who have given birth, they are not breastfeeding and they are probably not giving over the entire day and night to the baby, but this doesn't mean they don't feel overwhelmed by the changes a new baby can bring.

One study interviewed men whose partner was expecting their first baby. It highlighted how much men change, but they often feel different emotions from the mother. They also often feel that they can't or shouldn't talk about these emotions, as the mother has things so much 'worse'. Fathers tend to start to feel overwhelmed by responsibility. Many suddenly see their role as to provide for the family, and they start worrying about the security of their jobs and their earning power. Some decide that they need to do better at work and throw themselves into their jobs, which of course drives their partners up the wall becasue it looks to them as though he is 'escaping' from having to care for the baby.[20] Men can also feel overwhelmed by simply having a baby, with increasing research recognising that fathers can suffer from postnatal depression.

When fathers feel unable to help

Even when fathers desperately want to support breastfeeding, few know where to start. Given the issues we know that many new mothers face in understanding how breastfeeding works, what to expect and how to fix difficulties, how on earth do we expect fathers to know these things, especially when we exclude them from any chance of education? Surely, given that fathers are there in the middle of the night when mother and baby are crying, we should be giving them all the tools they need, not just another pint of beer.

When you look at the literature, most fathers state that they want to support their partner to breastfeed,[21] but at the same time many feel completely helpless when faced with helping out.[4] As you might expect, their concerns mirror those that mothers have – they don't understand what is normal or how to fix problems. Others fear that they will do the wrong thing, or even be perceived as 'taking over'. And, contrary to the view of the birth educators who send them off down the pub, fathers report wanting information on breastfeeding so that they can help more proactively.[22]

When fathers exacerbate problems

Sometimes, as with any support role, it is possible for problems and concerns to be exacerbated if the person supporting doesn't have the knowledge needed. We expect fathers to be there for their partners, but fail to give them the information they need. Fathers can be just as vulnerable to the concerns new mothers have, and if they feel helpless because they cannot actually feed the baby, this may intensify difficulties. For example, even the most passionate father may unwittingly exacerbate or create maternal concerns if he is asking 'Should he really be feeding again?'... 'Are you sure he's getting enough milk'... 'Are you sure he doesn't need a bottle'?

When fathers feel excluded by breastfeeding

Although fathers may state antenatally that they want their baby to be breastfed, sometimes they find that the experience is different from how they imagined. One of the most common 'complaints' among fathers in relation to breastfeeding is that they felt excluded; from feeding, or from their baby's life, as all the baby seemed to do was feed. Many believed that feeding was essential to bonding, and worried that they might miss out long term on bonding with their baby. Others are more vocal about this from the start of pregnancy, stating that they don't want their baby to be breastfed because they will miss out on doing feeds.[23]

Many cultures have strong beliefs that associate feeding and love in some way. And given that feeding is such an integral part of a young baby's life, it is easy to see how fathers can feel excluded. Some men were told that they should take on a support role; that it was their job to support the mother. But many didn't want that role. They wanted to be involved with their baby in every way. Unfortunately, this made them almost jealous of the mother and her perceived 'advantage'.[14]

When fathers feel embarrassed

Unfortunately, fathers can feel embarrassed by their partner feeding in public or in front of others. As one father who contributed to my research noted:

'At first I freaked out about her feeding in front of people. I couldn't stop thinking that she had her breast out in front of my father or my friends and that they were getting an eyeful.'

This naturally impacts on a mother's confidence and the likelihood of her doing it. She may feel that if her partner is embarrassed by her actions, the rest of the world must be laughing and pointing.

Alternatively, she may agree not to feed in front of other people, slowly damaging her milk supply.[12]

When fathers see breasts as 'theirs'

Sigh. Sadly this is a real issue. Some men continue to see their partner's breasts as sexual (and as their property) and resent her 'using' them to breastfeed a baby. This can be exacerbated if women are also having issues with soreness or sensitivity, or if she has had enough of having anyone near her breasts.

What helps fathers be supportive?

Plenty of noise is made about mothers' need for information and support around breastfeeding, but less attention is given to what fathers might need, other than recognising that they can make an important difference. Just applying what works for mothers is unlikely to suit fathers, given the differences in what they are actually doing (feeding v supporting) and more general differences between mothers and fathers. To understand this better I asked over 100 fathers, whose partner was breastfeeding, what helped them, or would ideally help them, to be more supportive of breastfeeding.[24] They had some great ideas.

In terms of the specific support fathers want, the findings from our research showed that in particular they valued 'facts' and detailed information about why breastfeeding was important. As one father put it, he didn't want vague generalisations such as 'breastfeeding was good for babies' health'; he wanted statistics to help them make an informed decision. Statistics, for example saying 'breastfeeding reduces the risk of X by five times', were much preferred over more general messages. This fits well with wider research showing that fathers generally want details and facts rather than general or basic information.[21] This sort of information, in terms of protection or economic savings, is readily available and could easily be adapted into information for new fathers.

A further key finding in our research was that fathers wanted to be given more information antenatally about what they can do to help breastfeeding. Aware – often from talking to friends who were already fathers – that breastfeeding was not always straightforward, fathers were keen to be taught about the basics of how milk is produced, efficient latching and how to solve problems. We found that men felt helpless when their partner had breastfeeding difficulties and they didn't know how to help solve them. Or they felt helpless and guilty when their partner was exhausted and sleep-deprived and they didn't know what to do. One father in our research suggested that even what seemed like obvious tips on how to care for your partner would be helpful, as when you are sleep-deprived you might not be thinking straight. He noted:

> 'One of the midwives told me that no, I couldn't feed the baby, and giving a bottle wasn't going to help anyone. But what I could do was care for my wife and in that way I was caring for my baby. By getting my wife to relax and rest on the sofa, find box sets for her and then cook her food and bring her drinks, I was actually feeding the baby – even if indirectly!'

This all chimes with previous research that showed that often men can feel helpless during pregnancy, childbirth and the newborn period, as they cannot solve their partners' problems. They are told they must be involved, and need to be supportive, but have little experience of what might help.[25] This is combined – although I'm generalising now – with men having a tendency to want to offer practical support and solutions to problems, which doesn't stop during pregnancy, birth and the newborn period.[26] Indeed quite a lot of research shows that men often view their ideal role in the breastfeeding partnership as finding solutions or fixing problems, meaning they feel disheartened when they cannot as they haven't been taught the right skills.[27] Of course, this can also contrast with the best support for breastfeeding, and what women often want – emotional support. In another research project, one midwife explained to me:

> 'I now tell dads that the best way they can support their partner is to look after them. Yes with cooking and so on but also just by being there. When she feeds, sit with her. Feeds can go on for ages but you can use that as an excuse to cuddle up together and watch a film just like before.'

A further finding in our research was that men really wanted to be recognised by professionals, and in health promotion literature, as playing an important role. Although the decision to breastfeed typically rested with their partner, and they viewed her as the most important person to support, they often felt that their emotions and experiences were sidelined. To some extent they felt that they were told they must play an important part in their baby's life, and that they must share equal responsibility for tasks, but their emotions and experiences were not recognised. This included being involved in things like antenatal education, or even simple visual representation in the leaflets about breastfeeding.

Can fathers be 'taught' to be better breastfeeding supporters?

Research interventions so far have had mixed success with teaching fathers effective ways of supporting breastfeeding, but that may be due to variation in the interventions used. I think that supporting fathers, as the rest of this book discusses, is only a small part of the picture. We cannot train fathers to solve all breastfeeding problems (in effect, simply moving the responsibility to them), but over time supporting fathers is part of the bigger jigsaw puzzle of supporting mothers and changing society.

One trial in Australia, in which expectant fathers attended an antenatal and postnatal support class, found that breastfeeding rates did increase at six weeks.[28] Another small trial taught fathers to identify and solve breastfeeding problems during the antenatal period and found that breastfeeding rates rose at six months.[29] Finally, another small trial inviting fathers to attend breastfeeding antenatal classes alongside their partner increased the duration of exclusive, but not overall, breastfeeding.[30]

Are there any negatives to involving fathers?

This is a difficult one. It is really important to listen to fathers and their experiences, especially given that society expects them to take a role in their baby's care. Moreover, their support can be vital for maternal wellbeing, infant development and of course breastfeeding. Involving and supporting fathers in breastfeeding by health professionals is also part of the broader domestic and international policy trend of 'Involved Fatherhood', which seeks to involve fathers in all aspects of their baby's/child's health and wellbeing.

Finding the best way to do this needs to be handled carefully. In a healthcare system with restricted and reduced resources, money must not be diverted away from supporting mothers. Rather, the economic benefit of fathers who are equipped to support breastfeeding should be recognised and valued, with additional resources offered (which then in turn saves money in the long run).

There is little cost involved in opening breastfeeding education up to men and thinking about the father's needs and viewpoint when discussing breastfeeding, with countries such as Australia actively involving men in the process.[31] However, delivery of this support needs consideration. Women may feel embarrassed at receiving breastfeeding education in a class with men, due to society's view of the breast as sexual,[32] or there may be cultural implications of their inclusion.[33] Additionally, men and women can hear information in different ways or have different preferences about information delivery or content.[34] Separate antenatal classes aimed at fathers have been viewed as beneficial.[35]

It is possible that too much control and involvement on the part of the father may have a negative impact on the mother–infant bond and thus breastfeeding duration. For example, one study examining level of paternal involvement and breastfeeding duration found that where fathers were highly involved in the early care of their infant, breastfeeding levels were lower.[36] Fathers wanting increased involvement may lead to feeding cues being missed, separation of mother and infant or increased bottle use, all of which may lead to reduced milk supply and breastfeeding cessation. However, this study showed a correlation – it is also possible that if a mother chooses to formula-feed, her partner then becomes more involved in infant care, and this might be one of the driving forces behind feeding choice.

So a potential negative side-effect of increased father involvement in the care of their baby is that they are involved in ways that damage breastfeeding. A recent study analysing data from the Millennium Cohort study in the UK found that when fathers were highly involved in their infant's care, breastfeeding duration was more likely to be shorter.[37] This data is cross-sectional, meaning that it looks at a snapshot of behaviour at any given time, so it is difficult to work out whether fathers trying to get more involved decreases breastfeeding rates, or whether in those families where fathers play a main role in early parenting, the mother is less likely to breastfeed. Fathers may increase their care of the infant for all sorts of reasons, including the mother being unwell, feeling overwhelmed or simply returning to work.

However, it is also possible that fathers, given permission to participate more fully in their babies' lives, also want to take part in the bits they see as fun and put pressure on the mother to allow them to bottle-feed the baby. Although as the baby gets older milk can be expressed and given to the baby with little overall effect on supply, if this becomes very regular it may damage breastfeeding. As one father put it:

> 'All he seemed to do was sleep, cry or feed. She was the only one who could feed him and that seemed to be the only time when he was awake he wasn't crying. In my mind she seemed to get all the fun. I wanted to take part in some of that.'

Another mother in a different project explained how she had wanted to breastfeed, but her partner had wanted to feed the baby and wasn't happy with giving the occasional bottle. As a 'compromise' they had agreed that she would express so that they could both bottle-feed the baby from birth. She found it incredibly difficult to combine expressing, caring for and then bottle-feeding the baby when he inevitably returned to work, and she eventually stopped breastfeeding.

In the UK parental leave laws were introduced in 2013 which allowed the mother to pass part of her maternity leave allowance to her partner. So far there has not been an analysis of how this has affected breastfeeding rates, but it is likely that some women will feel pressure to return to work earlier, if they are the main wage-earner, making breastfeeding more difficult.

Fathers, in terms of their attitude and approach to breastfeeding, therefore play a big role in how supported the mother feels. His attitude and behaviour can have a really big impact on her, yet many dads feel unprepared to support breastfeeding.

Same-sex couples and breastfeeding

Research is starting to emerge around the experiences of same-sex couples and breastfeeding. Of course, many of the issues relating to partners/fathers will apply, at least with some similarity. However, same-sex couples can also face additional challenges in getting the breastfeeding support that they need. Research more broadly exploring experiences of same-sex couples in the maternity care system shows that this can include subtle and more overt homophobia and the awful impact that can have on the care parents receive and their wellbeing.[38] One form of this is the existence of heteronormative assumptions or exclusion of the 'other parent', leaving couples feeling misunderstood, excluded and generally as if they are having a poorer standard of care and support.[39]

Looking specifically at breastfeeding, one core theme is that a lack of training around supporting same-sex couples can sometimes occur. In an article exploring her experiences as a gay woman breastfeeding her children, B.J. Epstein Woodstein discusses the challenges she and her wife faced.[40] Within this was the automatic assumption that she was in a heterosexual relationship, with health professionals referring to her husband, sometimes despite having met her wife, or had a conversation around her relationship. This brings us back to the concepts of trust and support between health professional and woman and how this affects experiences of breastfeeding support.

Another theme B.J. discusses is how breastfeeding can lead to all sorts of feelings between partners. The partner who did not give birth may feel jealous of what is seen as a 'quintessentially female act', particularly if she identifies as a mother too. In some couples, a woman who did not give birth may decide to induce lactation. Again, this opens up further potential challenges and need for support, both in terms of the practicalities of inducing lactation, and also the reactions and assumptions of other people. It also adds an additional aspect to the partnership of who will feed the baby and when, or potential for all sorts of emotions if one is finding breastfeeding easier than the other, or the baby seems to show a preference for one mother over the other.

Then there is the issue of often innocent but inappropriate questions that same-sex parents would rarely get asked. Starting off with intrusive questions around conception, this can lead on to questions about who is feeding the baby or how it all works. These questions may stem from genuine interest, but the impact on the parents can be very difficult.

As noted previously, the lack of research and publication (and training) on supporting same-sex couples when it comes to breastfeeding impacts negatively on care given. Health professionals may not have experience of induced lactation or how to support two parents breastfeeding a baby. Little is published on this skill and it does not, as far as I am aware, form a standard part of training for health and medical professions.[41] Taken together, there is a greater need for more research, skill and awareness around supporting same-sex couples with breastfeeding. This lack of evidence and awareness is likely to be negatively affecting feelings of support and ability to continue breastfeeding.

Action 9

✓ Educate partners and family to be the breastfeeding supporters they can be.

14. WE *STILL* HAVE RIDICULOUS ATTITUDES TO BREASTFEEDING IN PUBLIC SPACES

If you stop people in the street and ask them whether breast is best, they'll probably say yes. But that's where their support ends. Ask them whether they're comfortable with a mother breastfeeding any time, any place and they start to look a bit shifty... and the 'b' word comes in. 'I'm supportive of breastfeeding, *but...*' The truth is that they are supportive of breastfeeding in theory, but in reality? Not so much. And this is really damaging for the confidence of new mothers.

As a society we are not prepared for breastfeeding. We don't like to see it, and challenge it when we do. Often this is based on misunderstanding about how breastfeeding works and social conditioning to see the breast as sexual rather than nurturing, with a bit of good old British 'feeling a bit uncomfortable' when we do anything that might not be seen as polite thrown in for good measure.

Breastfeeding a baby in modern-day culture is therefore difficult. But that's not where the challenge ends. Modern life also brings with it social media and modern technology, and products that supposedly 'help' with breastfeeding, but actually have completely the opposite effect.

The internet might mean that social contact and information is constantly at the tip of our fingers, but what does that really mean for breastfeeding? Is it really helpful to have this information right there, all the time? And is it even the right information, written by people who truly want to help? Or is it misinformation? Trolling? Or even deliberately damaging?

'Breast is best... but we don't want to see that'

In March 2014 in north-west England, a young mother paused in the street while out shopping to breastfeed her hungry baby. Sitting on some steps, she quietly breastfed while eating her own lunch, with little skin exposed. She was probably thinking about what to have for dinner and giving little thought to what was going on around her. She was engaging in a biologically normal behaviour, as women and their babies have done across the world, for millennia.

The reason I can comment so exactly on the details of these few moments of her day is because, unbeknown to her, a passerby was so alarmed by the sight of her feeding her child that he not only paused to take a photo, but also posted it on a local Facebook page with the caption 'I know the sun is out n all that but there's no need to let your kid feast on your nipple in town'. His aim was to shame and ridicule, and although many criticised his behaviour, he also had plenty of supporters to echo his views.

This is not, unfortunately, an isolated incident. In 2015 the UK media was in uproar (again) about the issue of women breastfeeding in public (while apparently overlooking more important issues such as children not having enough to eat, disease and war). A woman was breastfeeding her 12-week-old daughter during a meal at Claridges (an upmarket London hotel) and was asked to cover herself up with a large napkin. A social media frenzy ensued, questioning whether women should be 'allowed' to breastfeed in public and, if so, how they should behave. Commentators included Nigel Farage (a far-right UK politician renowned for his racist, sexist, and homophobic comments), who suggested that although he supported breastfeeding, he felt that women should breastfeed in a corner rather than be 'openly ostentatious' when feeding their baby, as it might make others, particularly the older generation, feel embarrassed.

Others who felt that the debate needed their input included Boris Johnson (who was at that point simply a former London mayor and then later Foreign Secretary) and Jeremy Clarkson (a television presenter), who called on women to be discreet, with Clarkson adding that 'although breastfeeding was natural... so was urinating'. Clarkson has previously informed the world that men 'do not see breasts as part of the reproductive process... we see them as a plaything, a toy'. Bewilderingly, his comments on breastfeeding were printed by the *Sun* newspaper – a tabloid known for the now defunct 'Page 3' that featured bare-breasted models. So breasts are fine, just not when fulfilling their primary function.

Sadly there have been plenty of other examples. Mothers are frequently asked to stop breastfeeding in public, here and across the Western world. The *Huffington Post* in the USA, for example, carries a humorous yet depressing photo article depicting the numerous places women have been asked to stop breastfeeding, including schools, parks, malls, courtrooms, planes... you name it, and a woman has a tale of being stopped from breastfeeding there. A Google search shows the same pattern across the world. Typing in 'Woman stopped breastfeeding in public in… the USA… the UK… New Zealand… France… Australia' brings up almost identical stories. Women, you are *not* welcome to breastfeed your baby here.

A quick browse of the comments sections on online articles (I know, I know, *never* read the comments!) highlights a prevailing attitude that breastfeeding should not be seen in public. Even when an article is written with a pro-breastfeeding stance, derisive commentators always weigh in. And they say the same things. Over and over. In fact, the comments on the main tabloid websites are so predictable it's like a particularly depressing game of bingo, where the only prize is a sinking feeling that the average commentator has such illogical, perverse and deep-rooted views against breastfeeding, the female body and indeed women that Farage actually looks like better company. Ugh.

'Breastfeeding might be natural but so is urinating and I don't do that in public.'

One is a waste product that for health and safety reasons is disposed of in a separate area. Another is a product full of nutrients used to nourish a small baby. Let's play spot the difference.

'Mothers who breastfeed in public are just exhibitionists seeking attention.'

Yes, you're right. It's nothing whatsoever to do with a small baby needing to be fed. New mothers just want the opportunity to finally expose themselves in Starbucks.

'I don't want breasts thrust in my face when I'm drinking my coffee.'

I think perhaps a little fantasy is coming into play here! You actually want this to happen, don't you?

Heart-warmingly, these incidents have been met with a backlash. Social media has been flooded with outcry that women and their babies should be treated in this way. Breastfeeding protests have been organised. Journalists have seized the opportunity to speak out against those who were disgusted at seeing the natural act of breastfeeding. And politicians from opposing parties suddenly fall over themselves to condemn Farage and his comments and show their support of breastfeeding. (In the case of Farage, there was plenty of witty comeback – my favourite examples include someone suggesting the world would be a better place if Farage himself sat in a corner with a napkin over his head, an Exeter café putting up a sign saying that breastfeeding was welcome but UKIP supporters would be asked to eat in the toilet, and women posting photos of themselves breastfeeding in various acrobatic positions – #ostentatiousbreastfeeding).

Reflecting on all this for the second edition, I wonder whether things have changed in the last five years or so and actually I think they have. In 2018 Channel 4 *Dispatches* produced an episode called 'Breastfeeding Uncovered' (great minds think alike) exploring the issue of the challenges women face breastfeeding in the UK with a focus on feeding in public.[1] It feels like since then we have gradually become more and more accepting, with more women and celebrities posting selfies of breastfeeding and more positive imagery in general. Maybe the press have just reduced how much they try and sensationalise it. Or maybe there is a real difference. I know some women are certainly still anxious because of this dialogue. As I wrote at the time – 'are we really still talking about a woman's right to breastfeed in public?'[2] Recent research we did around women's experiences of breastfeeding through COVID-19 lockdown found that some felt more comfortable breastfeeding at home and some were now anxious about being able to go places and having to breastfeed in public. But it feels like we're moving in the right direction at least.[3]

What is it about breastfeeding in public that causes so much outrage? Breastfeeding is a biologically normal way to feed a baby. Research consistently shows the health and economic benefits. It is supported by policy at a global level and there is a continuous effort across the developed world to raise breastfeeding rates. So why is it even a question – let alone a topic of such emotive debate – whether a woman should breastfeed her baby whenever and wherever it needs feeding? Who gets to decide and make that moral judgment? And how does this impact upon women and their babies?

Think about the language used in these debates. Newspaper articles, health promotion, research (even my own writing) typically discuss the issue of 'women breastfeeding in public' rather than the issue of 'babies eating in public', which is what breastfeeding actually is. Women who breastfeed in public are not doing it for their own benefit, or to draw attention to themselves (despite what 'tabloid reader Bob from Brighton' might feel). It is neither a hobby, nor even really a choice; it is a biologically normal response to a baby needing to feed. It's what breasts were actually designed for. It's all about the baby. The baby eating, the baby's need to feed frequently and the baby's right to be breastfed – not the mothers' actions. Imagine for a moment the debate recast from that angle: 'Baby feeds ostentatiously in restaurant'... 'selfish baby demands to be fed'... 'Exhibitionist baby strikes again'. This shows what nonsensical madness it is. But, as in many areas of human behaviour, women are blamed and held accountable for others' actions. And the public feels it has the power to dictate to them how they behave, and to criticise, insult and mock them for their choices.

The debate about whether or not a woman can breastfeed in public is meaningless from a legal standpoint. In the UK women are protected by law. In England and Wales under the terms of the 2010 Equality Act you must not treat a woman unfavourably because she is breastfeeding.[4] In Scotland the law is even more specific; you must not stop someone in a public place from feeding a child under two with milk.[5] Similar laws protect women and babies in Canada, Australia, Europe and across the globe. Women should not be asked to stop breastfeeding, or to move, and they should not be made to feel uncomfortable or asked to cover up. This is because we want babies to be breastfed; it is a public health matter. It saves money. It cuts down on illness. It is not sexual, exhibitionism or akin to urination, no matter what the comments say. Ultimately babies have the same rights as everyone else – including the right to enjoy a meal in a public space. We shouldn't be talking about a woman's decision to do something, we should be talking about a baby's need to be fed.

Ignoring the legal protection women are afforded to breastfeed in public, and whether there should be any debate about it at all, it is not difficult to see how society's attitude towards breastfeeding can shape a woman's decision to breastfeed. It takes a very confident and self-assured woman to breastfeed in a public space when she knows her behaviour is a much-criticised topic of debate. If she feeds her baby, are people looking? What do they think of her? Is she exposing herself? Will someone confront her? Or take a photo of her and put it on social media? Throw in postnatal hormones, sleep deprivation and a feeling that life will never be quite the same and it is easy to see how bottle-feeding can seem a comforting alternative.

However, what is confusing is that society appears rather contradictory in its views about the acceptability of breastfeeding and breasts in public. On the one hand, the 'breast is best' mantra and pressure to breastfeed is strong. Only 1% of participants in a UK survey believed formula milk was a better choice than breastfeeding.[6] Similarly, in the USA, the annual Health Styles survey found that over 96% of respondents believed that breastmilk was the perfect food for a baby[7] and a global survey of mothers in nine countries including Europe, China and the USA found that over 98% agreed that 'breast is best'.[8]

This is what makes the public breastfeeding debate so surreal. It appears that although society believes that breastfeeding is best, we also believe it is something that should be done in private. We want women to breastfeed, but we don't want to see – or even think – about it happening, and we certainly don't want to consider the logistics of this or the impact it has on breastfeeding women. The proportion of individuals with this attitude is large. A YouGov survey in the UK found that 34% of the public agreed with Farage that women breastfeeding in public was embarrassing for others and should not be done.

This attitude that women should not breastfeed in public is echoed in the USA (57%),[9] Australia (30%)[10] and France – a country known for topless sunbathing – (44%).[11] One Australian telephone survey found that although most respondents were supportive of breastfeeding, 82% believed that formula-feeding was more acceptable than breastfeeding in public.[12] In the UK more people apparently believe it is acceptable for a woman to breastfeed her baby in a toilet than it is in a restaurant or on public transport.[11] Think about that for a moment – more people would like a baby to eat in a public toilet than to deal with their own feelings of offence if a baby is breastfed within five metres of them. And we're suggesting that it's breastfeeding mothers who have issues?

There are differences in 'who' is accepting (or not) of breastfeeding in public. At odds with Farage's claim that breastfeeding offends the older generation, those aged over 60 actually appear to be the most supportive of breastfeeding in public.[13] In contrast, a Canadian study found that nearly 80% of college students believed breastfeeding was an intimate act that should be kept private.[14] Is this a disturbing sign that the next generation will be even more disgusted by breastfeeding, or does it show that as people mature they become more tolerant? Sadly only time will tell.

Fathers, as you might expect, are more supportive than the general public. One US study found only 16% of fathers were against breastfeeding in public – but that still means almost one in five women will have a partner who would not want her to breastfeed in public.[15] And remember – these figures only relate to those who were brave (or daft!) enough to admit this in a survey. However, it is often women and mothers themselves – a group who you would expect to show the most compassion towards the needs of mother and baby – who reveal the most negative views. In a global survey, agreement that 'breastfeeding in public was perfectly natural' was actually highest among UK mothers, but still only 63%. One in three *mothers* believe a woman breastfeeding in public is wrong. *One in three.* And the UK is fairly liberal compared to the 57% of mothers in the US, 55% in Brazil, 35% in France and only 19% in China who agreed with this statement.[8]

It is bemusing that so many people hold simultaneously the belief that babies should be breastfed... but that we shouldn't see it. One Canadian study of university students found that although all students expressed a desire for their future baby to be breastfed, over two-thirds of the sample added conditions to this, such as that the woman should be discreet or feed in private.[16] Similarly, in an American sample, over 80% of college students planned to breastfeed their own baby, yet 65% believed that breastfeeding in public was not acceptable.

Again female students were more critical of breastfeeding than their male peers.[17] Even in an experimental set-up (where you'd think people would be alert to someone pointing out their bigotry, and at least pretend to be a bit more liberal), when participants were asked to examine photos of a woman breastfeeding and say whether they supported her behaviour, photos depicting a mother breastfeeding in private were rated far more acceptable than those breastfeeding in public. And in possibly the most contradictory study of all, Spear found that 91% of her US student sample believed that the US should promote a breastfeeding-friendly culture, while 78% simultaneously believed breastfeeding should only take place in private.[18] Yeah, but no, but yeah, but no, but yeah, but... oh, we don't know.

Finally, consider the public's attitude to other behaviours. Are we just offended by everything? Apparently not. A survey conducted by YouGov in 2014 found that only 19% of people in the UK support a ban on smacking children.[19] Nourishing your child – bad, assaulting them – good. *Excellent priorities, UK public.* Well done.[19]

And our rationale is...?

The obvious question is why, as a society, are we so disturbed by the sight of a woman breastfeeding her baby? What possible reason can there be for such heated debate? A Google search of 'Should a woman breastfeed in public?' returns over 31 million results. Thirty-one million separate debates on what should be a non-issue. Debates that are probably had over a nice cup of coffee or tea – with the addition of the milk of another species. Human milk – bad. Milk from an animal that lives in a muddy field – lovely, thank you. I'll pay a small fortune for a cup of it. Just to put this in context, if you put 'Should nuclear weapons be banned' into Google you get 1.1 million hits. 'Starving children in Africa' – 1.3 million hits. 'Cure for Ebola' – 15 million results. Although 'What do women want' does return you 113 million hits and 'Is Facebook down' – 154 million hits. This may be the reason aliens have taken a look and not invaded.

One possible explanation is that we are predisposed to be concerned about bodily fluids (although animal milk is just fine). Realistically this is unlikely to explain a significant proportion of our disdain; especially given the fact that breastmilk is a food made for babies (and not a contaminative waste product akin to urine). But it does make a good cover-up excuse for our real reasons. Although, in one survey of UK *Sunday Times* readers (in response to a news story of a mother being asked to leave a swimming pool for breastfeeding her baby), 65% believed it was acceptable to breastfeed her baby *by the side of* the pool... yet 64% believed it unacceptable to breastfeed while sat *in* the pool. Who knows the level of confusion one leg in and one leg out would have caused, but it does illustrate that some people have an irrational fear of breastmilk as a contaminative substance... although I presume they do understand that they're not the ones who are expected to drink it.[20]

The more likely explanation for our discomfort with public breastfeeding is what we as a society, consciously or subconsciously, associate with the female breast. Breasts are decorative, attractive and alluring – and associated with sexual gratification. Breasts are to adorn billboards, to boost sales of magazines and to enhance cinema ratings. But how does this affect breastfeeding, which should be a completely separate issue? Why can't breasts be fun and attractive and used to feed a baby at the same time? Legs can be attractive and still be used to walk. Eyes can be alluring yet still used to see. A mouth is completely multi-functional. But breasts... no, they cannot have a dual role. Breasts are sexual. Breasts are to admire.

This is the real answer. Breasts in our society are there for pleasure, and we don't want a small baby reminding us that they aren't there just for fun. Of course, not everyone has such black and white views about the role of breasts, but a significant proportion of society – or at least those who shout the loudest and have the time to write comments –

appears unable to see that breasts could perhaps be considered nice to look at, and also a handy way of ensuring the survival of the human race. Or have a private, sexual role, but also be used to feed a baby in public. And in most cases very little actual breast is on display. Yes, Bob from Brighton – most women breastfeed very discreetly indeed, and those who sometimes accidentally expose more breast are usually just getting to grips with it and would rather die of shame than think that you saw them (and enjoyed it).

So it's not even 'seeing' breastfeeding that we have a problem with. It's the very thought that it might be sexual. The social networking site Facebook neatly highlights the issue, persistently removing photos of babies being breastfed because they apparently contravene the 'decency code'. Many sexualised images remain uncensored on the site.

How on earth can we accept breasts in public if they are decorative, but not accept breasts in public if they are doing their natural thing? For those who objectify women and believe that they are there for sexual gratification, witnessing a woman breastfeeding is likely to lead to a negative response. 'Their' sexual breast is not only being used in a non-sexual way, but is being used to meet the needs of another. This perhaps explains some male disdain of public breastfeeding, but we know that women can be just as averse, if not more so. It is likely that some women have been so socially conditioned to view their own body in terms of sexual attraction that they feel that others using their body must be performing a sexual act. To them women who breastfeed in public – especially in front of their partner – are acting in a sexual way.

It's not that we hate seeing breasts in public. Breasts are fine in public if they're shown in a sexual way. It's just when they're used in a non-sexual way that they're accused of being sexual and suddenly that's bad. Yes, I know. It reads like a bizarre maths riddle.

Breastfeeding and the media

It is interesting that negative attitudes towards seeing breastfeeding become more extreme when considering breastfeeding in the media. It appears that breastfeeding may grudgingly be acceptable if an infant in real life really needs feeding (and is vocalising this rather loudly), but seeing breastfeeding outside of this context is frowned on. In a US study, only 48% of men felt it was appropriate to show a woman breastfeeding on a magazine cover, 37% on a billboard or poster and 46% on a family television show.[15] Yes, you did read that correctly. Breasts should not appear in magazines, on posters or on the television. Oh. Sorry. You mean *breastfeeding* should not appear. I understand your logic. Although actually… I don't. We'll get on to this particular hypocrisy in more detail later.

Breastfeeding mothers must also absent themselves generally from the television (presumably just erasing themselves quietly from any depiction of public life), with just 27% of US students feeling it was appropriate for breastfeeding to be shown.[21] A feature on *This Morning* (a UK daytime show with an audience of around 1.5 million viewers) recently discussed – and showed photos of – a penis enlargement at 11am on a weekday morning. Erections and all. Because that's natural, just biology. Oh, wait. I meant male biology, which is to be celebrated as a sign of power and prowess. Female biology is either for male pleasure or should be hidden. Presumably breasts doing their natural thing are scary to small children (or more likely overgrown children). Something tells me that if men could breastfeed and nourish a whole new human being with their milk alone for at least six months, breastfeeding would be perceived as a superpower, not a taboo joke.

If breastfeeding does actually get on to our screens, it is often in the context of it being problematic. TV soaps and dramas often have storylines in which women have trouble breastfeeding and use formula (usually giving them the opportunity to place a large can of some brand or other in the background), but seem unable to have a nice story about breastfeeding going well… or just normally. Otherwise, breastfeeding on TV is either about the shock factor (Look! A seven-year-old breastfeeding! This is wrong because… because… um… give me a minute) or about humour. Not women's humorous tales of others' disgust at them breastfeeding, but scriptwriters thinking it is hilarious to poke fun at breastfeeding mothers or create ridiculous scenes where breastfeeding is something weird to laugh at. A key sketch in the UK comedy *Little Britain* showed a mother breastfeeding her adult son every time he asked for 'bitty'. Ignoring the biological impossibility of this (mouth development means breastfeeding becomes difficult, if not impossible, after the age of seven or so), why is it acceptable to laugh at a vulnerable group in society?

Now consider for a moment the normalisation of formula milk and bottle-feeding in our society, and how many adverts for formula milk are seen in magazines, on television and on the internet, and how often an infant formula bottle is the default symbol for advertising feeding facilities and infant items. Wrapping paper, birth announcements and cards to celebrate new babies are covered in images of bottles. One midwife I talked to during my research for this book recalled how she had 'even been to a Christmas nativity play where the baby Jesus was fed with a bottle'. (I'm not sure whether Mary got given a free sample at her postnatal check, or whether she packed it on the donkey). Many children, and many adults, never see a baby being breastfed, yet are frequently exposed to media images of formula-feeding and bottles. One study estimated that only 29% of teenagers had ever seen a woman breastfeed,[18] yet it is highly likely that the majority will have seen bottle-feeding advertised, on television and in their local café. Little girls often get given a toy doll that comes complete with a bottle. Forcing prescribed gender roles on children is another pet hate of mine, but that might be another book.

Conversely, a doll that came with a vest for the child to wear, so they could attach the doll to the vest to 'breastfeed', caused a furore about sexualising young girls. Because breasts are sexual and by wearing that vest she may one day grow up to be… a mother who breastfeeds her baby (the horror!). These dolls were also seen as smug. Although it is the norm for a doll to come with a bottle, apparently attempting to equalise the situation by providing a breastfeeding version was, according to one *Daily Mail* feature writer, 'The Breastapo using dolls to brainwash our children', an example of 'Breast is best bigotry'. Ultimately we live in a formula-feeding culture that has little space, acceptance or respect for breastfeeding. Forget that at your peril.

We then have the many negative and downright nasty comments that appear all over our media. We all know never to read the comments section of a tabloid unless we are feeling brave, but one study examined the type of comments left on articles around women protesting their right to breastfeed in public. In 2014 there were numerous articles written about women being criticised for feeding in public and subsequently fighting back with articles, photos or nurse-ins. The research analysed 884 comments left on *Daily Mail* articles about this. People, hiding behind anonymity and a computer screen, described breastfeeding women as exhibitionists and lacking in self-respect. Somehow this moved on even further, calling women unattractive (as that's apparently how we try and hurt women), lazy (I guess it is easier to breastfeed sometimes) and bad parents (they mean bad mothers – again, how to try and hurt a woman). Women should feed inside and if they didn't then they should expect unwanted sexual contact or aggression from men. Righty ho. Where do you even begin with people who feel this way? Or perhaps they actually don't and it's all about taking the opportunity to criticise and control women.[22]

Fighting back

Of course, there are women who have the confidence and self-assurance to not only defy social convention and breastfeed their baby in public, but to openly and actively champion their support for breastfeeding. These breastfeeding activists, or 'lactivists', aim to raise awareness of the laws that protect breastfeeding women, and normalise both breastfeeding and breastfeeding in public. A common 'weapon' of the lactivist is to fight back against derogation of breastfeeding women in the press by organising 'nurse-ins' – where a number of women and their babies turn up to a location (usually where a woman has been told to stop breastfeeding) and simultaneously breastfeed their babies, knowing that they are protected by the law. Dr Kate Boyer, a researcher in the UK with an interest in social, cultural and feminist geography, extensively discusses the phenomenon, highlighting how women demonstrate against criticism of public breastfeeding by doing the very same thing: reclaiming their public space and territory and showing to the world that legally no one can stop them. Kate explains:

'Part of the challenge in increasing breastfeeding duration rates in the UK is the difficulties that women can encounter as they start to spend more time out and about in the weeks and months post-birth. Breastfeeding outside the home is uncommon in the UK: it's unusual to ever see it (outside certain affluent neighbourhoods in the South), and many women find it a really daunting prospect. Research also shows that it's not just fear of being 'told off' that's problematic, but that (seemingly) subtle, non-verbal forms of social disapproval like tuts and glares can also really put women off. Our culture is saturated with messages about who and what breasts are for, and feeding babies is almost never part of this calculation. Sadly, public reactions are a factor for women in the UK in decisions to switch from breastfeeding to formula. These demonstrations are about fighting back against all of this, by reclaiming the space that society tells women not to have and showing that mothers won't be put off by such attitudes. Of course, it's the more confident women who do this, but they can act as a source of confidence and hope for those who feel less able.'

Others use social media and humour as vehicles for fighting back against the negativity. For a particularly catchy tune, google *Ruin Your Day* by Sparrow Folk, a satirical song and music video ridiculing those who detest breastfeeding in public, including lyrics such as 'Everybody knows new mothers are exhibitionists – taking every chance they get to ruin your day with tits', 'Pretending their little ones need a comfort or a feed' and 'Because tits are scary, just like spiders... like being chased by a tornado'. Along similar lines is a parody on pop music hit *All About That Bass* called *All About That Breast*. 'I'm all about that breast, 'bout that breast, no bottle. I'm bringing boobies back… go ahead and use that beautiful rack'. Both are heart-warming and great for playing to those who are a little uptight.

In the last four years I think we have definitely seen a growth in positive images of breastfeeding being widely shared. I think this is going a long way in helping to normalise feeding and send the message that it is something that should be seen, and a woman can do it and not have to hide away in the house. Indeed, social media appears to be an increasingly common playground for sharing breastfeeding photos whether you're a celeb or otherwise.[23]

'Brelfies' were one example I talked about in 2016. Back then I was apparently hoping that 'brelfie' would become *the* word added to the *Oxford English Dictionary* in 2016 (sadly it wasn't). A brelfie is a term coined to describe selfies of mothers breastfeeding. Currently Google returns about 91,000 hits for the term and it has a Twitter hashtag.

Predictably, this defiance – be it a nurse-in, a music video or even an article online – rarely goes down well with those who are unsupportive of breastfeeding. The women who protest are portrayed at best as 'earth mothers' and at worst as strident man-hating feminists, who also hate all women who have ever even thought about using a bottle and probably all babies too. In fact the public have a number of common insults for those who champion breastfeeding, including 'breastfeeding police', 'breastfeeding nazis', 'breastfeeding mafia', 'nipple nazis' and 'militant lactivists'. It appears to be perfectly acceptable to associate women striving to promote and support a nurturing act with terrorist regimes, but *not* for a hungry baby to feed in public.

Brelfies also attract negative attention, being interpreted as sexual, or in some cases being perceived as smug, or as an attack on formula-feeding women (which seems ironic given the level of formula imagery in our press and social media). One tabloid newspaper published an article on the emergence of these photos with the headline 'Breastfeeding selfies are the latest trend for new mothers… but is it just naked exhibitionism?' We are back to sexualisation again.

Alongside this, over the last decade, a number of celebrities have released photos of themselves breastfeeding, which is great. Although, updating this in 2020, rather than instantly remembering the photos that Miranda Kerr and Caprice shared, I'm now feeling old reading articles about '20 celebrity mums who have normalised breastfeeding' and trying to work out who some of them are. I do however know who Ashley Graham, Chrissy Teigen and Kate Upton are. I'll be over here googling some of the others while you get on with the rest of the book.

On a serious note, one major change we have seen in the last four years in relation to breastfeeding celeb photos is them posting photos of themselves expressing milk. This has been in the form of formal photoshoots, posed photos at home or even while at work or in the car. Well done Rachel McAdams, Amy Schumer and Millie Mackintosh (also holding a glass of wine). And then there have been photos of famous dads supporting famous mums… the Rock famously feeding Lauren Hashian her dinner while she breastfed.

Some people take issue with these photos, arguing that they are only acceptable because the women are young, slim and beautiful, so they put further pressure on new mothers. Others are cynical, thinking that breastfeeding is being used to promote careers. But you know what? I think it's working. It might not be for everybody, but there is a definite increase in celebrities doing this and with the rise of social media and Instagram in particular over the last few years, these photos are visible and being seen.

There has also been a big increase in images or clips of breastfeeding mothers in adverts. Adidas used an image of a mother breastfeeding her baby in a tracksuit. Aldi featured a couple talking where she is casually breastfeeding. Jumping on the bandwagon? Yes probably. Making things more visible? Definitely.

Other adverts have made me raise an eyebrow though. One for Lloyds Bank had a horse galloping around, passing different people and families. The tune playing was Fat Boy Slim's 'Praise you'. If you know the lyrics you know they go '*We've come a long, long way together, through the hard times and the good*'. Maybe I've grown cynical, but when they played 'hard times' they cut to an image of a breastfeeding mother. Again, McCain chips did an advert of different types of mother (hmm)… the working mother (wearing heels obviously), the stay at home one (eating cake from memory) and then the 'doing it on my own mother', who was in a dimly lit room, looking stressed… breastfeeding her baby.

Then we had the bizarre incident of Dove – yes, the shower gel people – designing an advert saying '75% of people say breastfeeding in public is fine. 25% say put them away. What's your way?' I mean… what now? Why? Do they hold polls on other laws and splash them on shower gel adverts? Did they see other companies using breastfeeding images and think, I know what we can do…?!

The impact on new mothers

Unsurprisingly, society's attitude to breastfeeding affects how women feel about breastfeeding in public. And this affects whether they breastfeed at all. Countries that have very high breastfeeding rates such as Sweden – where breastfeeding *is* the normal way to feed a baby, are not worried about seeing breastfeeding women. Less than 4% of women believe that women should not breastfeed in public there.[11] This relationship is of course cyclical – the more supportive a nation is of breastfeeding, the more likely future generations are to breastfeed. And the more a nation sees women breastfeeding, the more 'normal' and accepted it becomes. And so on. Unfortunately, the UK and many other Western nations have this circle in opposition; the more unsupportive we are of seeing breastfeeding, the fewer women breastfeed, making breastfeeding seem even less attainable for future generations.

Mothers are very aware that there are individuals who do not support their choice to breastfeed in public, and that they could encounter 'Bob from Brighton' or one of his friends whenever they need to feed their baby. Even if, taking conservative estimates, only 30% of the population is opposed to breastfeeding in public, that's still one in three individuals. When that mother is sat in a coffee shop feeding her baby, she knows that four or five people, if not more, might be considering her actions as sexual, akin to urinating or selfish. And this knowledge has an impact. In 2009 a survey of over 1,200 mothers in the UK by *Mother and Baby* magazine found that 60% of mothers felt that the UK was not breastfeeding friendly, 65% found breastfeeding in public a stressful experience and 54% had directly received negative comments or actions.[23] A similar survey in 2014 of over 7,600 UK mothers found that 65% of mothers reported they had felt socially isolated when breastfeeding, 85% felt that society frowns upon mothers who breastfeed and 68% believed it was the cultural norm to bottle-feed babies.[24]

What all this noise does is instil fear in new mothers about their real or potential negative experience of breastfeeding in public, which in turn shapes their decision to breastfeed. Perceiving breastfeeding in public to be embarrassing or threatening predicts a lower intention and likelihood of breastfeeding at all.[25] For those mothers feeding their first baby in the early weeks, when breastfeeding might feel overwhelming and they might take longer to latch the baby on, the thought of doing this in front of strangers, in a public place, where they may be challenged, may make formula-feeding seem a much more comforting choice. Interestingly, many women who do breastfeed in public report that they have never experienced negative comments, yet they live in real fear that this will happen due to the stigmatisation of breastfeeding in public by the media.[26]

This fear and anxiety appears to be being exploited by the breastmilk substitute and bottle industry. In recent years there has been an increasing number of 'studies' led by companies who make bottles, teats and formula preparation machines into the experiences of women in relation to breastfeeding in public. A survey in 2020 for example, by Tommee Tippee, asked women about unwanted attention in public, including whether they received unwanted sexual attention. The headlines stemming from this included '*One in six mums say they've had unwanted sexual attention while breastfeeding in public*' which to me feels like a way of introducing this concern to new mothers rather than being supportive.[27] A new mother reading that may have never considered that she would receive such attention and subsequently be put off or made anxious. Tommee Tippee followed this up in 2021 with another campaign that included statistics about how uncomfortable women feel breastfeeding in public.[28] Perhaps they are just seeking to raise awareness, but luckily they just happen to make a whole range of products to 'help' women if they don't feel comfortable feeding in front of others…

A mother's choice

So – society has spoken. What is a breastfeeding mother to do? Essentially she has three choices: a) breastfeed and face the potential backlash, b) attempt to breastfeed out of the public's disapproving gaze, or c) stop breastfeeding and use formula.

Those who choose to breastfeed in public run the risk of encountering the disapproval of others, whether a glance, someone turning away or a verbal challenge. However, figures from the latest Infant Feeding Survey show that only around 58% of mothers who breastfeed took the risk and breastfed even once in public, and many who did so felt self-conscious.[29] Only 8% of mothers felt comfortable breastfeeding wherever they wanted. And the 58% figure is high compared to the 36% of Italian women who ever breastfed in public. In countries with far more positive attitudes, such as Sweden, nearly 80% of mothers with a baby aged six weeks old had breastfed in a public place.[8]

Although only around one in six women in the UK Infant Feeding Survey reported that they received negative comments about breastfeeding in public, far more feel the silent disapproval and this reduces their confidence and makes them unlikely to repeat the experience. Unsurprisingly, being made to feel uncomfortable feeding in public is a common reason for stopping breastfeeding.[30] Others feel that it is better for their own wellbeing to never breastfeed in public. But what exactly is a breastfeeding mother supposed to do if she can't feed her baby when she's out?

'Just feed it at home.' (Bob from Brighton says.)

Ah, OK. A very elegant solution. However, there is one tiny flaw with this argument – the natural physiology of breastfeeding.[31] As noted previously, breastfed infants feed very frequently. They also like a nice comfort feed and a rest, just like you and I like a nice cup of coffee and a slice of cake in a café. They're just joining in. And a mother who tries to ignore her baby's feeding cues is likely to end up with a baby who is inconsolable. Those who suggest that a breastfed baby can simply wait for a feed can never have met a breastfed baby. And they're presumably completely deaf. A breastfed baby denied a meal, when its mother's breasts are just inches away, will protest. Loudly. Do people seriously like the sound of screaming babies?

'Oh OK, just give it a bottle then.'

Many breastfed babies simply will not accept a bottle, particularly when close to their mother. Latching onto the breast and sucking milk from a bottle are two physiologically different actions and a breastfed baby often finds it very difficult to feed from a bottle. And anyway they miss the smell, taste and warmth of their mother's breast, and refuse to feed. Why should they have to have a bottle?

Even if a baby will accept a bottle of milk, many mothers would want to give expressed breastmilk in that bottle rather than formula. Unfortunately, expressing breastmilk can be a difficult and time-consuming process, with many finding they can only express a small amount.[32] And where are they going to find the time to express, and why should they? Would we really prefer women to be inconvenienced just so we don't have to think there might be a baby breastfeeding close to us?

'There's nothing wrong with using a bit of formula'

Not if this is what a woman genuinely wants, but she shouldn't have to make that choice based on others' views. And using formula alongside breastfeeding can decrease milk supply, as the body believes it is not needed, which increases the likelihood that a woman stops breastfeeding altogether. There is also the risk that the baby will decide a bottle is easier than having to put the effort into breastfeeding.[33] Moreover, if a woman skips a breastfeed to give formula milk, particularly in the presence of her baby, she is likely to experience painful engorgement, which increases the risk of infection or her milk being let down anyway. Do we really think that a mother being in physical pain and discomfort is worth it to spare the 'pain' of someone 'enduring' a baby being breastfed near them?

'In my day we just stayed at home – none of this feeding in public needed.'

Yes, mothers could stay at home all the time and become recluses until they become acceptable to the public again. But we know that isolation, exclusion and staying indoors all day makes postnatal depression more likely. It's already affecting growing numbers of women (and men). Should we condemn them to misery to spare the feelings of Joe Public?

Mothers who try to avoid breastfeeding in public stop breastfeeding sooner than those who manage it, because either the natural biological rhythm of milk production between her and her baby is damaged, or using formula seems a much easier solution. I guess this is what the objectors actually want: they see women stopping breastfeeding as their 'success' (obviously nobody has pointed out to them that the increased cost of treating illness in formula-fed babies comes from *their* taxes).

Is it not time for us to stand up, breastfeed 'ostentatiously' wherever we like, and put our politicians in the corner with a shawl over their head instead? In the words of Stephen Fry, if 'You're offended by that... well so f*****g what!'

ACTION 10

✓ Educate the public to stop being idiots, or at least do no harm.

15. A LACK OF PROTECTION FOR BREASTFEEDING WOMEN ON RETURN TO WORK

'Female MPs call for breastfeeding to be allowed in House of Commons.'

'Move may be 'ridiculously controversial' but it is necessary to get more women into parliament,' says Labour MP Jess Phillips.'

This was a headline in the *Guardian* newspaper in 2015. In the *Independent*, Simon Burns, a former transport minister, called it a controversial subject, stating:

> *'We have to be careful that, in pushing for a more realistic approach, we do not give the tabloid press the opportunity to ridicule us... I may be old-fashioned, but I share the view of the last-but-one Speaker of the House of Commons, Speaker Boothroyd, who... said that when she saw her checkout girl at Tesco's breastfeeding, she would allow it.'*

In April 2000, Julia Drown, a Labour MP for Swindon, asked for clarification about whether she would be allowed to breastfeed her baby in a committee room during a sitting of a Standing Committee. In a letter issued on behalf of the then Speaker, Betty Boothroyd, Sir Alan Haselhurst instructed that babies should not be taken into the Chamber or committee rooms, on the grounds that 'bringing refreshment into the [committee] room and the presence of persons other than members of the committee and specified officers and officials are prohibited'.

Would anyone like to help Simon (and indeed Betty) see the difference between breastfeeding in parliament and breastfeeding at a checkout? Not least the practicalities of scanning groceries and not accidentally packing the baby away with the shopping. And actually, perhaps parliament should be making changes. In response to Simon Burns's comment, newspapers reported the story of Tesco employee Victoria Williams, aged 25, who posted a photo of herself online, wearing her Tesco uniform and breastfeeding her son. The post went viral. Victoria explained that her 11-month-old son was ill and could not feed from a bottle. Her manager not only allowed her husband to bring her son to her at work to be breastfed, but also made her feel particularly supported in doing so, by providing her with a special feeding room and signs. Victoria wrote:

> 'I returned to work today and couldn't have asked for better managers. I chose a set time for my break and my husband brought my son to me. We were given a nice cosy office where the three of us sat and my manager made a poster for my door asking people not to disturb us. She also told me to take as long as I need, and make sure I have food and drink as well as just feeding my son. So many women dread going back to work while breastfeeding because companies can make it so difficult for breastfeeding mothers, but I couldn't be happier with the treatment I have received in my store on my first day. Well done, Tesco. Not only do we offer great customer service but you also train your managers to treat your staff the same way too. Loads of women who are still breastfeeding when they return to work get very upset and struggle to continue. I just think there are so many negative stories about breastfeeding, people getting told to cover up and take pictures down off things, so when it's something good we have to publicise it.'

Meanwhile, in Australia, where they are typically miles ahead of the UK in support and understanding of breastfeeding, politicians who are breastfeeding are allowed to bring their children into the chamber as part of new rules for a family-friendly parliament. And in New Zealand, everyone's crush Prime Minister Jacinda Ardern not only took her baby (and partner) into the chamber and breastfed, but also took her to the United Nations General Assembly in New York and breastfed at home while on live TV.

However, it is not just in parliament that women struggle to balance a career and breastfeeding. Helen Skelton, a TV presenter in the UK, recently discussed how difficult she found it to juggle her new role as a mother and attend meetings about work. She said: 'I breastfed Ernie in a production meeting in a sports news room full of a load of alpha males, who to be fair to them were brilliant about it.'

Women are clearly facing barriers everywhere about whether they can feed their baby in the workplace. Although perhaps the prize for the most bizarre exclusion has to be awarded to the organisers of a Scottish Government-led breastfeeding conference, who invited new mothers to the conference to hear their views on breastfeeding, then told them that babies were banned and there were no suitable facilities for breastfeeding at the venue! Ironically, the conference theme was 'Shifting the curve, sharing the challenge' – trying to understand how breastfeeding could be supported. Perhaps they should be looking closer to home to answer that one.

So what is going on? How does breastfeeding interfere with work anyway? Surely women with new babies aren't in the workplace? Actually, they are. Many new mothers return to their jobs within a few months of their baby being born for financial reasons or because they are concerned about the impact of having a baby on their career. In the UK we are fairly well protected by maternity leave laws. Mothers can remain on leave for a year after the birth, although only 9 months of this is paid, for many at a low rate. Unfortunately, it's usually the women with the least autonomy at work who have to go back early for financial reasons. In other countries such as the USA, paid maternity leave isn't mandatory, meaning that many mothers are back at work just weeks after having their baby. Concerns about having to go back to work and managing breastfeeding can stop some women from breastfeeding at all in the first place. So how the workplace deals with breastfeeding really matters.

How many new mothers are in the workforce?

The number of women with children who now remain in the workforce continues to rise. In the UK, around 38% of mothers aged 16–24 with a dependent child work, rising to 62% for those age 25–34 and 76% for those aged 35–49. Mothers who are single parents are less likely to work compared to those in a couple. Of mothers with a child under four, 41% of single mothers worked, compared to 78% of mothers in a couple. Of mothers with primary school-aged children the figures rose to 69% of single mothers and 84% of those in a couple. Lots of new mothers work. And as noted earlier, a third of new mothers are now the main wage-earner, meaning that they can't afford to give up work for a few years like many of their own mothers did.

Women often do go back to work during the first year. A recent NCT report showed that around 50% of women return to work when their baby is aged 6–9 months, with only around 6% going back before this time. Twelve months was also a popular time to return (15%), with only around 11% going back after this time. However, women from smaller organisations are more likely to return to work earlier. Conversely, in the USA most mothers who return to work after having a baby do so by the third month.[1] In the USA, where mandatory maternity leave does not exist, many women receive no paid leave at all, having to take sickness leave or holiday. In one study, a third of participants received no paid leave. By 9 months postpartum almost 60% of mothers have returned to work, 37% of them full-time.

Does work impact on breastfeeding?

Yes. Needing to return to work is a common reason for stopping breastfeeding – about a fifth of mothers in the UK who stop breastfeeding by four months give this reason, and it is the most common reason for stopping for those who stop breastfeeding between 4 and 6 months.[2] Stopping breastfeeding because of a need to return to work is reported in studies conducted in the USA, Spain, Singapore, Brazil and more.[3]

One large study of women in a health organisation in Australia found that although 98% breastfed at birth (suggesting high motivation), a quarter cited returning to work as the primary reason that they stopped breastfeeding. Nearly 60% of women had considered breastfeeding on return to work, but only 40% actually did so.[4]

If women go back to work early (before three months), they are less likely to continue breastfeeding. Women who go back at this point breastfeed on average for 4–5 weeks less than those who return later.[5] In the USA, women who received paid leave were more likely to start breastfeeding and still be breastfeeding at 6 months than those who were not. Longer paid maternity leave (in this case deemed to be over 12 weeks) was associated with a longer breastfeeding duration.[6]

However, there appears to be a dearth of high-quality routinely collected data on the number of women who breastfeed on return to work. I spent far more time than I should have trying to find this data, before concluding it probably didn't exist. Why? Because it's not deemed important? Because not many women do it? Because no one thinks about older babies being breastfed? Hausman declares this issue to be both political and feminist, suggesting that we should not simply be considering the health benefits of women continuing to breastfeed at work, but the importance of their personal experience of doing so.[7]

Why does returning to work affect breastfeeding?

This depends on what jobs mothers have, and how long they do them for. If they are full-time then they need to decide how they will carry on feeding. Will they leave work to feed their baby? This might be possible if there is childcare on site or close by, or if someone brings the baby to them. Otherwise they will need to express, so will need somewhere private to do that and a safe place to store the milk.

The problem comes when workplaces aren't set up to accommodate breastfeeding women, or don't feel that they should. Unfortunately, having to fight for their right to express or have breastfeeding breaks comes at a time when women are already under pressure; being a new mum, juggling caring for a baby and going back to work and dealing with getting back into their job. They may not have the energy, and they may not want to rock the boat.[8] Many new mothers worry that they will be judged on their productivity once they return from maternity leave, and feel colleagues are passing judgment when they leave on time, rather than working late. Is it any wonder, in this environment, that women don't want to push the issue of expressing? As one insightful paper worded its title 'taking the path of least resistance'.[9]

Furthermore, many women don't find expressing easy. Some women cannot express the volume of milk that they can give the baby when they feed directly from the breast. Some find they can hardly express any at all. For others it hurts – as we've seen, 15% of mothers have had a breast pump injury. It can also be time-consuming and yet another thing to fit in, when you're already trying to juggle motherhood with trying to give the impression that motherhood isn't affecting your ability to do your job.

Do employers need to consider breastfeeding?

In the UK, employer obligations around breastfeeding are a bit hazy. They are not allowed to refuse to support breastfeeding, but there are no requirements around what that support entails. They should make sure you have somewhere safe to rest, which should include a space to lie down. They also need to do a risk assessment to make sure that your environment is safe to work in.[10] There are guidelines that recommend a woman should have access to a private room to express milk (that isn't a toilet) and a fridge in which to store milk. However, these are guidelines and not laws and many employers do not follow them.[11]

Conversely, in the USA many states have issued legislation making it mandatory for employers to provide breaks for women to express, and breastfeeding rooms in which they can do so. However, what counts as a breastfeeding room can be quite creative: many women have posted photos online revealing the store cupboards with a chair they have been offered. One study showed that the vast majority of pregnant women or new mothers in one of four large public sector organisations were unsure of any employer policy or support for breastfeeding on return to work.[3]

Employers should realise that supporting breastfeeding is in their best interests. Studies from the USA, where companies often provide health insurance, show that breastfeeding can directly save the employer money. One study, which is now fairly old (so savings would be more today), showed that if babies were exclusively breastfed for three months the employer saved between $331 and $471 in healthcare expenditure per baby.[12] The US Breastfeeding Committee translated this into showing that for every dollar a company invested in supporting breastfeeding, they saved three dollars.[13]

For employers that don't directly fund healthcare, studies have shown that when mothers continue to breastfeed on their return to work they are less likely to take time off with a sick child. Other benefits to both employee and employer include increased morale, decreased staff turnover and increased retention of experienced employees.[14] In the USA legislation is in place to allow businesses to call themselves 'mother friendly' if they develop workplace policies to support breastfeeding, such as flexible work schedules, access to drinking water and private areas. Businesses designated mother friendly are more likely to retain women after pregnancy and recruit higher-quality staff. Stress levels are also lower and productivity higher.

In some ways, over the last few years we have seen a bit of an improvement in workplaces thinking about breastfeeding and how they can support it. The problem is that they don't always get it right. In 2020 I was asked to give a short presentation on women's experiences of breastfeeding and work for an exhibition in Cambridge, UK, on pre-conception, pregnancy, childbirth and care. As part of it I asked social media for some examples of how women had been treated helpfully or unhelpfully when breastfeeding and returning to work. Some of the 'almost but not quite' examples included being told to express in…

- … the toilet
- … a staffroom (with people eating their lunch)
- … a private room which had glass windows
- …a room with such thin walls the pump whirring could be heard everywhere

It is clear that many workplaces simply haven't encountered breastfeeding women, or had requests from mothers to express in the workplace. They try but just don't understand what is needed to support women.

What stops mothers from breastfeeding when they return to work?

Given the above you'd think all businesses would be looking at how they can support breastfeeding. Sadly, they're not. In one study in the USA, researchers examined breastfeeding support offered by 157 businesses. Most had little idea how breastfeeding could benefit the business, or why it might be important to support breastfeeding mothers.[15] Other studies showed that although employers would give the socially desirable answer that yes, they would support breastfeeding mothers, only a minority could state why.[16]

There is also the issue of breastfeeding being another 'elephant in the boardroom'. Employers may say that they support it... but they really don't want to think about it, or discuss the finer details. Yes, yes you can express breastmilk but please don't talk to me about breast pumps or milk storage. Some research suggests that workplaces are not only embarrassed by breastfeeding, but offended by it.[17] Feminist literature explores this idea further, suggesting that the female form, particularly in its nurturing and lactating state, is so far removed from the stereotypical male employee, that breastfeeding is perceived as offensive. Challenging these ingrained norms of how the typical employee looks and acts can be difficult for women.[18]

We will explore the concept of public revulsion at the very thought of breastmilk and breastfeeding in a later chapter, but it applies to breastfeeding in the workplace too. Once you start talking – and thinking – about breastfeeding, it raises the idea of 'bodily fluids' and the conscious or subconscious fear of contamination. Some go as far as to say that 'leaking bodily fluids', or breastfeeding, is viewed as a lack of control; after all, as adults we typically seek to limit or hide our 'leakages'. The fact that breasts are often labelled as sexual, rather than nurturing, adds another layer – a woman asking to leak sexual fluid around the workplace (and have time off to do it, of course) can be viewed negatively.[18] Others have suggested that some might make a further leap; the leaking of fluids can be seen as inconvenient and associated with illness and time off.[19]

This is nonsense, of course: breastfeeding is more akin to an employee bringing in sandwiches for lunch and storing them in the fridge than it is contamination, illness and lack of control. But I think for some, at least on a subconscious level, those feelings are there. Perhaps on a less emotionally deep level people simply associate breastfeeding with looking after babies and think that this is something that can be distracting from work.

Caroline Gatrell conducted a study exploring mothers' experiences of breastfeeding and their return to work. She focused on mothers with degree-level qualifications and professional roles, to examine the experiences of mothers who are typically the most motivated to breastfeed. Three of the 20 mothers she interviewed stopped breastfeeding before they returned to work, primarily because they could not face the thought of continuing to do so in the workplace. One quote she gives describes how women felt that they had to fit back into the male-dominated workplace, following the behaviour of the men in it:

> 'Breastfeeding? In school? Putting breastmilk in the staff fridge? You're joking. You can smell the testosterone when you walk in the door and you have to fit in, which obviously you can't do if you're breastfeeding.'

Notably, Gatrell discusses how among those who did continue to breastfeed, the sources of support they drew on tended to be outside the management of the organisation. The women looked to colleagues, friends and partners for informal and covert support. 'Covert' was a key word. The majority of women concealed their breastfeeding from those around them. Although some felt that their employer paid lip service to 'allowing' them to breastfeed, there was little support in terms of policies or facilities. Some reported that they were actively discouraged from breastfeeding, and were either subtly or directly told that they would not be allowed to express during work hours.[20]

I spoke to Dr Melanie Fraser, who recently completed her PhD exploring employers' experiences of supporting women to continue breastfeeding when they returned to work after their maternity leave.[21] One part of her work particularly struck me, in that employers were required to undertake risk assessments for women taking lactation breaks at work. Think about that for a moment – a woman continuing to breastfeed is considered risky, whereas not breastfeeding is not considered a risk. If an employer has to undertake a risk assessment for a woman to do something, does that increase the likelihood of them perceiving that behaviour in itself as risky? And that it should be discouraged in some way? And for a frazzled mum, returning to work while probably still being up in the night with a baby, does that risk assessment become just one more thing she has to do… or decide not to do? Melanie had a different take on this:

> 'Although it was not a part of my study, I was struck by the caring attitude of many of my participants (employers) towards all parents in the workplace. While I was concentrating on the situation facing breastfeeding women, it became apparent to me that managers were concerned to support all parents who are employees. The positive emotions associated with having a member of staff become a parent were balanced with a concern to promote the wellbeing and awareness of the stresses and strains of combining parenting and working, but therefore it seems to me that it would be appropriate for all parents to be able to access a risk assessment on their return to work.
>
> Fathers, adoptive parents and surrogate parents are all at risk of stress, fatigue, role adjustment issues and depression; all mothers may have birth injuries which impact upon their physiological health and mothers using an artificial breastmilk substitute face additional health risks. If the risks all parents are exposed to upon their return from maternity, paternity or adoption leave are addressed, one item to include within the risk assessment is the risk of early weaning. Managers would therefore be encouraged to assess and address the workplace factors that might encourage mothers to wean from breastfeeding earlier than they desire. Lactation breaks would therefore become a natural and normal part of the conversations concerning return to work.'

What works to support breastfeeding in the workplace?

Studies have explored the factors that help women to continue breastfeeding or expressing at work. Flexibility was a key factor in the Australian study above. Those who could have flexible working hours or flexible break times found expressing much easier. A minority (16%) were actually given paid lactation breaks, while 14% were allowed unpaid breaks. A private room also helped, although only 20% had access to a room designed for this purpose. Support was a further key variable; from both managers in the workplace and family and partner at home.[22]

Workplace interventions to make breastfeeding easier, such as breastfeeding rooms and breast pumps, led to women breastfeeding for longer.[23] In one intervention, companies offered breastfeeding classes during pregnancy and access to a breastfeeding consultant after birth. Almost 60% of mothers were breastfeeding at six months, despite returning to work on average at around 10 weeks.[24]

And if we really want to see what a difference a good breastfeeding policy can make, we just need to look to Kenya.[25] On realising more women were returning to work and having difficulties breastfeeding, the country changed the law. The Kenyan Breastfeeding Mothers bill enshrines in law a woman's right to breastfeed or express breastmilk at her work place. But they don't just pay lip service to this – they actually insist that every workplace has a lactation place to ensure this works. This includes a space that is:

- Shielded from view and free from intrusion from co-workers
- Clean, quiet, private and warm
- Not a bathroom or toilet

And has:

- A lockable door
- A wash basin
- A fridge for storing expressed milk
- A provision for an electric outlet and lighting
- A chair, table and a clean space to store equipment

Alongside this the employer also has to make sure the environment is safe for a baby and provide daily nutritionally balanced meals and snacks. They need to provide breaks up to 40 minutes in every four hours, longer with a medical note. Best bit? They're serious about this. If they don't comply with this they can get a fine of up to 500,000 shillings or go to jail for a year. Or both. Compare that to the cupboards, toilets and other random places where women in the UK have been asked to breastfeed.

So many breastfeeding mothers are also working mothers, who know that when the time comes to return to work they are going to need to juggle breastfeeding and work, or stop breastfeeding. For many the challenges seem too big, especially in the early months when they will have to express very regularly in order to get enough for their baby. Later, once the baby is also taking solid food, this requirement can drop, but some still find it very difficult. Others don't even start breastfeeding because they know they'll have to go back to work soon. If workplaces were better set up to accommodate breastfeeding, everyone – workplaces, society, mothers, babies – would benefit. So why can't we make this leap?

Action 11

✓ Support employers to be breastfeeding friendly.

16. INDUSTRY INFLUENCES ARE ALLOWED TO SPREAD INACCURATE MESSAGING

Since its invention commercial formula has been marketed to professionals and parents as a breastmilk substitute. At its peak in the 1950s, advertising of formula centred on the concept of 'science over nature', and aimed to show how a product designed for your infant must be far superior to what a woman's body could naturally produce. Parenting advice at this time generally focused on the idea that scientific advancements were best for babies, and that 'good' mothers would want 'the best'. Formula was promoted as an elite substance that the best parents would buy, and it was suggested that mothers who didn't use formula were uneducated, old-fashioned and even of a lower class.

We now know much more about the differences between breastmilk and formula, and that formula will never be 'close' to breastmilk. However, the formula milk market is currently the fastest-growing market in the healthy/functional foods category (energy drinks and probiotic drinks come next). In 1987 sales of milk formula were around 2 billion US dollars. By 2013 this was 40 billion. By 2019 it was 50 billion. Remember a billion is one thousand million. And that's nothing compared to its forecast growth – it's predicted to surpass 109 billion by 2027. These sales are made up of infant formula (39%), follow-on formula (25%), toddler milks (25%) and then specialist milks, such as those for low birth weight babies (11%). Half of this worldwide market is dominated by four companies: Nestlé, Danone, Mead Johnson and Abbott.[1]

What is particularly concerning is that the market is growing fastest in low-income countries in recent years. In 2018 Save the Children published their 'Don't push it' report, highlighting the extent to which industry was rapidly increasing sales in regions such as China, India, Indonesia, Mexico and Nigeria. Notably those countries attribute 236,000 child deaths a year to inadequate breastfeeding.[2]

China now makes up one-third of all global formula milk sales. Add in India and these two regions account for over half of global sales. This is attributed to the ending of the one-child policy in China, a growth in household income and urbanisation and marketing...

basically marketing then. To put this in context, the USA (the world's second largest market) accounts for only 11% of formula sales, down from 17% in 2010.[2]

In developing countries increasing sales of formula milk mean poorer health for babies.[2] The industry meanwhile thinks this is brilliant. A recent article from *Dairy Reporter* titled 'New market potential: huge growth opportunities for infant formula in China's lower tier cities' crowed about how innovative advertising campaigns were increasing sales in these 'lower tier' – so lower income – regions. The very areas where babies can least afford to be formula-fed.[3]

Advertising to grow sales costs the formula companies money. A lot of money. The latest estimates suggest that they spend around 6 billion US dollars per year – or in other words around 10–15% of overall profit – on advertising. One review points out that the amount spent on advertising in the UK is 10 times what the US government spends on promoting breastfeeding. Even more worryingly, companies are seeing the growth in sales in low-income countries and responding to it, in a cycle of continued advertising to increase profits.[4] Others have suggested that for every $30 advertisers spend on formula milk promotion, the US government spends 21 cents promoting breastfeeding.[5] These costs are passed onto parents through increased product prices.

Certain areas in low and middle income countries are often seen as 'untapped markets', or in other words breastfeeding is the norm so there's a lot of potential to disrupt that. In one of these regions, Myanmar, companies spent $480,000 on marketing in the first six months of 2015 alone. The report talks about how mothers are now seeing formula milk as better compared to breastfeeding and how everyone else is feeding their baby. Likewise, in Cambodia, two companies alone spent $34 million between them promoting products – 60 times more than the government spends on promoting breastfeeding.[2] And in 2013, 34 million US dollars was spent on advertising in Vietnam, compared to just 15 million US dollars in the USA. This was 61 times the amount the Vietnamese government spent on promoting breastfeeding.[4]

The WHO Code

You'd certainly be forgiven for thinking that formula companies were allowed to promote their infant formula to parents. However, they're not. In 1981, the World Health Organisation launched the

International Code of Marketing of Breastmilk Substitutes, which banned the promotion of breastmilk substitutes for babies under six months old. The Code was based on the knowledge that:

> *'inappropriate feeding practices lead to infant malnutrition, morbidity and mortality in all countries and that improper practice in the marketing of breastmilk substitutes and related products can contribute to this major public health problem.'*

The Code aims to contribute to

> *'the provision of safe and adequate nutrition for infants, by the protection and promotion of breastfeeding, and by ensuring the proper use of breastmilk substitutes, when these are necessary, on the basis of adequate information and through appropriate marketing and distribution.'*

The WHO urged governments across the world to enforce the Code, stating that:

> *'Governments should have the responsibility to ensure that objective and consistent information is provided on infant and young child feeding for use by families and those involved in the field of infant and young child nutrition.'*

The Code recognises that sometimes babies will need to receive infant formula and says that 'if babies are not breastfed, for whatever reason, the Code also advocates that they be fed safely on the best available nutritional alternative. Breastmilk substitutes should be available when needed but not be promoted.[6] According to the Code, companies:

- Must not advertise infant formula
- Must not use money off deals etc.
- Must not use promotional stands etc.
- Must not give free samples
- Must not seek contact with pregnant women
- Must ensure that any educational information states the superiority of breastfeeding
- Must not donate unless asked to do so – and only as long as is needed.

The drafters of the Code also went further and included rules for how companies were allowed to package their products. Companies must not idealise their product or use pictures of babies on the packaging. They must not claim that formula is better than breastmilk. Any claims they make must be factual and scientific. Rules on how follow-on formula, designed for babies over the age of six months (in the UK), can be promoted were also included in WHA Resolutions that have been added to the original Code over the years. (Follow-on formula is an interesting example of a product that exists purely to get around marketing restrictions. In the UK advertising restrictions apply to infant formula for the first six months, so manufacturers created 'follow-on' milk for babies over six months. In countries where marketing restrictions apply to all formula for the first year or two of life, or where there are no marketing restrictions, follow-on formula simply does not exist.) For follow-on milk:

- Adverts must not feature babies under six months old.
- There must be no risk of confusion between infant formula and follow-on formula.
- It is illegal to use advertising that makes direct comparisons between formula milk and breastmilk.
- It is illegal to blur the distinction between infant and follow-on formula in the promotion and labelling of formula.
- Advertising of follow-on formula should not discourage breastfeeding or compare follow-on formula to breastmilk.

In Europe some of the provisions of the WHO Code were adopted into the Infant Formula and Follow-on Regulations (2007) which determine what can be promoted and how.[7] Currently in the UK we follow these regulations. In these regulations, pictures and graphics on packaging must not idealise the product. This included:

- Pictures of infants, young children or carers
- Graphics that represent nursing mothers/pregnant women
- Pictures or text which imply that infant health, happiness or wellbeing, or the health, happiness and wellbeing of carers, is associated with infant formula
- References to infant's or carer's emotions
- Baby or child-related subjects
- Non-mandatory pictures or text which refers, directly or indirectly, to 'the ideal method' of infant feeding

Specific requirements are also made for follow-on formulas, including:

'Manufacturers must ensure that infant formula and follow-on formula are labelled in such a way that it enables consumers to make a clear distinction between infant formula and follow-on formula so as to avoid any risk of confusion.'

This includes making sure the term 'follow-on formula' is clearly featured on the packaging, in a font size no smaller than the brand name. Information on the labels should also state that the products are different. The colour scheme on infant formula packaging should also be completely different to that on the follow-on formula packaging (different shades is not OK). Finally, references to breastfeeding or breastmilk should not be made on packaging, as people might associate these words with feeding babies from birth... and follow-on formula should only be used from six months.

The reality

This all sounds tightly regulated, doesn't it? However, the Code itself is not legally binding. It is not a law, but a recommendation to Member States, which are expected to adhere to the aim and spirit of the Code and 'to take action to give effect to the principles and aim of this Code, as appropriate to their social and legislative framework, including the adoption of national legislation, regulation or other suitable measures'. In other words, every country should make their own laws to ensure the Code is adhered to.

A status report of Code implementation in 2018–2020 showed improvements in how many countries have, or have not, adopted the Code in their national legislation. Overall 44 countries had strengthened their recommendations since the last report. As of April 2020, 136 out of 194 WHO member states (70%) had legal measures to implement the Code. Out of those 25 were considered to have substantial alignment and 42 moderate alignment. The rest had 'some' provisions. Typically this means that countries may have legislation for some aspects e.g. prevent promotion of infant milks in healthcare facilities (79/194) but not others e.g. prohibiting educational material from industry (24/194). The regions with the best implementation are the Americas, Africa and south-east Asia, although substantial variation is seen within regions too.[8]

Although the WHO Code recommends that, even in the absence of national legislation, companies should adhere to the Code, some formula companies routinely break the Code and governments don't stop them. In 2010, 500 violations were documented across 46 countries. And those are just the ones that were reported and documented.[9] In developing countries many may be unaware of the Code and break it unknowingly. A survey of health professionals in Pakistan found that 80% were unaware of the Code, with 70% breaking it without realising.[10] Some governments have actively tried to prevent the Code from being introduced, perhaps because of the financial influence of multinational companies. In the Philippines the government was blocked from implementing its own legislation to enact the Code due to pressure from the industry.[11]

Some developed countries have either not adopted the Code, or allow violations of it. The USA – which did not sign up to the Code in 1981 when it was overwhelmingly approved by the World Health Organization – does little to regulate formula marketing. Studies from the USA find that free infant formula is considered a normal part of a hospital discharge pack, with one study finding that 91% of hospitals gave out free infant formula in a sponsored hospital discharge pack.[12] Another study found that 81% of mothers in a national survey reported having free formula in their discharge pack.[13] A further 55% of mothers reported receiving free formula in the mail.[14]

Ways in which companies get around the Code

The UK has enacted some aspects of the WHO Code. For example, it forbids advertising of breastmilk substitutes for infants under six months old, but this doesn't include food or products for babies over six months old. This means numerous loopholes remain, while mechanisms for monitoring and penalising infringements are far from robust. Here are some of the most common ways companies work around the Code to reach new families.

1. Advertising follow-on milk

The World Health Organization and UK Department of Health state that any infant milk other than infant formula suitable for 0–12 months is an unnecessary product. Follow-on formula differs slightly in composition to infant formula, but is essentially the same due to current compositional regulations for energy and nutrients (apart from iron). Babies can stay on infant formula until 12 months old when they can then move to cows' milk. There is no need for any other type of infant formula.[15]

However, under current EU law (which we follow at the time of writing in the UK), marketing of follow-on and toddler milks is allowed.[7] There is the possibility that we may be able to change this post-Brexit (I know, I know, let me have hope!). This ability to advertise follow-on formula basically acts as a gateway to advertise infant formula. Given that it is an unnecessary product which is pretty similar in content, it basically exists as a marketing tool.

And boy does it work.

The number of adverts for follow-on formula and toddler milks is closely tied to advertising laws. In the US, where infant formula advertising is allowed, adverts for other infant milks make up just 20% of adverts as there is not the same 'need' to promote these products.[16] Another study in Australia showed how regulations affect marketing. Researchers tracked the number of breastmilk substitute adverts that appeared between 1950 and 2010, looking at advertising before and after a voluntary agreement to not advertise infant milks for babies 0–12 months was put in place. Once the agreement came in, they saw a big increase in adverts for follow-on and toddler milks instead.[17]

Why? Because companies know that branding, and exposure to similar products, can enhance the sales of other products in that range. Brand advertising works; studies of other products have shown an increase in sales for a non-advertised but brand-related product when just one item is advertised.[18] People are also more likely to buy a product they have recently seen advertised, even though they have no memory of seeing that advert.[19] And mothers who report seeing formula adverts on TV are more likely to formula-feed.[20]

And it's working. Research from around the world shows how viewers often perceive these adverts for follow-on or toddler milks to be for infant formula suitable for younger babies. Studies in both Australia[21] and Italy[22] have found that pregnant and new mothers are regularly exposed to these adverts and frequently misinterpret adverts for follow-on formula to be adverts for infant formula. Likewise, in a recent research project we conducted for First Steps Nutrition Trust, exploring parents' views and experience of infant formula advertising, we found that two-thirds believed they had seen an advert for infant formula aimed at babies under six months. We know that this cannot be true due to advertising regulations: they had seen adverts for follow-on formula or toddler milks and perceived them to be for infant formula.[23]

Despite the Code's stipulation that packaging for follow-on milk should not be the same colour as infant milk, if you look at tins of formula and follow-on milk you will find that they are virtually identical, apart from the 'number'. The shape of the package and the graphics are often very similar, with a large focus on the brand name. Confidence in the brand is recognised and transferred from product to product. Many consumers cannot tell the difference between products in the range.[24]

The companies know that parents often don't know, or can't tell, the difference between follow-on milk and infant formula. This enables them to use the tricks that are banned in relation to infant formula to sell their follow-on product (and the infant milk by extension). For example, emotion is a key factor. One particular advert plays on a number of emotions, showing footage of a thoughtful father carefully making up a night feed while his partner sleeps soundly. The voiceover is him reading her a poem:

'I promise not to pretend I'm asleep when our baby wakes at 3am, or 4am, or 5am.

I promise never to say "my mother thinks you're holding the baby wrong"

I promise not to mention that sometimes when I kiss your beautiful neck it smells of perfume and baby sick.

I promise not to join in when any of my mates sing the theme tune from the Omen, although it is quite funny.

I promise to do at least my fair share of nappy changing and night feeding.

I promise to tell you often, how proud I am of you, and how you've made me the happiest dad on the planet. All this I pledge without any pressure from you, my lovely lovely missus.'

Awww, how sweet. However, the messages, both blatant and more subtle, are very carefully calculated. The father is shown happily making up night feeds while the mother sleeps (hmm – does that happen much in your house? Infant Feeding Survey data shows that even when babies are bottle-fed formula, mothers still do most of the feeding, suggesting that dads are paying lip-service to wanting to be involved in feeding). The poem refers to a number of things that apply to younger babies: the suggestion that there will be many night feeds and nappies to change at night, that she could be holding the baby wrong, that the baby wakes every hour. Many people watching might think this is an advert for infant formula. Feeding formula during the night is often associated with younger babies. The baby in the advert is suspiciously young-looking. Maybe they are technically six months old. The cynic in me wonders if there is a particular market in formula advertising opportunities for babies who are older than six months but look young.

Another advert plays on new parents' anxieties, exacerbating that feeling that you don't know what you're doing, and that you need an expert to help you:

'You have no experience but the job is still yours...
You learn as you go... doing whatever it takes
At SMA our follow-on milk... over the years we've really got to know mums and take it from us, you're doing great.'

Others more directly highlight fears about breastfeeding, while supposedly supporting it. One Cow & Gate advert showed a mother holding her baby and laughing, with the catchphrase: 'I'm thinking of getting a t shirt made – Danger! Sore boobs!' Humour is also often employed in advertising, but it comes with a bite – a not-so-subtle reminder of how much mothers have given up (and shouldn't they get dad to do something now, like the feeding?) 'You gave up your career, your social life and your figure. Then came baby's first word. Dada.' Others directly have a dig at breastfeeding promotion messages. One advert features a series of babies laughing, followed by captions such as 'Do I look as if my tummy is unhappy?' and 'Do I look like my diet's incomplete?'

And then we have the adverts that are barely about infant feeding at all. US formula company Similac (note the suggestion in the name that this milk is similar to breastmilk) produced an advert called the 'Sisterhood of Motherhood' in 2015 that went on to win awards. It was based around the concept of the 'mummy wars' and featured groups of different parents in a park basically having some kind of verbal fight about who is best. You had parents who were babywearers, who were breastfeeding, stay-at-home mothers versus those with prams, some who were bottle-feeding and some who had gone back to work. You get the picture – it was having a dig at this notion of different camps (which don't really exist outside of advertising).

Anyway, long story short – they're all arguing but then someone lets go of their baby's pram and it starts rolling down a hill. They all chase after it, catch it before something goes wrong and then realise what really matters. How you care for your baby? Doesn't matter as long as they are alive and happy. This includes how you feed your baby. Followed by a big logo and slogan for Similac.

It's a really emotive advert. By emotive I mean it brings a tear to the eye of those who don't realise what is going on, and deep rage to those who do. It's designed to stir up emotions, tell parents that things like how babies are fed aren't really that important, and advertise the product and company as the one that really cares about parents. If you can ignore the fact that it's trying to sway parents' decisions in order to fill the company's pockets, then it's a really clever advert. No wonder it won awards.

At this point many people will turn around and say '*Well this advertising doesn't affect me!*'. Maybe it doesn't. But it's certainly affecting someone out there, because otherwise the companies wouldn't put as much money and effort as they do into promoting their products. Other people will point out that advertising is everywhere, so why is this any different? Well, because it's about the nutrition of our most vulnerable population. What babies eat matters. When they can't be breastfed they must have infant formula. And it's all that they are eating. I really don't think this should be affected by the tricks companies use to try and promote their products.

Companies employ many tricks around additional ingredients and their implied impact on things like sleep, development or behaviour. Slogans, information or implied imagery can lead parents to think there are added benefits of buying one milk over another. One study in the US found that at least half of the 173 adverts they examined contained a statement around a specific benefit for health such as brain development, vision or the immune system.[25] In a similar study of websites that advertised formula in Australia, all had at least one health claim, with three-quarters also having a nutritional content claim such as having an added ingredient. Another common claim is that specific formulas reduce colic or other gastrointestinal symptoms, despite no evidence this is true.[26]

There are two issues here. One is that there are concerns that adding in too many additional ingredients could actually be a bad thing, overloading the infant's digestive system or worse, putting them at risk of illness.[27] High iron content, for example, is a worry. Infant formula has higher levels of iron in it than breastmilk anyway because less of it is absorbed. Parents often think 'more' is a good thing. However unabsorbed iron is a breeding ground for bacteria. Too much iron is actually not a good idea at all.[28]

Second, there is usually no evidence that these added ingredients work. If an added ingredient was found to have a positive impact, then it would have to be added in to all infant formulas under law.[29] You can't just go around adding loads of things to infant formula as it is better regulated. Many companies, however, are adding things to follow-on formula with no evidence that they work. This is another reason why sticking with infant formula is important. For example, claims made for Danone's 'Immunofortis' prebiotic ingredient were rejected by the European Food Standards Agency, which stated that there was insufficient evidence that it enhanced a baby's immune system as the company claimed. No independent scientific committee in the UK has agreed that there is any benefit from adding prebiotics (GOS/FOS) to infant formula.[30]

Parents often see these added ingredients and think a) they must be a good idea and b) they work. However, a recent paper in the *British Medical Journal* demonstrated that health claims made for infant formula can be misleading. Likewise, analyses of adverts for a range of infant milks have shown that many of the promotional claims and statements made are based on inadequate or misleading data.[31]

Another tactic is to use a 'probabiological' approach by making reference to a beneficial component found in breastmilk, e.g. prebiotics and then following that statement by referring to unspecified prebiotics in the formula product[32] – despite no clear evidence that the synthetic version is beneficial to health.[33] The use of 'human milk oligosaccharides' is a good example of this. Some perceived this synthetic ingredient to have come from human milk. The term was not allowed to be used under EU law, but due to a lack of stringent regulation, companies got away with using it for a while, meaning it became a commonly understood term. Companies are now using the acronym HMO, knowing people understand what it means and will buy the product anyway. Despite the minor issue that *even if* these HMOs were somehow beneficial, they've only managed to add a few to infant milk and not the 200+ that women produce in breastmilk (which vary in combination based on a mother's environment).[34]

This messaging works. Recent research with parents in the USA found over half believed that certain infant formulas are better for babies' digestion and brain development than breastmilk, with nearly two-thirds believing infant formula could deliver nutrition not found in breastmilk. Those who believed the claims were more likely to purchase infant milk products.[35] Likewise, in our recent research, when asked why they bought a specific product, many parents listed added ingredients or impact upon health or development. This was particularly true for those using follow-on products.[23]

Linked to all of this is the issue of price. A common marketing technique is 'increased value perception' – where customers perceive a higher-cost product to be better quality. All infant formula milks are very similar in content – as noted above, if a novel ingredient was found to be beneficial it would have to be added to all by law. All follow-on formulas are pretty similar bar those additional ingredients that have not been proven to be beneficial. The obvious question then arises – why on earth are formula milks such different prices? Some of the most expensive infant formula milks are up to two or three times the price of the cheapest. For example, based on 2020 current costs, the most expensive branded cows' milk powdered formula costs on average £16.74 a week compared to just £6.44 a week for the least expensive supermarket version.[36]

This matters. In our research we found that some parents were buying the most expensive milk because they believed it was better, while others were worried that they could not afford the most expensive ones. Some were buying more expensive milks and going without other things.[23] Indeed, in the Channel 4 programme "The Great Formula Milk Scandal' it was highlighted how some parents on a low income were struggling to afford formula for their baby, leading them to sometimes water down feeds, placing their baby at nutritional risk. The perception that more expensive formula was more advanced and better for their infant was in part driving this.[37]

On a final note, these adverts are now absolutely everywhere. Whereas they used to just crop up on TV and in magazines, some recent research we did has shown that they now seem to be all over the place. Women reported seeing them in magazines that had nothing to do with babies, on bus stops and in the cinema before children's films. There is also a growing targeting of mothers on social media, particularly during the recent COVID-19 lockdown when we found that a lot of women were struggling to get the breastfeeding support they needed.[38] Industry decided to set themselves up as breastfeeding specialists, advertising this to women on Facebook in particular. The problem was that this information was not always accurate or scaremongered about either COVID-19 or things like needing to eat a really balanced diet to make breastmilk.[39] We also saw specific targeting of breastfeeding mothers by companies with paid adverts.

When women clicked on 'why am I seeing this ad' the information said 'because you have an interest in breastfeeding'. It is against the WHO Code to deliberately target families, including on social media.

2. 'Supporting' pregnant women and new mothers

Most of the formula companies have a sideline in 'supporting' pregnant women and even running free breastfeeding helplines. How very benevolent of them! Of course they want to solve your breastfeeding problem and help you breastfeed for longer.

By supporting pregnancy in general companies are able to market their brand to expectant parents. And they use very persuasive techniques. Free branded gifts. A changing mat. A sunshade for the car. Nothing to do with milk whatsoever! Apart from the fact that their brand is there, in your everyday life. Free cuddly toy? An Aptamil polar bear? Or the Cow & Gate cow? For a few pennies they have given women something their baby carries around with them all the time. This also has the added benefit of the company being seen as the formula company which was helpful and 'cared'. Research has shown that if families who receive these free gifts or support go on to use formula milk then they are more likely to use this brand in future; the relationship foundations have been built and nurtured without ever directly promoting formula.[40]

Disaster situations across the globe give companies the perfect opportunity to step in and donate their product for free, in a seemingly generous way. We are also seeing an increase in donations of formula to food banks in the UK.[41] What should happen, in line with every global health policy in existence, is that mothers should be supported to carry on breastfeeding through disasters. The WHO Code states that 'for the majority of infants and young children in emergency situations, the emphasis should be on protecting, promoting and supporting breastfeeding'. However, companies see an opportunity to appear benevolent, while splashing their brand advertising everywhere.

Formula donations in these situations can be deadly.[42] While breastfed infants have continued access to the milk they need, alongside the protective immune factors of the milk and comfort of feeding, bottle-feeding carries an increased risk of unsafe preparation and infection in emergency situations. On a surface level a formula donation might seem like an obvious way to help, but actually undermining breastfeeding is the complete opposite of what needs to happen. Women need skilled breastfeeding support not breastmilk substitutes. Even in lesser emergency situations like using a food bank, staff do not have time or training to ensure appropriate products are given. Women who need formula should be directed to their health visitor, not a food bank.[43]

The companies are acting cynically when they donate formula. They know that when someone acts in a supposedly kind or benevolent way, others naturally make wider assumptions about them. They must want the best for babies and mothers, right? Or they wouldn't be helping. They're the kind and thoughtful formula company. When I move to formula… Oh, wait…

3. Targeting health professionals

In the UK (and elsewhere) the Baby Friendly Initiative has meant that companies can't access health professionals as easily as they once could. Companies used to give guest lectures or bribes through free social events. Now they have to come up with new and inventive ways to reach professionals and one of these is the funded study day. They know health boards don't have lots of money for training and to send staff to conferences, so they do it for free, just to keep those staff up to date and trained. (It's part of their kind and caring nature, see above).

These study days are often about something other than formula milk. They often seem to be about promoting infant health, or tackling obesity, or some other public health message. It might be about infant growth, allergies or wider wellbeing. Companies invite (and pay) experts to talk at these events, which gives them further credit, by 'reputation transfer'. Often these events are mistaken for academic or professional conferences. Formula milk is not discussed, but freebies from the event are branded with the formula company name and participants often sign up to mailing lists for further updates, without realising who they are giving their details to. Participants network with individuals. Companies will also buy space at academic conferences. Many paediatric conferences are sponsored, or have sponsored information stalls in an accompanying exhibition.[44]

However, 'there's no such thing as a free lunch', and the only reason formula companies get behind these events is that they know they will influence professionals. Some may see through this, and are hardened to their tactics, but the continued existence of the events tells us that some professionals go along to them. Some professionals may believe in the fake benevolence of these companies, believing that they want the best for infant nutrition and viewing them as experts. Others may feel indebted to the organisers, either consciously or subconsciously, because they value professional training which they may not normally be able to access.

If a mother sees that her healthcare professional has a branded pen or due date calculator, she may assume that the health professional endorses that brand. Subconsciously that brand is then embedded in her mind, and it may surface later when she comes to buy formula. We know this happens. In our recent research some women described how health professionals recommended specific brands of formula to them, or felt that brands were being endorsed in healthcare facilities.[23] Formula companies are also very aware of the benefits of being accepted and promoted by healthcare workers, seeing it as a means of endorsement and 'sanitising' of their brand.[40]

In countries without strict regulation of their activities, companies directly promote their products to health professionals and offer financial incentives for them to promote their products to mothers. A study in Pakistan found that over 40% of new mothers had their GP recommend formula to them.[45] In China this led to some health professionals violating privacy agreements and essentially selling new parents' details to the companies.[46]

UNICEF publishes guidance for health workers about conflicts of interest at study days provided by companies, which says: *Any health professional considering attending such a day, should ask themselves:*

- Whether attendance is really necessary for their education
- Whether it is compatible with their Code of Conduct and responsibilities to implement best practice
- How their attendance will reflect on their employing institution and its stated values
- Whether their name could be used to enhance the name and reputation of the formula company
- What effect their attendance could have on the families they serve.

If a decision is made to attend, the health professional should be highly aware of the true purpose of the day and make every effort to ensure that their attendance does not compromise the content, emphasis or tone of information imparted to parents.[47]

On a positive note, there have been great moves by some medical institutions and bodies to distance themselves from formula advertising. In 2019 the *BMJ* publicly announced that it would no longer be taking formula adverts despite losing £300,000 of advertising revenue.[48] The Royal College of Pediatrics and Child Health shortly followed, stating it would no longer take advertising revenue or funding from the formula industry.[49]

4. New markets of specialist formula milks

Another tactic closely related to relationships with health professionals is the rapidly increasing market for specialist formula milks available on prescription only. One of the most commonly promoted products is for cows' milk protein allergy (CMPA). Sales of this product have risen at a rate far higher than any natural increase in actual CMPA could occur – up nearly 500% between 2006 and 2016.[50] This means the NHS spends over £60 million annually in prescriptions for these products.[51] Meanwhile data on CMPA suggests nothing like the rise in cases this increase in sales should suggest.[52]

What is also suspicious is who is involved in the development of CMPA guidelines.[53] There are guidelines literally funded by industry and many of the authors across the guidelines have declared they have relationships (funding, speaking, research, etc) with the formula industry. Likewise, Allergy UK, which is a charity which provides information on allergy including CMPA, is partnered with Danone Nutricia. Other allergy websites have similar partnerships with industry. Many of these charities and organisations run training for health professionals on CMPA – events and training which are often sponsored by the formula industry.

One of the major issues is how many parents are worrying that their baby has CMPA and are subsequently receiving diagnoses from their GP (often with very little testing). If you have a look on some of the CMPA websites the problem is that many of the symptoms listed as being signs of CMPA can overlap with normal baby behaviour, such as being fussy and unsettled. Websites often give advice on how to exclude dairy from your own diet, which is a considerable undertaking and can seem unachievable. Formula – and free prescription formula at that – seems an appealing option.

5. Help from others, particularly on social media

The formula industry is sadly not alone in its marketing techniques. It has long relied on a variety of other organisations and celebrities to boost its reach. In terms of other companies, a common tactic appears to be to advertise and promote products that are related to formula-feeding rather than the formula milk itself, therefore cleverly getting around UK/EU law. Although the WHO Code states that things like bottles and teats should not be promoted, this hasn't been adopted into law, meaning companies can get away with it. These adverts boost the sales of the product but also work as brand advertising.

A really common marketing method appears to be to promote formula preparation machines, particularly the Tommee Tippee Perfect Prep machine. These machines, which act a bit like a coffee machine where you put in powder and water and a bottle of formula is produced, are increasingly common. In our recent research over half of parents who used formula milk reported using one of these machines. Aside from promoting a brand, these machines have safety concerns based on how hot the water is when it is mixed with the formula. It is important that water is at least 70 degrees to kill any pathogens in the formula powder but it is not clear that this machine does this.[54]

Promotion of this machine seems to be everywhere. During Breastfeeding Celebration Week in 2015, Babies R Us tweeted 'We know this week is National Breastfeeding Week but we also know that there are lots of parents out there that bottle-feed. Whatever your circumstances, we cannot recommend the Tommee Tippee Perfect Prep Machine enough'. In 2020, Tommee Tippee put on a breastfeeding event during World Breastfeeding Week, promoting all its products. It stole the title of the event from a long-standing breastfeeding celebration event in Northern Ireland – Breastival. The company also benefit from numerous celebrities and health professionals promoting the product including Mrs Hinch of house cleaning fame with 2.6 million Instagram followers.

Indeed, Instagram appears to be the place to promote follow-on formula milks. You can find many a celebrity posing with their box of formula milk in strange places, as if it just happens to be in their photo. Others have paid partnerships, tagging products or using hashtags. Sometimes these are pulled up. In 2018 watchdog OFCOM actually deemed Fern McCann's reality TV show breached guidelines through 'undue prominence to a baby formula milk' in the programme, or in other words she kept talking about it and placing it in shots.[55]

You then have celebrities who directly talk about how they love formula-feeding and brands. Famously in 2007, Jordan (Katie Price), the former glamour model, posed in a huge feature in *OK* magazine with her three-week-old daughter. She just happened to be feeding her in many of the shots, with a ready-made bottle of SMA, label clearly towards the camera. In an accompanying interview she said:

Interviewer: *Are you breastfeeding Katie?*
Jordan: *No. It's brilliant. I have 20 crates of teats and bottles – I don't have*

to sterilise or heat anything, you literally take the teat out of the pack, screw it on, throw it away. I don't care what people say – you don't have to breastfeed. They gave me a tablet that dries your milk so my boobs haven't leaked or anything.'
Pete adds: *Junior didn't breastfeed and he's turned out fine.*
Interviewer: *So why did you decide not to breastfeed?*
Jordan: *I don't want a baby drinking from me. The thought of it makes me feel really funny. I think only a certain person could handle my knockers.*

Incidentally, Pete seems to have changed his mind: when he had a baby with his new girlfriend Emily, who breastfed, he announced 'it's such an amazing thing and it has so many benefits.'

Industry also forms all sorts of other partnerships with the aim of promoting its reputation. These can include health organisations and charities. For example, the British Dietetic Association's corporate members include Danone, Abbott and Nestlé, while the British Nutrition Foundation partner with Nestlé and Danone too. They also reach other charity organisations. For example, the children's charity Barnardos has a long-standing relationship with Danone, which sponsors their 'Big Toddle' event for families. CEO Suzanne Connolly states that they simply sponsor the event and don't provide any products and therefore it is not an endorsement. However, we know that simply by association Danone will increase sales through brand advertising and by being seen to be a kind, caring company which is simply helping out vulnerable children and families.[56]

6. Investment in breastfeeding research

As mentioned previously in this book, there is an increasing tendency for the formula industry to fund research into breastfeeding. If you look carefully, many studies looking at outcomes of infant feeding or guideline development groups are closely linked to industry or involve scientists who have previously had funding from industry. This is problematic on all sorts of levels.

Firstly, we know that when industry funds research, the findings are more likely to be in favour of the industry than if the research was conducted by someone independent. One study found that out of 168 studies published by the food and drinks industry, 156 of them had findings that benefited the funder. One reason for this is that industry can own the findings and only allow publication if they are beneficial for them, so they can hide any findings that don't support their product. It may also be that researchers, needing funding and publication to advance their career, subtly end up influencing the findings towards that company.

When researchers have received funding from industry they should clearly state that they hold this conflict of interest, especially if writing about breastfeeding, formula-feeding or starting solid foods. However, often this simply doesn't happen or is inaccurate. One of the most horrifying examples I have ever seen is in a position paper about recommendations for follow-on formula milk, where the international group who wrote the paper pretty much came down in favour of it.[57] On this paper they have a clear conflict of interest statement that says:

'None of the authors reports a conflict of interest which would represent "a set of circumstances that creates a risk that professional judgment or actions regarding a primary interest will be unduly influenced by a secondary interest", as defined by the US Institute of Medicine'

But there in black and white, right next to those words, is the following (initials represent author names):

- Z.A.B. has received support as a member of the Nestlé Nutrition Institute advisory board advising on nutrition priorities and educational activities.
- W.C. has received support from Danone, Mead Johnson Nutritionals, and Nestlé Nutrition.
- S.C. received support from Biocodex, Danone, Nestlé Nutrition, and Pfizer Nutrition.
- M.E.G. acknowledges support from Abbott Nutrition, Danone, Mead Johnson Nutrition, Nestlé Nutrition, and Pfizer Nutrition.
- G.J.F. received an author's honorarium from Nestlé Nutrition.
- E.A.G. received support from Nestlé Nutrition. The University of Amsterdam and the Free University, Amsterdam, and its employee.
- J.B.v.G. have or have had scientific and educational collaborations with Abbott Nutrition, Danone, Hipp, Mead Johnson Nutrition, and Nestlé Nutrition.
- S.H.Q. received support from Danone. The University of Munich Medical Centre and its employee.
- B.Ko. have or have had scientific and educational collaborations with manufacturers of FUF, primarily as part of research collaborations funded by the European Commission and the German government, from Abbott Nutrition, Dairy Goat Co-operative, Danone, Fonterra, Hipp, Mead Johnson Nutrition, Nestlé Nutrition, and Pfizer Nutrition,

and receive grant support from the European Commission, the European Research Council, and the German Federal Government.
- *B.Ku. declares no potential conflict of interest.*
- *M.M. and the Women's and Children's Health Research Institute and the University of Adelaide have received support from the National Health and Medical Research Council (NHMRC), Clover Corporation, Dairy Goat Cooperative, Danone, Fonterra, Nestlé Nutrition, and Mead Johnson Nutrition.*
- *A.W. has received financial support from Danone, Mead Johnson Nutrition, and Nestlé Nutrition.*

So basically all but one author had received money in some form from companies who would benefit from that position statement, but none of them felt that they had a conflict of interest?!??!

7. And finally, promoting breastfeeding

Hang on, what? Why would a formula or bottle company promote breastfeeding? Maybe they're just being helpful?

Hmm. Over the last year in particular there seems to have been a major increase in the number of formula and bottle companies making adverts to promote breastfeeding, or at least promote breastfeeding *alongside* other modes of feeding. This is a clever tactic. On the surface they can say they are supporting breastfeeding, but actually as you'll have worked out from reading all the tricks I've already mentioned, they are simply promoting their products.

First, we know that brand advertising works. When a formula company makes a video or advert promoting breastfeeding, its brand name and colouring is still there. Consciously or subconsciously the brand gets advertised to whoever is watching the video alongside the breastfeeding information. Aptamil and their Aptaclub have been especially aggressive with this lately, particularly during the COVID-19 lockdown when women were struggling to find breastfeeding support (for more on the impact of the lockdown, see chapter 17). Social media marketing has meant that brands such as Aptamil can deliberately target their breastfeeding support posts at breastfeeding women.[58] Although the WHO Code states that formula companies should not be promoting their products to pregnant women and new mothers, they claim that they are simply providing breastfeeding advice to women who want it. In response to a news article challenging this, Danone (which owns Aptamil) simply responded that they do not promote their formula to those with a baby under six months old. Clever.

This type of promotion of breastfeeding can lead parents to think that the company cares about infant health and is being supportive. This means that when they come to purchase a breastmilk substitute or bottle, they are more likely to choose that brand.[40] Companies know that this works. For example, Tommee Tippee, the bottle and accessory company, made a very recent advert portaying women feeding their babies. It showed a realistic portrayal of all the highs and lows of breastfeeding including a lot of shots of breasts, milk and naked skin. Ironically it got blocked from Facebook for the perceived nudity, but it has been promoted widely as being supportive of breastfeeding. It is not an advert designed to support mothers and breastfeeding. It is an advert designed to sell products, but made in such a clever way that many people fall for it.[59]

An additional issue is that many criticisms have been made of the accuracy or wording of the messages in breastfeeding promotion by the formula industry. One website that has received attention is Danone's Aptaclub.[60] It has been criticised for being overly cautious about guidance, such as suggesting waiting for 2–3 hours after having any alcoholic drink to breastfeed so that the alcohol can leave your system. The wording on its website, as of 2 March 2021, states:

'Alcohol is processed differently depending on the person and so an exact time that the alcohol has left your system is hard to calculate. However, waiting about 2–3 hours per drink should allow the alcohol to be out of your system, both your bloodstream and your breast milk. Therefore, it is best to wait for 2–3 hours per drink before breastfeeding your baby, to avoid them ingesting any alcohol in your breast milk.'

There is also a section on 'Breastfeeding and diet' which makes several suggestions that a healthy diet is important during breastfeeding. This is absolutely true, but as we saw earlier, unless a diet is extreme, breastmilk content is not affected by the diet a mother eats. If her diet is poor, it is the mother who is likely to suffer and not her baby, as her body prioritises her milk. But the wording of the website suggests a much stronger link between maternal diet and milk content, which could well increase anxiety in women. For example:

'All of your baby's nutrition comes directly from your breast milk. That means every crunchy salad, curry or tuna steak you eat provides them with vital vitamins'.

'From staying well hydrated to eating a healthy balanced diet while breastfeeding, the nutritional choices you make enable your baby to get the vitamins and minerals they need to support their future health'.

This subtle use of language and suggestions matters, as it chips away at women's confidence.

Do companies honestly do all of this, or are you just being a bit paranoid Amy?

I've had this suggested to me in several different tones over the years ranging from the sympathetic to the angry and everything in between. Are we just paranoid? Exaggerating? Making it all up?

No.

We knew we weren't imagining all of this but in 2020 an eye-opening paper was published which I had to read numerous times to believe it was true.[40] The research team conducted interviews with experts who were working for, or had worked with, different formula milk companies. They asked them about the marketing tricks that they used. My worst fears about what they were doing were confirmed and actually exceeded. The paper, entitled 'Selling second best: how infant formula marketing works' highlighted the following tactics to persuade families to buy their product now or in the future:

- Using soft-sell techniques to build up supportive 'friendships' with new mothers such as using baby clubs and telephone advice lines to reach pregnant women and new mothers without mentioning formula. Using apps such as digital ovulation calculators and apps that bring new mothers together to chat to draw women in. Acknowledging that this develops feelings of kindness and trust of the company.
- Emphasising that 'breast is best' but 'not all women can breastfeed' to suggest they are simply meeting a need not trying to prevent breastfeeding.
- Trying to reach first-time pregnant mothers as they know brand loyalty persists. Referring to first-time mothers as 'the holy grail' as they know it will bring such a return on their investment.
- Targeting different mothers in different ways – splitting potential customers into blue, yellow and red mothers. Blue and yellow

mothers are the main types in western countries. Blue mothers apparently lean towards science and added ingredients while yellow mothers just like their baby to be happy.

- Continual development of new products to keep the brand active and vibrant.
- Developing specialist products to be able to engage with the medical profession – so that products will be promoted but also seen as evidence-based and supported by medics.
- Using emotion and positioning breastfeeding as a set of beliefs held by a minority group rather than scientific consensus.
- Talking about 'share of the stomach' and seeing breastmilk as a competitor for that.

Still think I'm paranoid? This is not about an informed decision to use formula milk, but a deliberate manipulation to persuade parents to use their brand.

How does all this affect breastfeeding?

In 1994 the World Health Organisation declared 'Those who suggest that direct advertising has no negative effect on breastfeeding should be asked to demonstrate that such advertising fails to influence a mother's decision about how to feed her infant'.

The impact formula promotion has in developing countries is devastating. Promoting a product that most cannot afford to purchase regularly or make up as safely as possible is disastrous for the health of babies, especially when those babies really needed to be breastfed in the first place. As Senator Edward Kennedy, chairman of the USA Senate Subcommittee on Health and Scientific Research, asked in 1978:

'Can a product which requires clean water, good sanitation, adequate family income and a literate parent to follow printed instructions be properly and safely used in areas where water is contaminated, sewage runs in the streets, poverty is severe and illiteracy high?'

In developing countries, the risk of dying from diarrhoea during the first five months of life is nearly 11 times higher if a baby is formula-fed. In Pakistan, the country with the highest rates, it was 21.3. Yes, 21.3 times more likely to die if given formula milk and yet companies still promote it.[61] Using infant formula in a region where water cannot be boiled, bottles cannot be sterilised and conditions are unsafe is very different to using it in a privileged household in the UK. The protection that breastfeeding gives is vital in countries with high infection, disease and infant mortality rates. That's before even considering the financial implications for families becoming reliant on infant formula and the unsafe alternatives they are given when this is not possible.[62]

Again some people will question whether formula adverts actually sell products. Well yes, of course they do… to someone out there, because otherwise companies wouldn't invest that money in promoting their products. In the USA, where free formula samples in hospital discharge packs are the norm, a Cochrane review showed that mothers who had such samples were less likely to continue breastfeeding.[63] Another study in the USA trialled what happened when one group of mothers received the usual advertising discharge pack, while another group received a pack with no advertising. Those who didn't see the advertising were 58% more likely to breastfeed exclusively for six months.[64] Finally, another study showed that women who received commercial discharge packs were 1.4 times less likely to be breastfeeding at 10 weeks than those who didn't.[65] Why? Again, because it creates awareness of products. Brand recognition. Feelings of support and loyalty. Easy access when things are tough and there's a free sample in the cupboard. Normalisation.

There is some progress in trying to change all of this. In 2016, SNP MP Alison Thewliss, chair of the All Party Parliamentary Committee on Infant Feeding and Inequalities, campaigned to get a law passed in parliament around the advertising and promotion of feeding products for babies and children. It cleared its first parliamentary hearing and the bill was published in February 2017.[66] It called for new legislation to:

- Introduce plain packaging for all formula milks;
- Establish a body, totally independent of industry, to test all products and verify the claims of manufacturers prior to them being licensed for sale;
- Ban the use of misleading terms such as 'follow-on' or 'growing-up' formula milks;
- Stop companies from circumventing existing laws by introducing a ban on identical packaging for stage two and subsequent products;
- Prohibit formula companies from advertising in health journals and magazines;

- Bring forward tougher penalties for companies who flaunt the legislation, including greater financial fines and prison sentences for company CEOs;
- Ban advertising of formula milks on TV, social media, the internet and through parenting clubs.

Somewhat unsurprisingly, the British Specialist Nutrition Association, which represents Abbott, Danone Nutrica Early Life Nutrition, Mead Johnson, NANNYcare and Nestlé, was opposed to the Bill. Unfortunately, due to the strange nuances of parliament, a long agenda for the day and a lack of time meant that the bill was not debated and subsequently the process ended. One can spend a lot of time reflecting on parliamentary regulations and the ability of MPs to simply fill up time and prevent things being discussed.

Advertising of formula products matters, and the companies know it or they wouldn't be doing it. Brand advertising targets parents who may base their decision on how to feed their baby due to trust in a brand they know and recognise. Huge potential is there to damage babies' health for profit. And the costs of all the advertising and exploiting the loopholes in regulation is added to the cost of formula milk – so parents who buy formula are paying for it.

I'm not going to suggest that formula doesn't have its place and should only be available on prescription. But it shouldn't be advertised. Why does it need to be? It's an essential infant product for those who are not breastfeeding. Take away the influence of industry, make a generic product with everything that is needed (there really is little difference between formulas, despite what industry tries to tell people) and make it cheaper and more affordable for those who need it.

What about other products promoted by industry?

Industry is not just trying to persuade breastfeeding mothers to introduce formula milk to their babies. It is also trying to capitalise on the process of milk production and breastfeeding, by creating products that supposedly 'help' breastfeeding yet at best appear unnecessary and at worst may well be damaging a woman's ability to breastfeed her baby.

It's fairly safe to say that technology is now a major part of our lives. YouTube states that over 300 hours of new videos are uploaded to its site every minute, with estimates of the total number of videos uploaded in total passing one billion. Technology also seems to get more advanced by the minute. Would we really have thought 10 years ago that we would all carry the internet in our pocket? A quick search of iTunes or the Google Play store will offer you an app for almost anything. Apparently there are over 1.6 million apps currently available to download. We're wearing smart watches that tell us if we're stressed. And late night TV continues to try and sell us the most random products that we're all absolutely convinced we need, at least in that moment.

But how does this all fit with breastfeeding? Isn't technology the absolute opposite of breastfeeding, its antithesis even? All breastfeeding really needs is a pair of boobs, some good support and a lot of time (and cake). Does it really need intervention from manufacturers, scientists and engineers? And do the products they develop really help, or might they do harm?

In recent years the market has been flooded with devices that claim to support breastfeeding. However, given that we know how breastmilk is produced, and that we have survived as a species for millennia without the internet or technology, what good are the devices? Do they actually support new mothers to breastfeed or simply part them with their cash?

The danger of breastfeeding products

Countless products are now apparently 'essential' for breastfeeding. A quick google brings up an article entitled 'Fifteen products that make breastfeeding easier'. This heavily sponsored site suggests nipple shields, breast shells, nipple cream, a cushion, baby weighing scales, a breast pump that costs 300 dollars, specific bottles, a breastfeeding cover, breast pads, silicone breast pads that don't give you visible nursing pad lines (because we needed something else to worry about), herbs to boost your supply, gel pads for engorgement, a nursing top, a breastfeeding wardrobe and a magazine subscription! I'm exhausted just reading that, but what's more worrying is that the blurb next to every 'essential' item describes a breastfeeding problem – sore nipples, engorgement, low supply. Or the wording damages confidence by making references to your 'post-baby tummy' and the visible nursing pad lines (acronym VNPL?).

The problem is not just one website. Amazon for example has over 4,000 products available when you search breastfeeding. *Mother and Baby* magazine actually has an award category for the best breastfeeding products. Predictably, the 'short list' showcases a wide range of potential products you could buy, and there isn't really anything short about it. Typing 'What do I need to buy to breastfeed' into Google brings up 16 million results. If anyone can hack a redirect to a page that simply says 'nothing'... or perhaps 'chocolate', then that would be great, thanks.

These products plant seeds of doubt in a woman's mind that something will go wrong and breastfeeding is difficult. Secondly they create a need or reliance on products that aren't necessary. And finally, they can be off-putting. The products on the first website alone added up to over £500. Just for the first batch of them – and that's without the brand-new nursing wardrobe. Suddenly it's starting to seem a lot cheaper to formula-feed... hmm, it's almost as if the formula companies designed these products... oh wait. (More on that later.)

Going back to that Google search for 'What do I need to buy to breastfeed', many of the pages brought up are thread upon thread on parenting websites with anxious mothers asking what they need to buy to breastfeed. 'Help!' shouts one. 'Baby is due in a month and I've bought nothing to breastfeed'. Another states 'Confused! Do I need to buy a breast pump, bottles and steriliser if breastfeeding?'. Well done technology and advertising, you've convinced us we need stuff that we don't.

Some mothers do find some products useful. Breast pads can help if you leak a lot; a pump can be useful if you need to express regularly. But the way in which these products are promoted suggests they are necessary, when they are not. The Unicef Baby Friendly Standards recommend that mothers be shown how to hand express milk, because this can help build confidence and prevent engorgement. But increasing numbers of new mothers now purchase a breast pump as a matter of course, rather than in response to an individual need to express milk for their baby. In the UK, where mothers have longer maternity leave and are less likely to need to express in order to go back to work, many mothers will never need a breast pump.

One study interviewed lactation consultants about breast pump use. Common responses included the fact that increased technology around pregnancy, birth and breastfeeding meant that more and more mothers wanted 'control' over the breastfeeding process and believed that technology was the answer. Breast pumps enabled them to see and measure how much milk they were producing, although actually this could have a negative impact on confidence, as most women don't express as much milk as their baby naturally drinks directly from the breast. As we know, this can lead to concerns about milk supply. Which, if your pump is produced by a formula company, is exactly what they want you to think, isn't it?

Breast pumps and breast pads aren't the main issue here. What is more concerning is the sheer number of unnecessary products being advertised – at a significant cost and often formula-company branded.

Breastfeeding apps

There are some really good breastfeeding apps available. I'm talking about the ones with useful information and links supporting breastfeeding. But the breastfeeding app market appears to have been flooded with apps that offer the 'opportunity' to closely scrutinise exactly how much your baby is feeding and growing. Others allow you to track every last interaction with your baby in order to monitor your routine. Knowing what we know about on-demand breastfeeding, sleep and growth these apps seem like a fundamentally bad idea.

More worryingly, the app market is a lovely loophole through which those who are invested in getting babies to stop breastfeeding can reach parents. Have a look and see how many breastfeeding apps have been designed by formula manufacturers. Take the Similac Baby Journal App, for example, which states:

> 'We used to have baby books, now there's an app for that. Similac Baby Journal allows you to keep a detailed log of everything your baby does each day. Track each breast-feeding session by tapping the right or left breast on the diagram and then starting the timer. The diaper changing section is so detailed that you can choose the color and consistency of your baby's stool with the touch of a finger. Graphs that show your baby's development and behaviors over time can then be exported and emailed to a pediatrician. You can also see tips from the makers of Similac and other moms and dads.'

That sounds like a recipe for disaster. Anxious parents keeping track of the exact amount of time their baby feeds. And the exact consistency of their nappies, which until now I had no idea was a thing that needed to be monitored. Thanks Similac. How did we survive as a species without this app? Or maybe there are hieroglyphics about baby poo consistency if you look closely enough. Why do we need to know exactly what a baby does each day? Do they need timesheets to get paid or something? Another app, called Baby Connect, states:

> 'Baby Connect allows moms on the go to have a full picture of what's

going on with their baby at all times. You can record nursing, pumping, and bottle-feedings as well as sleep, development, and even the baby's mood. The app also stores important medical information like doctor visits, blood type, allergies, and current medications. When you're away, your caregiver can use the free web interface to log information as well. Data can be automatically synchronized between accounts online, so everyone involved in the baby's care can have access.'

These baby apps are clearly popular, with new mothers often asking on parenting forums about the best ones, so they can time and monitor feeds. There is clearly significant anxiety there – and, more worryingly, an assumption that an app is needed to record how much a baby feeds. Thankfully the responses to these questions can be sensible and urge caution about the technology. As one poster noted:

'The best app for this is your baby. Look at her and see what she wants.'

Having said that, I do like this poster's style:

'There are some benefits to timing feeds. I do it so I can complain to DH how long I have been pinned to the sofa, so he brings drinks and chocolate.'

Breastfeeding apps might work for some, particularly if a baby has been losing weight and the mother is anxious. But the assumption that they are needed in order to judge intake is what worries me. That writing it all down somehow means it has happened, and if you don't the baby didn't really get fed. The anxiety caused if one day the baby decides not to feed as much, when this can be perfectly normal. The potential to compare data with others. The obsession it could create. For me at least, simply starting to measure something makes me think about it (and worry about it) more. My family can tell you about my new-found anxiety over our gas and electricity consumption since getting a smart meter. We are lucky enough not to have to really worry about our usage (from a financial perspective at least) but as soon as we got that meter, I became anxious. It's currently switched off and the anxiety has disappeared. The more I think about it, the more I wonder how much these apps affect the confidence of even the most laid-back mothers. We need to tread very carefully.

Other than apps, there are some products that are marketed to breastfeeding mothers that no new mother needs. These include overpriced nutritional supplements and milk monitoring technology.

Breastfeeding nutrition

The concept of specialised nutrition for breastfeeding women is relatively new. Not content with promoting formula milk, the formula companies have started to design specialised nutrition products for breastfeeding women. The marketing insists that new mothers need these products, which come at a high price. Formula companies should not promote their infant milks to health professionals in the UK, but they are allowed to promote their breastfeeding nutrition products, which of course carry their brand name. Recently I was handed an information pack that a health visitor had received all about supporting nutrition during pregnancy and breastfeeding, and surprise surprise, the pack was full of leaflets advertising nutrition products.

Do we need specialised breastfeeding nutrition products at all? No. A quick glance at the label reveals that the only thing 'special' about these products is their price. One type of breastfeeding cereal bar is promoted as providing vitamin D, folic acid, omega 3, iodine and iron, 'dedicated to the nutritional needs of pregnant and breastfeeding women'. The adverts state that 'Good nutrition whilst breastfeeding can optimise not only your health, but the health of your developing baby now and in later life'.

A pack of five cereal bars costs about five pounds. Yes, a pound for each cereal bar. And you're meant to eat one every day you're breastfeeding. Add that up for the two years or more the WHO encourages, and the manufacturers must have gigantic pound signs flashing in their eyes. The bars may contain essential vitamins, but women can get these through a normal diet or even by taking cheap vitamin supplements that cost just pennies a day (or are free if you qualify for the Healthy Start scheme). While I'm on the subject, the same is true of specialised breastfeeding vitamin supplements, priced at £10 to £20 per pack. Cheaper equivalents, without the word breastfeeding on the packaging, do exactly the same job. These 'breastfeeding' products are designed to make money by inducing anxiety. By making women doubt their own bodies. It's a way of somehow making money out of breastfeeding.

I'm not sure how many women actually buy these bars. It concerns me that women may think they are essential, and decide that actually it might be cheaper to formula-feed than worry about their own diet.

And no one needs these bars. Women in low-income countries eating very basic diets produce excellent quality breastmilk. There's really no need to worry about the content of your breastmilk – but you can see why the companies who stand to profit from the product would try to persuade you otherwise.

Measuring breastmilk intake

While you're still rolling your eyes at the breastfeeding bars, let me introduce you to MilkSense. This is a device that claims to tell you how much breastmilk you are producing. The recently launched 'personal breastfeeding monitor' can apparently tell you how much milk you have stored in each breast and how much milk your baby consumes with each feed. The device, which looks like some kind of spoof sci-fi gadget, offers you stored information about the time baby last fed, the side they fed from and how much they consumed. Detailed information is then compiled to measure and track baby's feeding and growth over time and to measure 'breast productivity' at different times of the day. Notably it describes this data as 'vital information for your specialist'.

When I first heard of this I thought it couldn't possibly be real. April Fool's day was coming up, and I thought it must be an elaborate joke. Sadly, it's no joke. The advertising for the device deliberately aims to undermine normal breastfeeding and to sow seeds of doubt in a mother's mind. Promotional information about the monitor actually asks new mothers:

'What if babies could tell you how much they actually feed?'

They can! Wet nappies. Dirty nappies. Smiling babies. Frequent feeds. And so on. Mother Nature works brilliantly if you let her. The website then goes on to say:

'Choosing which method to feed your baby is an important decision in a family. Whether it is breastfeeding or bottle-feeding, moms need to know that they are helping to nourish their baby properly, so that they can develop, grow and thrive. MilkSense is passionate about breastfeeding and understands the importance that breastfeeding has on the long-term health and wellbeing of your child. MilkSense is the world's first breastfeeding monitor that measures how much breastmilk mom produces and how much milk baby consumes. It has no contact with your

baby, and does not interfere with natural breastfeeding. MilkSense helps sustain breastfeeding efforts by increasing your confidence regarding milk production and consumption, increasing efficiency of your time and tracking feedings so there is no need for additional apps or diaries.'

MilkSense also states that it was designed based on the needs of 'hundreds' of mothers. Given that 700,000 or so babies are born each year in the UK (and 130 million globally), the needs of 'hundreds' of mothers might not be representative. But the advert is likely to reach far more than 'hundreds' of mothers, and has the potential to be damaging. We don't need to measure how much milk is in a breast, and given that breastmilk is continually produced, I don't see how that is possible. What it is doing is creating new anxiety for mothers, damaging their chances of breastfeeding while relieving them of their money.

Milksense was shortly followed by the creation of 'Momsense' (which to me sounds like nonsense, but there you go). This machine is essentially a set of headphones and a sensor which you fit just underneath your baby's jaw. The device claims to use the sensor to detect how often your baby swallows (their ear/jaw wiggles when they do) and sends this information to an app on your smartphone where it supposedly turns this data into estimating how much your baby has drunk. The headphones are for you to listen to all of this via the sensor. The product states it uses 'advanced algorithms' to work all this out. Reviews on Amazon are very mixed, with the main criticisms being predominantly that babies don't like it and it simply doesn't work. I mean, how could it? And would you like something stuck to your jaw as you eat?

And finally you then have Coroflo. This is essentially a nipple shield with a sensor in it to measure how much milk flows through it. It comes with an app that records the length of feeds and volume of milk consumed, comparing this to your individual baby and others. As I write the company has received over €4 million in funding including from the European Commission under its Horizon 2020 programme. It was runner-up in the 2018 Irish Times Innovation awards.

As far as I am aware there is currently no independent research into Coroflo's efficacy. As noted earlier, nipple shields can be problematic in reducing milk flow or interfering with latch. They have their place as a potentially useful tool, but encouraging unnecessary use seems, well, unnecessary.

Overall my main concerns around any device that claims to

measure milk volume are:

- How do we know it is accurate?
- How do we know if a feed using these devices is the same as a feed without?
- If they are accurate, how do we know that amount of milk was the 'right amount'?
- What happens to our hormones, particularly stress and oxytocin, when we use these devices?

Breastfeeding is about so much more than just milk transfer. It's about comfort, warmth and connection. It's a way of mothering and calming a baby. What happens to all of that when you have to stop and use a device? If we are really struggling with low milk supply, perceived or otherwise, let's stop and fix that rather than bringing in an added layer of complexity.

Breastmilk content

Finally, a number of companies will now analyse your breastmilk content. For a price, of course. One company, called Happy Vitals, will test the nutrient content and supposed 'toxicity' of your breastmilk. Different packages (with ever-increasing prices) are available depending on what you want to test for. Their website states that:

> 'Happy Vitals provides families with the tools they need to monitor and improve the long-term health of their children. With our simple and easy-to-use tests, mothers can learn for the first time about the nutrient make-up of their breastmilk, improve their diet and nutrition, and safeguard against exposure to heavy metals and other toxins that are harmful to a child's growth and development.'

That's nice. But it's completely unnecessary. Science shows us that there is little variation in breastmilk content between mothers. However, apparently Happy Vitals:

> '...helps you visualise your biological health, so you can easily make improvements through diet and lifestyle tweaks. With our test results in hand, mothers have a better understanding of their health and nutritional needs, and how those needs can improve the health of their child. Our

tests also help mothers safeguard against exposure to harmful toxins and chemicals in the environment that may be passed on to their child.'

For $170 you can have the levels of fat, protein and carbohydrate in your milk tested. But that's just the basic package – and no one wants that, do they? – so for $270 you can also have immunity and key vitamins and minerals tested. And for $660 you can test for all those nasty toxins swimming in your breastmilk trying to make your baby ill. Never mind that this isn't true. Happy Vitals claim:

'Most people are unaware of heavy metal toxicity, and its irreversible consequences, until it is too late. Heavy metal exposure during pregnancy and breastfeeding can cause impaired cognitive function in children, including low IQ and behaviour problems, learning disabilities, and other cognitive disorders. While modern living makes the complete avoidance of heavy metals impossible, limiting exposure to these toxins is critical to your health and the health of your family.

In addition to our most detailed nutritional assessment package, this premium package includes tests for Heavy Metal Toxins, conveniently takes samples of your child's hair/nails and tests for the four most harmful metallic poisons. Results may provide families with the information they need to help take action to reduce exposure and limit the potential negative impacts for mother and child.'

Thank heavens for Happy Vitals, eh? How have we survived until now? Yes, there are some toxins in breastmilk. There are toxins in formula milk. Toxins are everywhere. They cannot be avoided. Toxins in breastmilk are at such a low level that they are insignificant. In fact, walking down the street exposes a baby to far more toxins than anything else. Depending on where you live, this exposure will be 25–135 times higher. Yet we walk down the street without a thought every day.

Indeed, 'chemicals' are everywhere. One great piece that often does the rounds on social media notes:

'IT CONTAINS MORE THAN 4,000 CHEMICALS AND IT HAS SPREAD INTO EVERY HUMAN BODY ON EARTH.

Among its components are formaldehyde, acetone, ethanol, ketone bodies, dihydrogen monoxide, tryptophan, urea, dehydroeplandrosterone, hexosephosphate P, and at least 20 kinds of acids.

Nearly every chemical constituent will, in certain concentrations, kill children and adults. Chemical compounds within it are also used in yoga mats, explosives, warfare, and industrial applications.

It is now so pervasive that every human baby is born with high concentrations already in his or her tiny body.

Healthcare workers, pharmaceutical companies, and governments will spend billions each year to maintain or increase its presence in citizens.

It's your own blood.'

Science can be amusing. Geeks who do science and write this type of stuff definitely are. Did you know that 100% of people who have died have drunk dihydrogen monoxide? In other words, water. Chemicals are part of us. But Happy Vitals don't make comparisons, or consider toxicity levels. They just look at whether the chemicals are there or not and then scaremonger. For a price.

Four years on from the first edition, other companies have also developed this idea. Lactation Lab looks at calories, carbohydrate, protein, fat, calcium and vitamins. Alongside scary-sounding things like arsenic, cadmium, lead and mercury. It's easy to think things like arsenic are inherently poisonous at any level, but in fact low levels can be found in food and water (although in countries with higher levels, particularly in water, this is a predictor of all sorts of illness). Incidentally, research has shown that even when mothers are exposed to arsenic, such as through drinking water that has high levels, the levels in their breastmilk are extremely low. Formula-fed babies actually have up to eight times the exposure through levels in formula milk and water.[67] But no one is testing that, are they?

Finally, while I'm on the subject, those tests you can buy to measure alcohol content in breastmilk? They'll pretty much give a positive reading if any alcohol at all has been consumed. Again, not helpful (unless someone is really that drunk they can't remember they've had a drink) and anxiety-inducing.

Breastmilk-like breastmilk substitutes

An emerging market is also building around the concept of formula milks that are marketed as being 'like breastmilk'. I don't mean like previous adverts for formula milks that were banned for claiming to be the 'closest to breastmilk', but rather investment in companies that are claiming to produce a product that is *just like breastmilk*. One of these companies is called 'BioMilq', a start-up led by two women who want to produce an alternative milk for women who are struggling to breastfeed.[68]

The company is essentially using techniques to grow breastmilk in a lab. Scientists use the epithelial cells that line the mammary glands in the breast to culture a milk. When these cells are grown and nurtured, they appear to secrete milk. The initial stages of developing the product were based on cells taken from cow mammary glands and as the technique was developed the team started using human breast cells. These cells are available for sale as medical products, and are usually used in breast cancer research.

So far, experimental techniques have led to milk being secreted from these cells that contains some of the same proteins and sugars found in human milk – which differ from those found in cows' milk-based formulas. The company hopes that eventually they will be able to develop their product so that women have the choice of buying this milk if they cannot breastfeed. Given the process and likely cost of the milk, the company is currently promoting the idea of the milk as something that a woman who is struggling to make enough breastmilk could top-up with rather than use formula. It also seems like it might be an intensive process for women. The idea long term is that a mother will be able to use her own epithelial cells in the process. She will visit the lab in pregnancy, and epithelial cells will be collected from her breast. These cells will be cultured in a solution that enables them to multiply and ultimately secrete milk. This milk will then be sent back to the family.

On the one hand this is an interesting innovation and could potentially be an option that women might find useful. But I have a lot of questions and concerns. First of all, the concept of a milk matching breastmilk in terms of some proteins and sugars is great, but it still does not match breastmilk. There are so many other components in breastmilk, such as antibodies, good bacteria and factors that support development that are not present in this milk. The company recognises this and states that it will not be possible to replicate things like antibodies in this milk. The risk is that people may think that the milk is more like breastmilk than it actually is.

The second concern that I have is that the company has received over $2.5 million in funding from Breakthrough Energy Ventures, which is Bill Gates's investment firm for climate change. Don't get me wrong, I'm fully supportive of female entrepreneurs in particular getting such funding to develop their science and tech ideas. But wouldn't it be amazing if we could access similar funding for interventions to actually support women who are struggling to breastfeed in the first place? In a world where breastfeeding support gets ridiculed, dismissed and its funding cut, it is painful to see that a tech alternative can get funding, rather than investing in a better understanding of why women's bodies are not working as expected in the first place.

When technology does work

More positively, technology can be useful in supporting new mothers to breastfeed. One study used a randomised controlled trial to set new mothers up with usual support, or additional access to a breastfeeding monitoring system. This site did ask women to monitor how often they breastfed, how many nappies their baby went through and any problems they were having, but this information was used in the context of providing support. If women breastfed fewer than six times a day, the system sent them information about the importance of frequent feeding. Conversely, if they breastfed more than eight times a day they got positive notifications about how well they were doing. On top of that, if they inputted information that was suggestive of a particular problem, they got sent links to specific problem-solving tips. Overall, those who used the system were more likely to be breastfeeding at one, two and three months.[69]

Another team of researchers in Australia set up an online forum that gave women direct access to a lactation consultant to whom they could ask questions, and a forum to talk to other mothers. They found that women who used the system were more likely to exclusively breastfeed for longer.[70]

So technology has its place, if it's there to genuinely support mothers and reduce their anxiety, rather than deliberately exacerbate it in order to sell a product.

Action 12

✓ Regulate industry to prevent the promotion of unnecessary and potentially harmful products.

17. HOW HAS THE COVID-19 PANDEMIC AFFECTED ALL OF THIS?

This is a bonus chapter of sorts. Or perhaps whatever the opposite of bonus is. A chapter I never imagined writing, but which certainly exposes the weaknesses in our society's systems and how this affects mothers and babies. As I'm writing this, it's still an evolving situation. In February 2021 it's almost a year since the first cases of the novel coronavirus known as COVID-19 reached the UK and the first of several lockdowns was implemented. And the impact of the pandemic on mothers, babies and families is inescapable.

Hopefully you are reading this in a brighter future where social distancing is a distant memory and the parts of life we have missed so much have been revived. If you are, I hope that the promises of politicians and policymakers to invest in families and children came to fruition and there is funding and opportunity for them to catch up on what they missed out on (and any trauma they experienced). Unfortunately, even at this relatively early point, we already know from research that precautions to reduce the spread of COVID-19 impacted negatively on many new families, although the picture is a little more complex than saying it was a terrible time for all.

Research into families' experiences of perinatal care during the pandemic has been mixed. The *Babies in Lockdown* report (a collaboration between Best Beginnings, Home Start UK and the Parent-Infant Foundation) explored the experiences of pregnant women and parents with a baby under 24 months during the first lockdown.[1] The authors found that:

- 68% felt lockdown affected their pregnancy or baby
- 34% felt their baby's interaction with them had changed
- 47% reported their baby had become more clingy
- 26% felt their baby cried more than normal
- 25% were concerned about their relationship with their baby
- 61% had significant concerns about their mental health
- 87% felt more anxious as a result of COVID-19

Some, on the other hand, felt very little change, with some even feeling better due to a slower pace of life or being more removed from difficult family connections. However, reflecting a pattern found in lots of pandemic-related research, the report found that experience was not equal. Younger parents (who tended to be less financially stable) and those from Black, Asian and minority ethnic families were hit the hardest.

But what was the impact on breastfeeding?

Women's breastfeeding experiences during COVID-19

During the first lockdown in May 2020, I conducted a study with Dr Natalie Shenker exploring women's experiences of breastfeeding during lockdown.[2] It included over 1,200 mothers who had breastfed at least once since the start of the first lockdown in March 2020. We found that overall women had very mixed experiences, strongly dependent on their living situation at home. Some had a positive time, some reported that they didn't really feel affected and some described very negative experiences indeed. More on those specifics later in the chapter. In terms of actual impact on feeding we found:

- 58% of women in our study were breastfeeding exclusively
- 22% were mixed feeding
- 19% had stopped breastfeeding

What we were particularly interested in was how the pandemic had affected those experiences. When we looked at how early women had stopped breastfeeding or started using formula milk, we found that in both cases this was pretty early on in their feeding journey, suggesting initial issues that they couldn't get support for. The average age for women to start using formula milk was when their baby was 2.7 weeks old, and the mean age for them to stop breastfeeding was 3.1 weeks. Unfortunately, those decisions were not often made through choice. Many introduced formula or stopped breastfeeding before they had planned or were ready to do so – although some mothers did say they were breastfeeding or delaying formula longer than planned.

Of those mothers who had stopped breastfeeding:

- 13.5% described themselves as ready to stop feeding
- 4.7% stopped breastfeeding when planned
- 64.8% had planned to feed for longer

- 19.4% did breastfeed for longer than planned

Of those who had introduced formula:

- 68.7% stated they had never intended to do so
- 13.5% of the participants introduced formula earlier than planned
- 3.6% breastfed exclusively for longer than intended

When we started to explore why mothers stopped breastfeeding, the typical reasons of pain and difficulty emerged. However, 70% of mothers attributed their shorter breastfeeding experience to a lack of face-to-face support during lockdown. When asked if they felt they had more or less support than usual during the lockdown, 4% felt they had more, 22% about the same, 67% felt they had less, and 7% were unsure.

Support was directly affected by the lockdown. Although lack of support is a common reason given for stopping breastfeeding outside of the pandemic, more women who gave birth after lockdown started reported a lack of support compared to those who had given birth before it began. Breastfeeding support is important throughout an infant feeding journey, but the most intense support is often needed in the early weeks as mothers are getting to grips with feeding. We found that for those who gave birth during the pandemic, 38.2% felt they had enough practical support and 34.4% enough emotional support. Conversely, 42.3% of women who gave birth before the pandemic felt they had enough practical support and 38.8% enough emotional support.

Similar figures emerged in the *Babies in Lockdown* report. Although many mothers did initiate and carry on breastfeeding, half of those who were using formula had not planned to do so. A quarter felt that they did not get the breastfeeding support they needed. Likewise, in another study in the UK, mothers who were breastfeeding during lockdown described how they found a lack of breastfeeding support, particularly face-to-face, really challenging. Often practical problems were solved by trying to express milk or giving formula.[3]

In the US, one study compared breastfeeding outcomes for women who gave birth with COVID-19 and those who did not. Although the number with COVID-19 was small, those with the infection were less likely to be breastfeeding at six weeks, despite equal initiation rates to those who did not have the infection. It is likely that some of the factors surrounding birth affected this. Those with the infection were more likely to have a caesarean section and not have a birth partner – two things we know are associated with more challenging experiences.[4]

How did women's experiences of feeding differ?

What was striking in both our research and the *Babies in Lockdown* report was that women's experiences of feeding during the pandemic (or indeed generally caring for their baby) were not equal. We had a split of around 41% who found the experience of lockdown had a positive impact upon feeding experience, 30% neutral and 29% negative. Notably, when we looked at specific ways in which lockdown could affect feeding experience, different women interpreted those factors in different ways. For example, of those mothers who gave birth during lockdown:

- 21% found having to stay home had a positive impact, while 57% found it had a negative one
- 16% found not having close family visit positive, while 60% found it negative
- 31% found the experience of having no visitors positive, while 55% found it negative

We then explored women's experiences in more depth, asking them to describe how lockdown had affected breastfeeding and caring for their baby. For those who had a positive experience it was clear that many of the barriers talked about in this book that subtly (or not so subtly) affect breastfeeding experience had been lifted, reduced, or disappeared altogether. For example, some women talked about:

- More time to breastfeed. With nothing else to do apart from care for their baby (or go for yet another walk) some felt that they had more time to focus on their baby and really get to grips with breastfeeding. Women talked about sitting at home with their top off, getting that latch just right.
- Fewer visitors. We saw in earlier chapters just how influential other people's views and experiences of breastfeeding can be. Some women pointed out that because no one was allowed to visit, this meant that not only could they stay at home uninterrupted, but they could also avoid other people's unhelpful behaviour and views.
- Supportive partners with more time at home. Those who a) had a

supportive partner and b) that partner was furloughed or working from home, felt that their partner could help support them with getting breastfeeding off to a good start.

- Not having to worry about getting to grips with breastfeeding when out and about. Nowhere was open, so anyone who felt nervous about breastfeeding in public didn't have to face that challenge until they felt more confident.
- Found it easy to access support online. Women sometimes preferred to be able to video call for support in the comfort of their home rather than visit a clinic or private practice.

However, other women found the situation very difficult, feeling that it negatively impacted their breastfeeding experience and led to them stopping before they were ready to do so. These women tended to be more likely to experience:

- A struggle to find the support they needed. Either they could not access, did not know about or struggled with online support methods. Women in this group often talked about not being able to access the healthcare support they needed, with support given over the phone or socially distanced.
- A lack of access to specialist support when needed. Tongue-tie services in particular appeared patchy, with some women being told their baby could not be treated, leaving them in considerable pain and difficulty.
- A poor relationship with a partner who was at home more, especially those who were unsupportive of breastfeeding.
- A partner who was working as a critical worker and out of the house even more, with added concerns about safety.
- Feeling isolated and alone, not just in terms of breastfeeding support, but from family, friends and other new mothers.
- A feeling of intense focus on breastfeeding. With little else to do some felt that all they did was breastfeed, so they felt overwhelmed and like they couldn't escape from it.

Unfortunately, existing inequalities played a central role in women's experiences. Mothers who had a more positive experience were more likely to be living in more privileged circumstances. They lived in safe areas, with large enough homes, gardens and green space to walk in. They had plenty of devices on which to access the internet and could afford (and were able) to access high-speed connections without worrying about eating up data. These women tended to have fewer financial worries.

Conversely, those who were struggling were more likely to be living in cramped accommodation, in higher-level flats and with no access to a garden. They often lived in areas with little green space. Financial and relationship difficulties were more common, alongside finding it difficult to practically access online support, particularly over video messaging. One factor that was particularly concerning was that women from BAME backgrounds were more likely to stop breastfeeding, despite data we looked at early on in this book that shows how on average women from BAME groups breastfeed for longer than white women in the UK. This came back to support: women from BAME groups reported less access to practical support than white women.

It was clear that different women were having very different experiences. For some lockdown led to a more supportive and nurturing environment, which is of course great. But for others, the situation was far more challenging. It is easy to understand how in those circumstances breastfeeding can become difficult and feel unmanageable. Alongside cultural messaging that things will be easier if you bottle-feed, the chain of stressful events that culminates in stopping breastfeeding, often before a woman is ready, is easy to see in hindsight.

What other factors affected women's breastfeeding experiences?

It was clear in our research and that of others that women's direct experiences of breastfeeding support and the early days of getting to grips with feeding affected whether they continued breastfeeding or not. But as we know, although practical and emotional support is a really important part of helping women breastfeed for longer, it's not the only factor. Numerous other things play a role too. And these started having an effect on breastfeeding in their own way during the pandemic. What were they?

1. Incorrect information, including from medical professionals
Even outside pandemic times, worries about the 'safety' of breastfeeding are common. As we've seen in previous chapters, anxieties over medication, diet and lifestyle choices can all affect breastfeeding

decisions. Unfortunately, COVID-19 was added to that list. Although things got much better as the pandemic progressed, particularly at the start there was a lot of misinformation and anxiety around whether breastfeeding could somehow transfer the illness to babies.

In our research one in six mothers reported that they were worried breastfeeding was unsafe. This led to some women stopping breastfeeding as a precaution, with over a fifth of those who stopped breastfeeding during lockdown giving this as one reason that contributed. A lot of mothers who were anxious were affected by misinformation on the internet, with friends and families fuelling rumours and anxieties. However, some mothers in our research (around 5%) were told directly by a health professional that breastfeeding might not be safe or that they would not be 'allowed' to breastfeed if they had symptoms. Although 5% is fortunately a small percentage of mothers, if you multiply that across a population of 700,000 mothers giving birth in the UK each year then that adds up to a lot of mothers potentially being let down.

At the start of the pandemic, given that COVID-19 was a novel virus, there were no data initially available on whether the virus could be passed from mother to baby during pregnancy or postnatally through contact or breastfeeding. Unfortunately, this led to misinformation and overly cautious approaches, meaning that mothers with symptoms or a positive test were separated from their baby after birth or told that breastfeeding would be harmful.[5]

One of the concerns was that somehow the virus would pass into a mother's milk and into the baby. However, we knew from limited research with mothers in China who were diagnosed with COVID-19 that no transmission of the virus into their milk was found.[6] We also knew that there was no evidence of transmission during similar viruses such as the Severe Acute Respiratory Virus (SARS-CoV) outbreak in 2003.[7] As research emerged it showed that COVID-19 did not pass into breastmilk[8] and didn't even necessarily pass from mother to baby in other ways. One case study from Australia found that when a symptomatic mother took suitable precautions (e.g. mask-wearing and handwashing), her infant did not contract the illness.[9]

On top of this we knew that breastmilk can help protect babies from other illnesses. It is full of live immune properties that help boost a baby's immune system at the best of times, but we know that when a mother becomes ill with an infection she can produce antibodies in her milk against future infection which she then passes to her baby.[10] Although during the first lockdown it was too soon to have research to show that this would happen, it was a logical conclusion and in previous epidemics, such as SARS-CoV, women who were infected were found to produce antibodies in their milk.[11] Later research would show us what we expected – that milk from mothers who had COVID-19 contained antibodies to help protect their baby.[12] We also learnt that babies rarely appeared to be seriously affected by COVID-19. When they did catch the virus, their reactions were typically mild.[13]

This lack of information and general panic led to over-caution. Unfortunately the American Academy of Pediatrics initially recommended separating mother and baby in case of suspected infection[14] – guidance that thankfully changed to keep them together.[15] Globally mothers and babies were routinely separated in China, Malaysia, the Philippines, Indonesia and more, with breastmilk substitutes sometimes recommended.[16] Although public health organisations in the UK, such as the UNICEF UK Baby Friendly Initiative, Public Health England and the Royal College of Obstetricians and Gynaecologists, quickly responded with reassurance that breastfeeding was safe and the mother-baby relationship should be protected, there were cases of this not being followed. The spread of events across the world also invoked fear, leading to separations 'just in case'. Unfortunately we know that separating mother and baby goes against everything we know about supporting breastfeeding and promoting stable newborn behaviour.[17]

All of these discussions around safety and breastfeeding were, as always, one-sided. Every discussion appeared to hinge on whether there was any risk of transmitting COVID-19 to a baby without ever considering the opposite: the impact of not breastfeeding on mother and baby. We know that breastfeeding helps protect the health of mother and baby in other ways.[18] Furthermore, if we reflect on the earliest chapters in this book, we know that breastfeeding protects maternal wellbeing. It reduces the risk of inflammation, enhances sleep and moderates stress.[19] We know the devastating impact it can have on mothers psychologically when they cannot meet their breastfeeding goals.[20] The issue highlighted just how much all of this is often ignored in conversations around breastfeeding 'safety'.

I'd like to say that this misinformation has gone away, but as I write it is still occurring. Just as the virus itself mutates, so it appears does the communication of misinformation. In late 2020 the first vaccinations against COVID-19 were developed and because breastfeeding mothers were not included in their trials, the initial messaging was that the vaccine should not be given to pregnant or breastfeeding women or those trying to conceive (although no such message was given to men about their sperm).[21]

This led to women worrying that they would have to stop breastfeeding prematurely to have the vaccine, particularly if they were healthcare professionals. Or they considered not having the vaccine as they wanted to continue feeding. The guidance at the time simply said breastfeeding women could wait until they finished breastfeeding to have the vaccine – as if that would be in a week or so, rather than the many consecutive years women can be pregnant or breastfeeding.[22]

In the UK, a group of experts led by grassroots medical organisations passionate about supporting breastfeeding (including Breastfeeding for Doctors, the Hospital Infant Feeding Network and the GP Infant Feeding Network) were involved in getting this changed. Their work was based on expertise and research from other vaccines that showed there was no evidence to suggest the vaccine would pass to (or affect) a breastfed baby.[23] The government updated the official advice to state:[24]

'There is no known risk associated with giving non-live vaccines whilst breastfeeding. The Joint Committee on Vaccination and Immunisation advises that breastfeeding women may be offered vaccination with any of the currently authorised COVID-19 vaccines.'

This was supported by statements from different breastfeeding organisations, including the Academy of Breastfeeding Medicine:[25]

'During lactation, it is unlikely that the vaccine lipid would enter the blood stream and reach breast tissue. If it does, it is even less likely that either the intact nanoparticle or mRNA transfer into milk. In the unlikely event that mRNA is present in milk, it would be expected to be digested by the child and would be unlikely to have any biological effects.'

And the US Infant Risk team:[26]

'As for breastfeeding, little or none of these vaccine components would ever reach the milk compartment, or even be transferred into human milk. Even if they were, they would simply be digested like any other protein by the infant. It is our opinion that the present group of vaccines

are probably going to be quite safe for breastfeeding mothers. The infant may even gain a small amount of maternal IgG in the breastmilk, which may even be beneficial.'

However, even as I write there are still cases of women being told that they cannot breastfeed and have the vaccination. Medical misinformation, a lack of consideration of the importance of breastfeeding for population health, and a disregard for the importance of women's health and their bodies (especially when it comes to breastfeeding) all continue to play a role.

2. The impact of birth and postnatal care experiences during COVID-19

In earlier chapters we saw how birth and postnatal care experiences can physiologically and psychologically affect infant feeding. Unfortunately, the COVID-19 pandemic also had a significant impact on women's experiences of pregnancy, birth and postnatal care. Changes made to who could enter hospitals, supporters and social distancing had some horrific knock-on effects on women, with some hospitals over-interpreting guidance and exacerbating these negative effects.

Many antenatal and postnatal care appointments were carried out online, and face-to-face appointments rapidly changed to include physical measures. Pregnant women and new mothers unsurprisingly really struggled with this. Research with 1,451 pregnant women and new mothers found that although most understood why virtual appointments were necessary, 62% found it impersonal and that it affected their interactions with their health professional, particularly around mental health issues.[27] Communicating in this way was particularly difficult for those with hearing impairments. Others talked about how they didn't want to necessarily say things in front of their partner, but there was little privacy at home. Another fear was that things would be missed over a phone call. This was a particular fear among women who had a previous stillbirth.

Women also felt more anxious due to their interactions with staff and experience of any hospital or clinic-based appointments. Some felt some staff were more concerned about any risks of COVID-19 than they were about their pregnancy health. Others worried about what would happen if they had symptoms of COVID-19, including whether they would be 'made' to have a caesarean section or be separated from their baby. Some felt worried about contacting the hospital when they needed to for issues such as reduced foetal movements. And two African Caribbean women in the study explained how they had been told they were more likely to die from COVID-19 by their health professionals, but were not told why or what would happen to help protect them.

This atmosphere of fear increased anxiety in women, which we know can have an impact on their birth experiences. A study from Italy found that pregnant women were more likely to describe their feelings around birth using words such as fear, uncertainty and sadness.[28] Although women would express some fear when thinking about childbirth pre-COVID-19, this was more often alongside feelings such as joy and excitement, which significantly reduced during COVID-19. Pre-COVID-19 fear was often based around the pain of childbirth, but post-COVID-19 fear was more closely related to sadness, loneliness and restriction.

There were also numerous changes to how care was delivered, which seemed to differ between hospitals, health boards or simply who was working that particular shift.[29] The charity Birthrights, which is dedicated to improving women's experiences in pregnancy and birth, reported a significant increase in women contacting them worried about how their birth would be affected.[30] Some of the changes we saw included:

- Women being alone for scans and other appointments
- Partners not being allowed into the hospital until the mother was in established labour
- Partners being sent home straight after the birth
- Doulas not being allowed at the birth (or a choice to be made between partner and doula)
- Restrictions on water births
- Restrictions on home births (or women being told they risked an ambulance not being able to get to them if necessary)
- Restrictions on maternal request caesarean sections
- No visitors on the postnatal ward
- Restrictions being made on 'visiting' babies in neonatal care
- Wearing masks during birth or postnatal care

Unsurprisingly, this affected women's experiences of birth. In our infant feeding research one of our most distressing findings was the impact on mothers who had a baby admitted to neonatal care. We found that some of these mothers were separated from their baby and had their 'visits' restricted. I put 'visits' in inverted commas as no one should consider a mother a 'visitor' to her own baby. They are a dyad that should be treated as one person. Although the number who were restricted was thankfully low, the impact was extremely high. Over 80% of mothers restricted from seeing their baby stopped breastfeeding in the first six weeks compared to around 10% of those who could freely be with their baby in NICU.

Likewise, in the *Babies in Lockdown* report, over a third of respondents felt that their care during birth did not go to plan. In particular, aspects such as needing to be induced but not being allowed to have their partner with them until they were in established labour, or having to go back to the ward alone, really affected women. In another study with 885 women in the US, 61% did not feel they were adequately supported during birth, with 20.5% feeling unsafe at the hospital.[31] In our infant feeding research 15% of women without any symptoms at all were told to wear a mask when holding or feeding their baby in the hospital, increasing their anxiety and affecting their interactions with their baby.

Increased anxiety around care during birth is likely linked to a devastating trend globally in an increase in stillbirths seen last year.[32] Although data showed that premature births reduced[33] (potentially due to lower air pollution, less commuting and home working) stillbirths increased in some countries, although data is not completely clear yet at this point. This was thought to be in part because women were not wanting to go into hospital unless necessary due to fears around infection, worried about putting pressure on the system, or wanting to stay with their partner as long as possible. In our infant feeding research we found that some mothers were not seeking support with breastfeeding when they needed to, either because they were worried about accessing healthcare and becoming infected, or because they were worried that they would place an additional burden on an overstretched health service.

Mothers who had symptoms of COVID-19 during birth often had even more challenging experiences. Despite the World Health Organization recommending that mother and baby be kept together even with symptoms or a diagnosis of COVID-19, practice often differed significantly from this.[16] This included separation and preventing women from breastfeeding, despite evidence showing low transmission rates between mother and baby and milder symptoms if transmission occurred.[34] Weighed against the known harms of separation and preventing breastfeeding, guidance was that keeping mother and baby together was more protective.

One recent study to emerge from the pandemic examined maternity care practices specifically in relation to those who had confirmed COVID-19 infection (or symptoms of) when they gave birth.[35] The experiences of 357 mothers from around the world were examined in relation to skin-to-skin care, breastfeeding and keeping mum and baby together. They found that for those who gave birth with symptoms:

- 61% did not have skin-to-skin for at least an hour after birth
- 29% had their baby taken away without holding them after birth
- 29% were not breastfed directly at birth
- 40% did not stay with their mother in arms reach

They compared this to mothers who did not have symptoms at birth (but were in the study because they developed symptoms later on):

- 50% did not have skin-to-skin for at least an hour after birth
- 14% had their baby taken away without holding them after birth
- 6% did not directly breastfed directly at birth
- 9% did not stay with their mother in arms' reach

That is a big difference in experiences and of course it had consequences: babies who did not have skin-to-skin after birth, who were not directly breastfed and did not stay with their mother, were less likely to be breastfed (even when strength of maternal illness was taken into consideration). Understandably, being separated from their baby was very distressing for mothers. This reflects the experiences of mothers in our infant feeding research: 16% of women with COVID-19 symptoms were told that their baby could not stay with them after birth.

These decisions, as we know from previous chapters, go against what we know helps get breastfeeding off to a good start. Anxiety increases the risk of birth complications, which in turn increases the risk of breastfeeding complications. Women understandably wanted to get home to their partner as soon as possible after birth, meaning they often missed out on breastfeeding support in those early hours. In our infant feeding research 21% of mothers received no breastfeeding support at all in the hospital, with a quarter saying they had no information about things like expressing milk. This was also reflected in the *Babies in Lockdown* report, with mothers being sent home quickly without any sort of feeding plan. Feeding support was then given over the phone if needed.

3. Impact on postnatal care experiences

We know that consistent, high-quality practical and emotional postnatal support with feeding and caring for a baby is really important in supporting mothers to breastfeed for longer.[36] However, sadly the pandemic significantly impacted upon the care women received postnatally. Many health visiting appointments were moved to video or phone calls, with mothers in both our infant feeding research and the *Babies in Lockdown* report stating that they had not seen a health visitor face-to-face at all. Postnatal midwifery appointments were often rushed and focused on basic checks rather than having time to talk about how women were feeling or spend time helping with feeding queries. Again, although women recognised why this was necessary, many struggled with digital appointments, especially with specific feeding difficulties or in talking about their mental health.

Others worried about reaching out for support when they needed it. In our infant feeding study we found that women were reluctant to ask for breastfeeding support when necessary, either through fear of face-to-face contact or not wanting to overburden the health service. Another study of pregnant and new mothers produced similar findings – women reported difficulty in accessing services or not wanting to bother anyone. It was clear that these fears had been stirred more than necessary by the media.[27] In the *Babies in Lockdown* report women echoed this, feeling that when they did approach professionals sufficient support could not be given. Without this support women turned to formula when they didn't want to.

Infuriatingly, but perhaps not unexpectedly, the breastmilk substitute industry saw this gap in postnatal care and women's anxieties as an opportunity to promote their products, under the guise of offering breastfeeding support. In our infant feeding research, 80% of breastfeeding mothers saw targeted adverts from the formula industry on social media, despite it being against the WHO Code to directly target mothers with a baby under six months old. When we looked at why women were receiving these adverts (by clicking on 'why am I seeing this advert' on Facebook) one of the reasons given was because women had an interest in breastfeeding. These adverts were often for breastfeeding support, but with heavy branding in the background which we know serves to promote products. Complaints were also made by mothers about how inaccurate or overly cautious information was.[37]

In other countries around the world with more lax following of the Code, companies really took the opportunity to promote themselves. In India Danone supported a YouTube channel called 'Voice of Mums' that advised women with COVID-19 to maintain a distance of at least six feet from their infants and to stop breastfeeding until they had been free of fever for more than 72 hours and free of other symptoms for at least seven days and had two negative PCR results. As we saw earlier this is completely against guidance from the World Health Organization. Companies also stepped up donations of formula milk to communities, despite this again being against the WHO Code.[38]

Isolation was another big theme. Reports have emerged of parents talking about how their baby has never seen another baby face-to-face, or met extended family members. We know how important extended family and community support can be for women during the postnatal period. With face-to-face baby groups closed and restrictions on visiting, many mothers reflected on how isolated they felt. Some talked about how they regretted having had a baby during this time, feeling robbed of their maternity experience. Of course, some women had the opposite experience, feeling protected from interfering or unhelpful family members, or feeling relieved at the pressure of not having to socialise. As with many experiences during this pandemic, the variation in how families have been affected is important in considering how we move forward from here.

Understandably, as the pandemic progressed, reports of increases in perinatal mental health issues did so too. Numerous studies have already been published examining the impact of isolation and everything it brought upon new parents, mothers in particular. One study in Canada compared pregnant and new mothers' rates of depression and anxiety before and during the pandemic. They found that pre-pandemic 15% of mothers were displaying symptoms of depression and 29% significant symptoms of anxiety. However, during the pandemic this rose to 41% showing symptoms of depression and 72% with anxiety. That is a huge leap.[39]

Likewise, in the UK COVID-19 study of women with a baby under 12 months old during the pandemic, 56% reported feeling down, 59% lonely, 62% irritable and 71% worried – although simultaneously 70% felt that they were coping. Again, having a lower income and concerns about money to the point of worrying about not being able to afford food negatively affected maternal mental health.[40] Another study with mothers with a baby aged 0–12 weeks in the UK found a similar effect:

43% of women had a score indicating depression and 61% indicating anxiety. One of the strongest predictors of depression and anxiety was the degree to which women felt lockdown had affected their mental health. Changes were mainly negative and stemmed from losing social support from family and friends.[41]

This all happened within the wider context of how lockdown, home schooling and working from home affected women, particularly those with older children. Although of course there are exceptions, far more women took on the role of home schooling and caring for children and the home to a greater extent during the lockdown. Families being at home more meant that more housework was needed, which women tended to take more responsibility for.[42] Working mothers were five times more likely to have reduced working hours than men – with the gender gap in working hours growing by 2–50%.[43]

All of this again runs contrary to what we know is important for postnatal care. It isn't just about practical breastfeeding support, but rather how we support women and new families to adapt to life with a new baby and recover from birth. Social support, connection and care is vital in helping that transition to motherhood and for many women it has been disrupted.

Moving forward

Changes are slowly being made as we move through the pandemic, although guidelines around what is 'allowed' in terms of contact have differed between countries in the UK, causing confusion. During periods of stricter lockdown allowances were made for families with a baby under one to have more contact with family or friends in a 'bubble'. Some socially distanced baby groups were allowed to continue.

But moving forward it is vital that we recognise the damage that has been done to new families. Support will be needed in healing the trauma that families will have experienced around birth and postnatal care, including those who have not been able to breastfeed for as long as they wanted to. More broadly, investment must be made in babies and children who have missed out on socialising and opportunities for development that we know are so important in the first year. Based on this a group of charities are calling for the UK Chancellor to invest in a 'Baby Boost' stimulus package to enable an increase in targeted support and interventions based around health visiting, specialist services and charities to support families in recovering from the damages of lockdown and social distancing.[44] Here is their request –

let's hope the government listens:

Dear Chancellor,
We are writing to urge you to ensure that this week's Spending Review allocates vital funding for the youngest children.

The pandemic has resulted in worrying numbers of babies and young children being exposed to stress, trauma and adversity which, if not addressed, could have a significant impact on their wellbeing and development:

- *The Chief Inspector of Ofsted has reported that between April and October, there was a 20% rise in serious incidents of harm to babies compared to the same period last year.*
- *Recent research has shown that almost 7 in 10 (68%) parents felt the changes brought about by COVID-19 were affecting their unborn baby, baby or young child. Many families with lower incomes, from Black, Asian and minority ethnic communities and young parents were harder hit by the pandemic.*
- *When parents experience stress and trauma it can have an impact on their babies too. A range of emerging evidence suggests that the pandemic and lockdown has had a negative impact on parental mental health, due to the traumatic experience of experiencing labour and birth alone, the pressures of lockdown and a lack of support for families.*

The Government's response to COVID-19 has included support for many vulnerable groups in our society, but not the youngest. There is a narrowing window of opportunity now to address the impact of the pandemic on the most vulnerable young children.

Earlier this year Government announced £1bn new funding for schools to close gaps in achievement caused by COVID-19. This equates to around £112 per pupil. A Baby Boost could provide the same amount of funding for the babies of 2020. This would equate to £68m. It would enable local commissioners to fund interventions such as targeted support from health visitors, specialist services and charities, to help babies and families recover from the harms caused by the pandemic.

Alongside action as part of the COVID response, there is a need for more substantial investment in early life. We welcome Government's longer-term commitments to this agenda, including the Leadsom Review, the refresh of the Healthy Child Programme and the increase in the value of healthy start vouchers. Decisions made about the restructure of Public

Health England must also keep the needs of the youngest child in sharp focus. Any new policy commitments must be supported by substantial and sustained investment to rebuild our Health Visiting workforce and enable effective, whole-system action to give every baby the best start in life.

Babies can't wait. Therefore we urge you to take action now to include babies in the COVID recovery, alongside committing to longer term strategic investment in the three-year spending review.

Yours sincerely,

Sarah Hughes, Chief Executive, Centre for Mental Health
Jeff Banks, Director, A Better Start Southend
Neil Leitch, Chief Executive Officer, Early Years Alliance
Anna Feuchtwang, Chief Executive, National Children's Bureau
Melanie Armstrong, Chief Executive, Action for Children
Alison Baum, Chief Executive, Best Beginnings
Peter Grigg, Chief Executive, Home-Start UK
Peter Wanless, Chief Executive Officer, NPSCC
Dr Cheryll Adams CBE, Executive Director, Institute of Health Visiting
Angela McConville, Chief Executive, National Childbirth Trust
Dr Beckie Lang, Chief Executive, Parent-Infant Foundation
Mark Hodgkinson, Chief Executive, Scope
Dr Nick Waggett, Chief Executive, The Association of Child Psychotherapists

18. HOW CAN WE MOVE FORWARD AND PROTECT MOTHERS AND BABIES?

I did not want this book to simply be a list of all the barriers mothers can face when breastfeeding their baby. One of the key aims of my research is to understand how women who want to breastfeed can best be supported to do so. Personally, I believe that we focus far too much on encouraging mothers to start breastfeeding, then forget all about supporting them to continue. Or we tell them it's great, when that's not the full picture. Of course, supporting women to start breastfeeding is important: if they don't start, then they can't continue. But often public health messages try to persuade those who don't want to breastfeed to try, while we then let down those who are trying to continue. This is important in itself. How can we stop it?

I started to explore this question in 2012. I spent a lot of time reading and writing about the challenges women experienced when breastfeeding. I spent a lot of time working with mothers who hadn't met their breastfeeding goals to try to understand why. It occurred to me one day that this was only part of the jigsaw. We were missing a lot of women out: those who had straightforward and enjoyable breastfeeding experiences. They do exist, but they tend to be busy with other stuff, not ruminating on breastfeeding! So could I find them? And what could their experiences tell me?

A key finding of my research was that no one was really happy with public health messages about breastfeeding. So I decided to run a study asking women what helped them to breastfeed, and how they felt breastfeeding education, promotion and support messages could be changed. I set up an open-ended questionnaire, then went away for a couple of weeks, hoping I might get a few answers. I nearly fell off my chair when I came back and found nearly 2,000 responses! Clearly this was something that women felt really passionately about. Might we have an answer?

I sat and actually read every single answer. I couldn't move. Here were hundreds and hundreds of women telling me their experiences and their ideas in such an eloquent way. Eventually I analysed the data for publication and for that I had to reduce the sample, selecting a representative response from 200 participants. I couldn't perform a proper qualitative analysis on them all. But I read them. Every single one. I would love to simply cut and paste all the responses here (maybe that is another book!), but I will summarise what I found.[1]

Firstly, women weren't against breastfeeding being promoted:

'We definitely need to be telling new mothers about why breastfeeding is so good. It is important that they learn about the differences between breast and formula and make an informed choice. I think this should play a larger role in antenatal education but also be extended to everyone else. Everyone needs to know why breastfeeding is so important for mums to stand a chance of making this work.'

But it wasn't that simple…

'You have the ideal behaviour, the gold standard that we should be aiming for. But we have to realise that not everyone can do that. Yes we want it (they want it) but we want them to do lots of other things like not smoke or drink too much. Realise that just feeding for a few days is an achievement for some, or some will want to give formula too. Understand some mothers need to go back to work. Support, understand, enable. Nagging never works. Make breastfeeding seem non-threatening, non-embarrassing and normal and by taking a step back we might actually just get where we want to be.'

From the responses it was clear that women really wanted breastfeeding to be promoted and they felt that organisations such as the NHS should be providing education about breastfeeding during and after pregnancy. Overall around 90% of those who responded felt that it was important to promote breastfeeding, with 80% believing that this promotion had the power to affect a new mother's decision to breastfeed. As one mother noted:

'Before I got pregnant I hadn't really thought about how I would feed my baby. I didn't know anyone who had a baby and my only experience of feeding was, in hindsight, through the formula companies. I thought formula was perfectly normal and fine (and made your baby giggle!) until I heard more about why breast is so good so we really need this information in case others are in the same situation I was.'

So far so good. However, the good news ended there. Around 80% of respondents were unhappy about how breastfeeding was promoted or the information they received from NHS sources:

'I think a fresh approach is needed as the relentless positivity around breastfeeding does a lot to put people off.'

So I set out on a long and involving journey into understanding mothers' experiences of breastfeeding promotion. What did they really want? What worked? What didn't?

Breast is not best

The anti-'breast is best' theme was meant to be a small section, but it demanded its own space and I think it deserves it. Many respondents to my questionnaire wanted to see the 'breast is best' message done away with. Three little words seemed to provoke such outrage. And rightly so. As many were quick to point out, yes, breast is best. We've figured that out. But now what? How does that actually help us? Around 80% of mothers commented on or complained about this phrase – that's a lot of disgruntled women.

'Telling people is one thing but only the start of a very long journey. I think you'll find that most people actually know breast is best now and want to breastfeed. It's not as easy as just doing what's good though or we would all be shockingly healthy and sin free!'

Many rejected the phrase because breastfeeding *isn't* 'best'... it's just normal. Implying that breastfeeding is a superior behaviour is problematic. Saying its 'best' makes it sound like something you need to struggle to achieve... while formula milk is perfectly good enough. 'Best' makes it sound like the icing on the cake. A choice that a certain type of person might be able to make. A gold standard. Something to be idealised... when in fact it's just what bodies are designed to do.

'Breast is best but this puts breastfeeding on an unobtainable pedestal for some people. This then makes infant formula seem to be reachable, normal and something that has all the stuff needed for babies. Instead breastfeeding should be marketed as normal and perfect.'

This idea plays right into the hands of those who would prefer women not to breastfeed. Who honestly does everything right? Eats their five a day? Stays away from chocolate? Just has the occasional alcoholic drink? Goes to bed dutifully at 10pm each night rather than staying glued to a screen because someone is wrong on the internet and needs telling (or there's a particularly funny video of cats)? No one. Even if you manage the diet stuff, the cat videos will still get you.

'Most people are happy to settle for less than the best. The same way most people don't buy premium ranges in supermarkets, they are happy to settle for average or normal, which is what formula is assumed to be in my area'.

Some women commented that 'breast is best' sounded as if it was made up by the formula companies. Given that I don't know any health professionals or breastfeeding supporters who actually use this term any more, I suspect they may well be right.

'It is possibly the single most damaging message to use to "promote" breastfeeding. It sounds like it's been taken straight off the side of a can of infant formula. If breast is best, it is special, above and beyond requirement, so infant formula becomes normal. If breast is NORMAL, it is necessary, anything else is substandard'.

If breast is best, does that mean mothers who breastfeed are best?

The 'breast is best' message also had a darker side. It fuels the 'mummy wars' that appear to be at the heart of many breastfeeding debates. As we've seen, some women won't be able to breastfeed. Some will have to take medications, or have health issues that prevent them from breastfeeding, some will decide that their circumstances mean they need to formula-feed, others will be so battered by negativity and pressure that they will end up formula-feeding despite their intention to breastfeed. What does that make them? Many mothers in my study raised the point that if breast is best, yet they do not breastfeed, does this mean they are not the best mothers?

'Breast is promoted as being best. So if you breastfeed you are the 'best' mother and doing the 'best' for your baby and making the 'best' choices. If you can't breastfeed where does that leave you? A not good enough

mother? A bad mother?'

It's easy to see why mothers feel like this, especially if they are upset about having to stop breastfeeding and exhausted to boot. What the 'breast is best' message does is falsely idealise breastfeeding while condemning those who want to breastfeed but cannot for whatever reason. Women feel guilty, anxious and angry and this leads to a perceived divide between 'the best' and 'the rest'.

'I had a doctor ask me why I didn't want to do the best as a mother for my baby. I was distressed enough at stopping in the first place but his comments broke my heart.'

If we're not going to call breastfeeding 'best', what do we call it? I think this is a key question that we should all think about. 'Normal'? Does that make women who don't breastfeed 'abnormal'? Is there any language we can use without upsetting someone? Or do we need to stop thinking about language and concentrate on understanding why such emotion and personal blame is attached to infant feeding decisions?

Breast is best and the language of breastfeeding

Another idea that came out of the responses to my questionnaire was consideration of how to pitch breastfeeding from a 'biological norm' perspective. Diane Weissinger wrote an excellent article explaining how our language made formula seem like the norm.[2] She challenges our tendency to talk about 'benefits' or 'advantages' of breastfeeding, rather than considering the 'risks' or 'damage' of formula-feeding. This idea was popular in the responses. Women thought that breastfeeding, as the biologically normal thing that a body 'expected' to do, should be the default. Anything that differed from this 'caused' any difference in outcomes. Women felt that public health messages should be flipped to present the risks of formula in this way.

'We need to start talking about the disadvantages of artificial feeding, both to babies and to mums, in the way that we advise against certain things in pregnancy such as smoking, alcohol use, etc.'

'Breastmilk does not reduce the chances of a child being obese etc.,

formula increases the chance of them being obese. We may be sparing some feelings by flipping reality on its head but in the long run we are only hurting ourselves (and making the formula companies a nice big profit!).'

'*We have created adequate substitutes for lots of human functions and processes which in many cases are sophisticated and life-saving. We can transplant hearts, give blood transfusions, donate a kidney. But no one suggests this is anything but something to use when nature does not work. OK so heart disease and milk feeding are not in the same league, but we certainly don't talk about having our own hearts as being 'best'. The underlying message is the same – we should be incredibly grateful for the science that has created formula milk, but it should be marketed as the solution if the normal does not work, not an active choice.*'

In theory this makes a lot of sense. In other areas of health promotion, comparisons are made with the biological norm. Messages surrounding smoking cessation are not cast in terms of the benefits of *not* smoking; they highlight the risks to health of deviating from the biological norm. However, if you look at the breastfeeding literature it typically talks about the benefits of breastfeeding. Even the World Health Organization states that 'Exclusive breastfeeding for 6 months is *best* for babies everywhere', while the NHS ran a breastfeeding campaign entitled 'Off to the *best* start'.

I once had an argument with a reviewer of a paper in which I wrote about the 'risks of formula-feeding'. Their response was 'I'm not sure what this author is talking about when they refer to the risks of formula. As far as I know there are no risks to formula-feeding and if they want to use this terminology then they must show the evidence of these risks'. I argued for a bit, but was too new and naïve an academic to risk my paper being rejected. My review of the literature reveals that most academics appear to feel the same. I have only found one paper that includes the word 'risk' in its title – a 2010 paper by McNiel and colleagues entitled 'What are the risks associated with formula-feeding? A re-analysis and review'.[3]

However, this is science and academia – journal articles are essentially written for other academics and researchers. How should public health messages be worded? I am really torn. Factually, and logically, I believe our language should reflect the truth: that breastfeeding is the biological norm and the health risks of substituting it with something else should be communicated. Might we see increases in breastfeeding rates if the wider population saw formula-feeding as a risk, rather than breastfeeding being a little bit 'extra'? Might others be quicker to support a mother's choice if they understood that formula carries risks, rather than being 'good enough'?

At present the general public certainly doesn't perceive formula as risky. In a study in the USA researchers asked people whether they agreed with two statements. The first was 'Breastfeeding is healthier for babies', and the second was 'Feeding a baby formula instead of breastmilk increases the chances the baby will get sick'. Whereas most people agreed with the first statement, far fewer agreed with the second, despite them actually saying the same thing. How we phrase things certainly seems to be important.[4]

But what about the not-at-all minor issue of women's emotions? In a perfect world I would prefer women who are currently struggling with breastfeeding, or who are upset about stopping breastfeeding, not to have to hear about the 'risks', but I want future populations to have adopted the more accurate language. Surely, if we have magic machines that measure breastmilk, we can manage a little blurring of consecutive realities? However, how do you manage use of language? Does a mother who has struggled to breastfeed and cannot do so, or who is being pressurised by others to formula-feed, really need to hear about 'risk'?

Risk is so emotive. Infant feeding is so emotive. New mothers are a bundle of emotions. And their decision to breastfeed or not is affected by so many factors. Is a decision to formula-feed her 'fault'? No. It is far more complicated than that. Fault implies blame and an active, rational choice from many possible options. Similarly, risk implies a gamble – a deliberate gamble – with her baby's health. Risk is also such a damning word. Yes, on a population level formula-fed babies are at higher risk of illness, but giving your baby formula doesn't mean they will definitely suffer, although the chances of it happening are mathematically higher. Risk sounds so harsh and cold.

I don't know what the answer is. Every time we provoke an emotional reaction we risk(!) creating divides. Maybe we need to work on the issues of emotion and guilt before we decide how we are going to talk about breastfeeding in the future. In this book I have been at pains to avoid labelling or any suggestion of how women should behave. Throughout I've tried to understand and support those who want to breastfeed, and consider the responsibility of others in enabling that. I do not want to tell you to breastfeed, or question your decision to feed in any other way. Most of all I do not want to add fuel to the fire of the concept of mummy wars or breastfeeding battles, not least because I believe that putting this fire out is essential if we are to normalise breastfeeding and support new mothers.

What do women really want?

The first finding in my research was what mothers did *not* want – no more breast is best! However, mothers had very clear ideas about how they *did* want breastfeeding to be promoted. Here are some of the main points.

Breastfeeding is more than just about health

Many mothers reported that during pregnancy and antenatal education they were given plentiful information on the health impact of breastfeeding, but there was less emphasis on other potential benefits of breastfeeding, including those not so obviously health-related. Mothers asked why they weren't told about convenience, lower cost, ease and closeness.

> 'Breastfeeding is about so much more than health. It is about cuddles, and closeness and bonding. It saves time, costs nothing and you can never forget to take it out with you. Why don't we emphasise these things more?'

Perhaps this is because the NHS – understandably – might focus on health rather than our finances and convenience? Yes and no. The problem is the complexity of the message. If the NHS gives you a simple public health message, that breastfeeding protects your baby from X, Y and Z, when the reality is more complicated that message is queried and held to a standard it wasn't meant to support. Just because formula-fed babies are at higher risk of an illness, doesn't meant that all formula-fed babies will get ill. Nor does it mean that no breastfed baby will get ill.

> 'Although there are health differences between breast and formula-fed babies they are not guarantees. Breastfed babies can still get ill, so if mothers are sold the idea of breastfeeding on health benefits alone and then their baby gets sick it can make them feel like they did it wrong or that it wasn't actually that good and they might as well formula-feed as

their friends who did have really healthy kids.'

In an environment where there is so much emotion and blame circulating in relation to breastfeeding, and there is too much emphasis on health and breastfeeding, mothers can face a backlash. Many respondents noted that people had been quick to judge them when their breastfed baby did fall ill, suggesting that if breastfeeding 'worked' then their baby shouldn't ever have had an illness.

> *There is a lot of defensiveness amongst some mothers who do not breastfeed at the idea of breastfed babies being healthier. I had a number of people pointedly notice that my breastfed baby had a cold/bit of dry skin/sticky eye saying that they thought breastfeeding was meant to stop all that and their formula-fed baby didn't have it.'*

We know that illness isn't black and white, and that in life you can't go back and compare the consequences of a different behaviour. Illness is a continuum – a bit of dry skin may have been a lot of dry skin if the baby was formula-fed. We'll never know. Respondents noted that some seemed to view breastmilk as a medicine or health product. Another idea was that moving the focus away from the health implications of breastfeeding might help people to see the more immediate and tangible benefits of breastfeeding:

> *'I think sometimes people don't think much about the health benefits of stuff, especially as they see lots of children who were formula-fed and fine, but tell them about how much cheaper it is, or they will get their figure back quicker or how they don't need to make up bottles in the middle of the night and you'll probably appeal to them?'*

> *'What worked for me second time round was knowing that a tin of formula costs £9 a tin and by 4/5 weeks you'll be buying more than a tin a week. Hit people with the reality of what it'll cost them to formula-feed. Promote the ease and convenience of breastfeeding once the early days are over.'*

Recognising that every feed matters

Breastfeeding was often perceived to be promoted in an either/or dogmatic way, with the implication being that if you weren't going to exclusively breastfeed for six months, you might as well formula-feed.

'If you really want to boost breastfeeding, you have to abandon this black or white stance. I know exclusively breastfed is much better than mixed feeding. But there are so many rules now. No bottles before six weeks, no formula ever, ever – no wonder people give up. Whereas in reality, if mums felt that they could introduce a bottle earlier, or even give a formula-feed now and then, the chances are the baby would still go back to the breast without a problem, and the mum is then much more likely to continue breastfeeding for longer. It's a spectrum, with exclusive breast at one end, and exclusive formula at the other. But it's promoted as a black or white choice and most mums end up failing to keep all the rules and giving up the whole thing.'

I'm not going to say that the WHO advice to breastfeed exclusively for six months and then up to two years and beyond is wrong. Nor am I going to say it is physiologically unachievable. But right now, in our culture, where formula-feeding is normal, is it achievable for the majority? I'll go as far to say it's probably not. Could it be in the future? Yes. I believe that one day in the future breastfeeding will be normal and all women who want to breastfeed will be supported to breastfeed for as long as they want.

But right now only around one in six mothers is exclusively breastfeeding at three months. We 'fail' WHO standards on the *first day*. So why do we keep on, almost dogmatically, telling people that this six months of exclusive breastfeeding is the target? Would it not make more sense to incrementally move towards it? It was clear in the responses that many women felt that breastfeeding had been presented as an either/or. You were either a formula-feeder or a breastfeeder and there was nothing in the middle. Looking at the statistics for the UK, 19% of new mothers never breastfeed and 1% breastfeed exclusively for six months, so the vast majority fall in the middle somewhere. But they also feel like failures. How on earth do we have a situation where such a majority group feels like a failure?

Some suggested that the WHO recommendation discouraged mothers from breastfeeding, and in some cases from even trying at all, because the challenge of breastfeeding exclusively for six months seemed too difficult and they didn't realise that there was a middle ground. Mothers were left feeling that unless they breastfed exclusively they might as well not bother. Apart from this being inaccurate – exclusive formula-feeding carries a greater risk than partial breastfeeding[5] – it is damaging to women's intentions and wellbeing.

Although no respondents thought that the WHO message should be ignored, they felt that wider discussion was needed, to consider how a woman might fall somewhere in the middle. Women needed to know that there was still reason to breastfeed even if the infant was mixed fed, and that breastfeeding for even one day was better than not at all. A common suggestion was that if mothers adopted a 'one day at a time' approach they might end up feeding for longer than they originally intended. Mothers liked slogans such as 'every breastfeed makes a difference', or 'every drop counts'.

'It is all too much. It is overwhelming as a first-time mother who is exhausted by the birth to feel she must now feed this baby exclusively for the next six months. Although we do need to tell mums that it is important, give them some credibility. Tell them the guidelines but explain how all breastfeeding counts. You might have a mother who baulks at the idea of six months, but six weeks or even six days seems achievable for her. That is better than not at all. Take it step by step, doing the best they can. Who knows, once she has breastfeeding established she might end up doing it for two years after all – like me!'

Alongside this there should be recognition for women setting and meeting their own breastfeeding goals, whatever they might be. New research shows that mothers who don't meet their breastfeeding goals are more likely to experience postnatal depression, and my own work consistently shows that readiness to stop breastfeeding is a predictor of wellbeing. Instead, mothers who knew the facts but made an informed decision to stop at six weeks, or who incorporated an occasional bottle of formula, were left feeling guilty or that they had failed their baby.

'We all want the best for our children but that needs to take place within our day to day lives and sometimes that means giving an occasional bottle of formula or stopping at four months old. Stop making us feel like we have failed when we have actually done a good job!'

Mothers make the decision to introduce formula alongside breastfeeding for many different reasons, and although they need to be aware of how it can affect their supply, continued breastfeeding alongside formula milk has fewer risks than stopping breastfeeding altogether. Mothers felt that if discussions could be a bit more open, and give them the information and tools they needed to make an informed choice, more women might initiate breastfeeding and breastfeed for longer. Recognising their efforts, rather than focusing on what they didn't achieve, may help reduce feelings of guilt about stopping breastfeeding.

Make a breastfeeding plan

'Driving a car is great. It gives you so much freedom. You can get from A to B and not have to rely on the vagaries of public transport. Now, here's your driving test examiner – off you go! What? What do you mean you haven't had any lessons? Driving a car is great! We all think you should do it. Off you go...

Time for your algebra exam. If you get this right there are so many benefits. What? You don't know how to balance equations? But algebra is great. You must learn algebra, it's really important.'

Breastfeeding is biologically normal. That doesn't mean it is straightforward. Many new couples eagerly attend antenatal classes to prepare for childbirth (also biologically normal), which is only the relatively short start of a journey of caring for a baby. However, many pregnant women spend hours reading about labour and making a plan for the birth. They think about what might happen, and the strategies they would like to employ to cope. But what about breastfeeding? Many breastfeeding classes cover the ubiquitous 'breast is best' message, followed by advice about how to latch a baby on. Nothing about what it is really like to breastfeed. Nothing about how frequently a baby feeds, how they need feeding lots at night or the importance of responsive feeding. For many of us, our own baby is the first baby we ever truly care for. We are unlikely to have grown up around lots of siblings being breastfed, and with fewer and fewer women openly breastfeeding and talking about it, we are unlikely to have ever really understood it.

As a consequence women have babies that need feeding. Now. And likely again in an hour or so. And an hour after that. Many mothers in the survey discussed how they struggled with breastfeeding in the early days, or felt that breastfeeding was not as they had expected. Many lacked experience of caring for a baby or knowing what it was like to breastfeed. Their desire to breastfeed was high, and their intention to do so was strong, but their knowledge? Lacking. When faced with a newborn, many struggled with latching the infant on, pain or just wondered whether they were doing it 'right' or not. Was their baby getting enough milk? Should they feed them at night? Surely they can't need feeding again? An overwhelming feeling of being unprepared was common.

So how should we present this to new mothers? It has been suggested that if we present breastfeeding as 'problematic' or 'challenging', it could put new mothers off and perpetuate the 'myth' that breastfeeding is difficult. But this seems condescending. Giving birth is difficult. Being a parent is difficult. Feeding a baby, in any way, can be difficult! Give women some credit. Many of the things we want in life are difficult in some way, but being prepared for them (by revising algebra, or taking driving lessons) enhances the likelihood that we will be able to do it. Breastfeeding should be no different.

Secondly, the idea that emphasising the challenges of breastfeeding perpetuates the myth that it is difficult is untrue. When a woman says breastfeeding is difficult and she had to stop, most of the underlying reasons are nothing to do with the act itself being difficult. It is a lack of the knowledge underpinning how breastfeeding works that leads it to be seen as too difficult. If women knew the importance of responsive feeding and what normal breastfed baby behaviour is then they would be more prepared to breastfeed. We gloss over the realities of breastfeeding, even though women have little experience of what breastfeeding is really like, and are then surprised that they struggle. We effectively shield mothers from the idea of potential difficulties, demands or inconveniences to encourage them to breastfeed, but it has the opposite effect, leaving them shocked and concerned that because these issues haven't been mentioned, something must be wrong.

'It was all so positive. Breast is best for your baby. Breastfeeding will help you lose weight. Breastfeeding will make bonding with your baby easier. Breastfeeding is a wonderful experience. Perhaps all that is true but it is in no way the whole picture. When I then found it difficult, at times demanding and my baby appeared to want to scream rather than snuggle serenely at my breast I felt like a complete failure and embarrassed and guilty that I felt that way to boot.'

'I think more honesty is needed. The majority of women find it difficult and painful to start with but being told that if you are doing it right will mean you experience no problems just leaves loads of woman feeling like they are doing it wrong. I think it insults mothers to think that they will only do what is easiest. I think that even if you told mothers that this will be a long hard slog for the first few months they would still breastfeed as every mother wants what's best for their child. They would simply be *better prepared.'*

Specific issues that mothers wished they had known more about before they had their baby were things like honest information about pain, potential infections and how normal it can be for babies to feed all the time.

> *'Honest, real information about how hard it can be to latch on, things you can do to help latch, most common issues and solutions to those. How it can hurt, its normal to struggle at the start, information about growth spurts, more information on how milk production actually works so mums can then make informed decisions on feeding and know if they do something like top-up with formula then how it will impact their supply.'*

> *'It would have helped to have been honestly told that it's not a piece of cake and that you have to learn it and that it's normal to hurt/feel uncomfortable for the first few weeks; that "it's natural" doesn't mean "it's easy and will just happen". More information about potential problems would be useful. I have various friends who failed to breastfeed for various reasons, baby not latching on properly, tongue-tied, etc. They were made to feel guilty and didn't get much support, which I think is wrong.'*

This supports stuff we already know. Sheehan studied this in 2006[6] and I'm sure if I dug further back I would find research showing that mothers have been asking for this information for much longer. We also know that mothers who are more confident and informed about breastfeeding, breastfeed for longer. It's not rocket science. So why aren't we doing it? Why are we not spending time teaching mothers to breastfeed?

Redesign the image of breastfeeding

It is also important to get messages that target the mother right. If you look at promotional materials for breastfeeding, although they are getting better, many portray a certain 'type' of mother; older, educated, middle-class and often almost deliberately flashing a giant wedding ring. This seems counter-intuitive, given that this group of mothers usually breastfeeds for longer anyway. Mothers in my research said that these pictures and promoted lifestyles needed to be far more inclusive. Breastfeeding needed to be 'sold' as attractive to all groups, emphasising how it fitted in with lifestyle and other commitments. Mothers felt that a message that showed mothers of all ages breastfeeding and combining it with looking after other children, a social life, education, hobbies, activities or a career would help fit the idea into their lifestyles, rather than it being viewed as something that was restrictive and for a certain 'type' of mother.

> 'Often the pictures in manuals are rather 70s and hippyish and contribute to a stereotype that breastfeeding is for frumpy earth-mothers. I would like to see more mums like me – young, lipstick-wearing professionals – and a recognition that breastfeeding can be combined with a social life and a high-status career.'

Using celebrities who were open about breastfeeding was thought to be a good tactic for helping to normalise breastfeeding and to appeal to younger girls who might be thinking about how in future they might feed their baby.

> 'Angelina Jolie breastfed twins for 3 months, Dannii Minogue breastfed before shows on X Factor. Use strong role models like this to show those who won't try that it is not that difficult.'

Target a wider audience

A current concept in supporting families is the 'team around the family'. At its heart is the notion that everyone who works to support a family – in health, education and social care – should work together to enable the family to be the strongest it can be. A similar approach can be applied to breastfeeding, in that those around the mother should be working together to enable her to breastfeed for as long as she wants. As discussed earlier, partners, friends, family and wider society all affect her decision and ability.

So why, when it comes to breastfeeding promotion, does everything seem to be targeted at the mother? No man is an island… and nor are breastfeeding mothers and babies. They are affected by the actions of others, and wider social, economic and environmental factors. Given that most women want to breastfeed, shouldn't we focus on getting everyone else to help her (or at least stop criticising her)?

> 'You can tell women that breast is best until the cows come home. But if their partner believes differently and the mother-in-law is trying to give the baby a bottle, who do you think is going to win? Tell mums by all means but also tell their wider family – get the message out there in a way

everyone will buy into it.'

'I found the hardest struggle was trying to educate the mother-in-law – get the family on side and breastfeeding becomes a lot easier!'

Respondents' ideas about breastfeeding promotion went further. Many suggested that promotion needed to be more general – and, given the attitudes towards breastfeeding in public we've already discussed, this is a critical point. The general public must be made aware that breastfeeding is an important thing to support, or at least be told to stop criticising it and believing their comfort is more important than a baby being fed.

Mothers in the survey felt it was important to target society as a whole, so that new mothers would feel confident in their decision to breastfeed. By encouraging greater acceptance of breastfeeding, it would become more commonplace, visible and expected. Future generations of mothers would feel supported, as breastfeeding would once again be the social and cultural norm. Ideas for targeting wider groups and increasing acceptance included incorporating breastfeeding into school curricula, billboard campaigns and having breastfeeding featured in television programmes.

'The only thing you can do is make it more normal and accepted. If everyone grows up seeing pictures of it, seeing it on soaps etc. and seeing people doing it, it will be a normal natural thing to do.'

'I'd like lots of images of breastfeeding to surround us and to live in a world where mothers could and did breastfeed openly in public. I'd like to see pictures of babies at the breast instead of babies with bottles.'

Advertising campaigns aimed at the general public were seen as important. Mothers raised the very valid point that formula companies bought significant screen time, even if they were supposedly advertising a product for older babies, whereas there was an absence of breastfeeding promotion in a format that got anyone's attention.

'Australia does some good adverts on TV which are very widely seen and help to counter formula promotion. PLEASE stop the TV ads for formula as they're so misleading and PLEASE promote breastfeeding on TV. Breastfeeding welcome signs are also brilliant.'

'Formula companies advertise by showing bouncy, happy babies rather than just them sucking on a bottle. Maybe we need to see how we can promote breastfeeding in other ways than the more traditional.'

Talking about younger children, a number of respondents also raised the idea that breastfeeding should be firmly on the curriculum in schools:

'Maybe have breastfeeding mothers go into schools and talk about it. I'm rather horrified by the number of small children who see me breastfeeding and have absolutely no idea what I'm doing.'

'Go into schools. Talk to the children before someone else gives them the idea that breastfeeding is something to be ashamed about and formula milk is normal.'

Could schools handle this? I have a feeling many are not ready. One friend explained to me how her child's teacher had asked whether anyone's parent could bring a young baby into school to show the reception-aged children, as they were learning about babies. A few put their names forward and two mothers went in. Both of those mothers were bottle-feeding. Those who were told thanks but no thanks were breastfeeding. Perhaps this is coincidence. However, another friend, who asked if she could take her breastfed baby in to show the children how babies were fed, was told she could not as it was a sexual behaviour. I'll just leave that there for a moment. Yes, some people responsible for educating our children believe that breastfeeding is too sexualised for a young child to see. And then we wonder why our teenagers are horrified by the idea of breastfeeding...

Young children handle the idea of breastfeeding very well, although many have simply never seen it. When I breastfed my own children in public I often got asked 'What you doing?' by a small child who had wandered up. Children know what they see, and children who have been bottle-fed, whose siblings are bottle-fed, know about bottle-feeding. There is no need to explain differences in feeding practice at length to random small children, but introducing children to different ways of feeding is important.

What about breastfeeding support after the birth?

'I was on the verge of giving up and then a friend gave me this number and told me to ring it as they could help me. I spoke to this lovely woman who just listened to me cry for a bit and then gave me some advice that made such a difference. It changed my life and that isn't an exaggeration. I owe her so much.'

Cries for more support jumped out from my survey of new mothers, but the concept of support is nothing new. Many mothers felt that they had been so strongly encouraged to breastfeed – built up, pressurised even, and then after the birth… tumbleweed. Breastfeeding is normal, yes, but as described earlier, not necessarily easy. And learning how to breastfeed is an important stage of caring for a baby. But, sadly, for many mothers that skilled support is not there.

'The breast is best message is good but in the absence of practical support it is really just words! It means nothing to "know" it's best, to read it on posters etc. when you cannot physically manage to get through the physical and emotional trauma and nobody will help you! The message is great but mothers who encounter problems and are begging for help need far more than just lip service! We need to know what problems to look out for, how to get support and, more importantly, that support should be forthcoming when we ask for it!'

It is this lack of support, after months of being told that 'breast is best', that makes mothers feel miserable about stopping breastfeeding. Many felt that the promotion of breastfeeding had succeeded in raising their desire and determination to breastfeed, but had not equipped them with information and support to do so, leaving them feeling guilty and upset when they stopped.

'They seem to spend so much effort telling everyone to breastfeed, how important it is, how they must do it etc, etc. Then once you actually have the baby they just leave you to get on with it! Of course mums then struggle, give up and feel guilty… guiltier than they would have if they hadn't been told just how good it was.'

'I am deeply disappointed with the NHS. The breast is best message means that if you have to or choose to formula-feed you are vilified, no advice or support provided and you feel you are poisoning your child. I

had minimal help despite my baby starving as I made minimal milk. I was bullied into breastfeeding. My baby lost weight, was readmitted to hospital and formula was withheld by midwives. I expressed every three hours for weeks with no help or support while unwell. The promotion is unrealistic and makes mothers who cannot feed feel like failures.'

Sadly a number of mothers told the same story: they were failed by a lack of trained health professionals after the birth. Many felt angry that health professionals were not following through with their promotion of breastfeeding. They felt that although antenatally the message was clear that they should breastfeed and avoid formula, when they actually experienced difficulties or needed support, the solution given was to introduce formula or to stop breastfeeding:

'I needed more specialist help in the hospital rather than just a printed sheet to take home with me and also I felt that the midwives/health visitors that saw me at home did not help me with the issues I was having. Eventually I went to a drop-in clinic that had an expert advisor there and she was brilliant. All of the midwives should be able to advise like that. Before that I went to the breastfeeding advice drop-in at my local children's centre and the midwife there said "Well I don't know why you are so worried about breastfeeding, and I am not an expert, so I can't really help you".'

'It was almost funny. They spent the whole pregnancy enforcing the breastfeeding message and refusing to talk to me about formula-feeding as breast is best. And then postnatally, when I had problems and looked for help, almost the first suggestion was 'Why don't you try a bottle?'. I almost expected a comedian to jump out and tell me I was in some kind of satire show.'

So what is actually going on with breastfeeding support? Why are mothers not able to access the support they need? Surely building mothers up to breastfeed and then not supporting them to do so is at best a pointless waste of resources and at worst deliberately harmful? Thankfully, not all the responses were so bleak. Positive stories did emerge, with mothers recalling how they had talked to breastfeeding peer supporters and expert health professionals who did help them. So what does work?

'I went to this great class. We covered why breastfeeding is so important

and how to do it but also what it was really like to breastfeed. Some local peer supporters came in and actually fed in front of us (which was the first time I had seen a baby feed) and talked about problems they had and importantly how they got over them. They then gave us details of how to contact them and groups to go to once the baby was here. We felt part of something and like we knew what to expect.'

'One of my friends told me she found it really difficult and often wanted to give up in the early days but to come and speak to her if I felt like this. I thought she was being a bit melodramatic at the time but when, at a few weeks in and I had barely slept since the birth, I found myself about to ask my husband to get formula I remembered her words. If she hadn't said that I might have asked him to go get it as I might have thought it was just me.'

Peer support (which the government is cutting funding for) always comes up when you ask women what they want.

'Peer support was absolutely vital to me breastfeeding. I'd never have done it without meeting other mums who were going through the same thing. I really wouldn't have. I was so tired and fed up but I'd go along to group and there would be all these friendly faces and someone would make me a cup of tea and I just knew it would all be alright again.'

'Seriously – peer support is so important. You need to know what you are doing is normal, especially if everyone else around you has formula-fed and is telling you that baby should be on a bottle or sleeping or whatever it is that your baby isn't doing.'

I spoke to Dr Heather Trickey, who is an expert on the issue of peer support, about what works best:

'It is overly simplistic to think of breastfeeding peer support as a single intervention which either works or does not work, and which can be evaluated in isolation from delivery context. Given the considerable heterogeneity in models of peer support that exist across the UK and the small proportion of possible interventions that have been trialled, it is conceivable that the right intervention, with the right population, in the right context, employing the right mechanism, towards the right outcomes has not yet been evaluated. The conclusion that peer support is "unlikely to be effective" in the UK seems premature.'

The conclusion to all this is inescapable. We need to invest in different layers of breastfeeding support for women. This includes professional and peer support, but also educating the general public on how to support breastfeeding women.

19. HOW DO WE HANDLE SUPPORTING *ALL* FAMILIES?

'I don't understand how we have ended up in this situation with so much emotion and bad feeling attached to how we feed babies. The message we are currently giving to new mothers has not increased breastfeeding, but it has increased guilt, division and anger. I don't know anyone who would knowingly say "you know what, breast is best but I can't be bothered with that". Decisions are much deeper and often have a long and emotional story behind them. We need to work out a non-confrontational way of telling everyone just how fantastic breastfeeding is, but following through by supporting them. Actually help new mothers to breastfeed. Recognise achievements no matter how small. Make breastfeeding seem normal again. Stop the criticism and pressure and bit by bit by taking a step back we might actually just get to where we want to be.'

This really is the ultimate question. How do we promote and support breastfeeding, without further damaging women who are uncomfortable about their breastfeeding decisions? I pondered this question back in 2016 for the first edition, and apparently wasn't quite so sure what needed to be done. However, later that year I undertook some research to answer that very question – how can we better support women who wanted to breastfeed but were unable to do so for whatever reason?[1] The research was part of a larger project on how women feel when they are in this situation. They talked about the emotional impact of not being able to breastfeed for as long as they wanted, highlighting the sheer breadth and depth of their grief, anger, guilt and other emotions.[2] What was particularly pertinent was that the emotions they felt were due to two main things. First, not being able to breastfeed, but second, how they were treated when that happened.

Their words provided an important plan for making things better for all women – whether they are breast, formula or mixed feeding. And putting that plan into place is so important. Some people might do a double-take at this point. What? You want to put effort into supporting formula? When women who are breastfeeding are being let down at every level?

Yes, absolutely.

The number one reason for this is that supporting all women and families is important. Everyone deserves information, kindness and respect, however they feed their babies. Being pro-breastfeeding is not the same as being anti-formula – and anyone who thinks otherwise is not helping anyone. What I want to see is informed choice. Genuine informed choice. So everyone has information, free from industry influence. And then they have the support they need to make their infant-feeding decisions happen. At the moment we are a very long way away from choice, informed or otherwise. Women often end up wanting one thing and being forced into another, so supporting everyone is really important.

Another reason is that we need to do better at getting this first point across, because so much time is wasted and people hurt in the process due to debates getting completely out of control. You know the type. Sunday afternoon on Twitter. Someone posts something innocuous about supporting breastfeeding women and all hell breaks loose. Everyone ends up somewhere between pissed off and upset. Or both. And we don't actually get any further with helping anyone. I want to see a world where 'we need to support breastfeeding women better' is taken as the factual statement it is and not a criticism of anyone's decisions or suggestion anyone's baby isn't okay.

So what ideas did women have about making things better?

1. Better support for breastfeeding

Notably, the most common thing that women suggested was that they wished there had been better support for breastfeeding in the first place. The fights you see on social media suggesting we shouldn't invest in breastfeeding are one-sided and made up of a minority of voices. Most women realised that if we wanted to make things better for the future, we needed to invest in making sure the next generation of women had a much higher chance of being able to breastfeed.

This included more skilled support, better training for all health professionals who could influence infant-feeding decisions and better identification and support for breastfeeding complications. When complications arose, they wanted specialist pathways and someone who knew what they were doing and could help. When things really weren't working out they did not want to be told that 'lots of women can't breastfeed'. They wanted it to be treated as other medical issues are – tests, diagnoses and interventions. Not simply a statement that their body was not working. They wanted recognition of a problem – a label as such – rather than inference that they hadn't tried hard enough.

As part of this women called for more research into the breast and breastfeeding, more specialist training and ultimately more funding. There should be referral pathways and treatments available, not leaving this entire area of health to rely on volunteers.

2. Better antenatal education and honesty around breastfeeding

Just like in the previous chapter, women wanted more information that was realistic and actually prepared them for breastfeeding. They didn't want flowery encouragement or a suggestion it was the easier option. They wanted facts, knowledge on how to spot complications and avenues for support. This was also important for them when they stopped breastfeeding as they then weren't made to feel like there was something wrong with them because 'breastfeeding is easy and idyllic'.

3. Changes to language used

Again, that pesky 'breast is best' message came up. But other phrases also made women feel guilty or like they were failing their baby. These included:

- Suggestions that infant-feeding decisions were a 'choice' e.g. choosing to formula-feed when very often they were nowhere near a free choice.
- Use of the phrase 'give up breastfeeding' – as if they'd just decided to chuck it in the bin one wet Thursday afternoon.
- Anything that uses the word 'failure' anywhere near a mother. Women do not fail to breastfeed, they are failed.

Women also talked about trying to make sure that promotion messages were accurate and didn't villainise formula milk. There is no need to continually say 'breastmilk is great because it contains X… and formula doesn't'. Promotion strategies in particular that suggested formula-feeding was akin to giving a baby a Mars bar or McDonalds were particularly hated. This was all embedded in wider over-exaggeration of the protection of breastfeeding (and by default the risk of formula-feeding) when actually, as noted earlier, it is about risks and odds, not a definitive death sentence (in countries with access to clean water and sanitation).

4. More recognition and support for the emotions not being able to breastfeed can bring

Women wanted better support in managing stopping breastfeeding. They wanted a chance to tell their story and debrief and receive additional specialist support if needed. They wanted recognition that they were grieving, and their emotions were serious. They wanted to know where to find this support and who would give it non-judgementally. Women wanted someone to see their pain and difficulty and acknowledge it, rather than pretending it didn't matter or exist. Just a few kind words made all the difference. Part of this was helping women to value what they had achieved rather than what they had not.

Many brought up the phrase 'fed is best'. Some said they found the phrase comforting, feeling that it emphasised that the main thing was that their baby was fed, and that they were caring for their baby despite not meeting their own expectations. However, many others raised the fact that the phrase, even though often said with good intentions, actually made them feel a lot worse. To them all they could hear was that no one cared about how they felt and that the main thing was that their baby was fed… their emotions didn't matter and to feel anything negative was wrong, as this suggested they cared more about themselves than the baby.

This is so important. Saying that you value breastfeeding is not saying that you would rather your baby starve. You can be simultaneously very grateful for formula milk and grieve breastfeeding. One does not cancel the other out! To me telling mothers 'fed is best' can feel like the equivalent of telling a new mother that all that matters is she has a healthy baby. Of course everyone wants a healthy baby. But again, these things aren't an either/or situation. We don't have to pick one. A woman and her baby both matter.

5. More practical support for those who use formula

A lot of mothers said that they felt there was no real information or support for formula-feeding, e.g. picking a milk, making up a bottle and how much to give their baby. Somehow women are falling through the gaps as both UNICEF Baby Friendly and the NHS are clear on the information and support women should have and have detailed guidance online. Somehow this information is not reaching some mothers. One area in particular women wanted support was for mixed feeding – something that keeps coming up. Again, this information is out there but it doesn't appear to be reaching women. Why?

Others highlighted the lack of social support for mothers who were not breastfeeding. They wanted more groups where all feeding was supported. One mother talked about being told she could no longer attend a breastfeeding group as she had to stop breastfeeding and was absolutely floored by this. Some felt that information for other activities such as baby massage was accessed through breastfeeding groups meaning that they missed out.

The idea of mixed feeding support groups always leads to debate. Some feel that breastfeeding women value that safe space and in a world with limited funding that must be preserved. Others think that given many women both breast and formula-feed, a mixed group could be a good idea. Some who have no intention of breastfeeding may change their mind if they see others do it. Conversely, few breastfeeding women are going to be swayed to stop breastfeeding just because they see it in a group – it's not like they never see bottle-feeding outside of baby groups!

6. Better value for mothers

Finally, alongside smashing the patriarchy and bringing down capitalism, a core feeling was the idea of better valuing mothers. If we loved and cared for and respected new families, we'd go a long way to improving things for everyone. Really, that just sums up about everything in this book doesn't it? Job done.

20. SO, WHAT CAN WE ACTUALLY DO ABOUT THIS? WHAT CAN *I* DO?

Bringing all this together, I wanted to suggest a clear action plan for what we can do as a society and individuals to make things better. I hope by now we have a good understanding of what is influencing our infant-feeding decisions in the UK and around the world. To recap:

- ✓ Action 1: Invest in woman-centred, one-to-one care during pregnancy and birth to get breastfeeding off to the best possible start.
- ✓ Action 2: All hospital, neonatal and community services should adopt UNICEF Baby Friendly standards and practices.
- ✓ Action 3: Invest in expert support for all breastfeeding women right from the start of breastfeeding.
- ✓ Action 4: Tell all new parents and those around them about normal feeding and sleep, and support them in other ways to get more rest.
- ✓ Action 5: Tell parents and those around them about normal patterns of weight loss and weight gain in breastfed babies, and why this doesn't mean that they are underweight.
- ✓ Action 6: Bin all the rubbish baby care books.
- ✓ Action 7: Give new mothers the emotional and practical support they need, every step of the way.
- ✓ Action 8: Stop this ridiculous body image pressure on new mothers and come to terms with our own illogical sensitivities and prejudices about human milk and the female body.
- ✓ Action 9: Educate partners and family to be the breastfeeding supporters they can be.
- ✓ Action 10: Educate the public to stop being idiots, or at least do no harm.
- ✓ Action 11: Support employers to be breastfeeding friendly.
- ✓ Action 12: Regulate industry to prevent the promotion of unnecessary and potentially harmful products.

Although we can all do our part in contributing to some of these, such as supporting the new parents that we know, many of these actions require higher-level investment and commitment. They require the government to recognise why breastfeeding is important for society and to implement the structures that would enable more women to breastfeed for longer. Some of these things are only in their direct power – investing in more midwives, health visitors and lactation specialists for example, or cracking down on industry advertising. In 2017 I wrote a review paper[1] considering what steps the government should focus on in order to try and move things forward and create an environment that enabled change. It focused on five key areas:

- Investment in health services
- Population-level health promotion
- Supporting maternal legal rights
- Protection of maternal wellbeing
- Reducing the reach of the breastmilk substitute industry

These five points cover many of the broader action points above, taking the perspective that if we invest in supporting new mothers right from the start in terms of practical support, mental health, legal rights and simply valuing them, then we will come a long way. They basically say that if we support women better, rather than putting barriers in their way, they will be able to breastfeed for longer.

A number of initiatives in recent years are focusing on similar steps. These include:

1. The Global Becoming Breastfeeding Friendly project[2]

This project led by Yale University supports countries to identify whether their country has a breastfeeding-friendly environment and to set steps to improve it. It asks countries to rate themselves across a series of measures, considering whether they are doing those things well or whether there is room for improvement. They include:

- Breastfeeding advocacy
- Political will
- Legislation and policies
- Funding and resources
- Training and programme delivery
- Promotion

- Research and evaluation
- Coordination, goals and monitoring

The idea is very similar to my research paper above –if we invest in the structures that we know support breastfeeding, we will move forward. However, we need government recognition and buy-in to do that. The UK has taken part in the exercise, including separate projects for the different nations. At the time of writing the Scottish report is available, but look out for the others soon.[3] Scotland scored fairly well – we suspected they would compared to the rest of the UK as they generally have greater active investment in supporting breastfeeding such as setting up their own infant feeding survey, as mentioned earlier, when the UK-wide one was cancelled. Their key areas for improvement are around breastfeeding promotion and legislation and policies.

2. UK World Breastfeeding Trends Initiative (WBTi)

In 2016, the UK WBTi report was launched. The WBTi is a tool to examine how governments are supporting 10 key indicators that we know support breastfeeding.[4] It helps countries identify what they are doing well and where they could make improvements, allowing countries to compare themselves on these set ratings around the world. The indicators (scored neatly out of 10 and the UK scores for 2016 in brackets after) are:

1. National policy, programme and coordination. Is there a national infant and young child feeding strategy, a national coordinating committee and a national coordinator, as recommended in the Global Strategy? [score – 1]
2. Baby Friendly Initiative. Do all mothers have access to accredited Baby Friendly maternity care? [score – 7.5]
3. International Code of Marketing of Breastmilk Substitutes. Are the provisions of the International Code and subsequent World Health Assembly Resolutions (the Code) enacted in national legislation and fully enforced? [score – 6]
4. Maternity protection. Do women have adequate paid maternity leave and breastfeeding breaks? [score - 6.5]
5. Health professional training. Are all health professionals who work with mothers and babies adequately trained to support breastfeeding? [score - 5.5]
6. Community-based support. Do all mothers have access to skilled

breastfeeding support from health professionals and others in the community? [score – 7]

7. Information support. Is there a comprehensive national information, education and communication strategy, with accurate information on infant and young child feeding at every level? [score – 5.5]

8. Information support. Is there a comprehensive national information, education and communication strategy, with accurate information on infant and young child feeding at every level? [score – 6.5]

9. Infant and young child feeding during emergencies. Are guidelines in place to provide protection to infants and young children in case of emergency? [score – 0]

10. Monitoring and evaluation. Are monitoring and evaluation data regularly collected and used to improve infant and young child feeding practices? [score – 5]

Overall, to save you the maths, that's a score of 50.5/100. Could do better UK, could do better. The rest of the report explores data for the four nations, including adding in feeding practices indicators to give a score out of 150. These are:

- Early initiation of breastfeeding within 1 hour of birth
- Mean percentage of babies 0–<6 months exclusively breastfed
- Median duration of breastfeeding
- Bottle-feeding: percentage of babies of 0–12 months fed with bottle
- Complementary feeding: percentage of babies receiving solids by 8 months

Overall scores for the four nations are: Scotland [102.5], Northern Ireland [102], Wales [88], England [80.5]. Again, the simple message is that governments need to make investment in policy, practice and legislation that creates the environment that enables more women to initiate and continue breastfeeding. None of those things are about pointing the finger at individual women, but rather giving them the support they need.

Are governments paying attention to this?

Governments are listening to these recommendations… partially. Recently Wales developed an All-Wales Breastfeeding Five Year Action Plan,[5] which I contributed to alongside great colleagues in public health, policy and academia. This plan sets out strategic aims and steps to meet these, with the aim of supporting more women to breastfeed.

Strategic Approach 1: Health System

1. Supporting families to make informed decisions about how to feed their baby.
2. Enabling mothers who have opted to breastfeed to do so successfully for as long as they would like to do so.
3. Creating and sustaining an environment that supports breastfeeding in the healthcare system.

Strategic Approach 2: Population Level and Whole System

1. Supporting the population to make informed choices on infant feeding.
2. Influencing social norms – towards breastfeeding being seen as the normal way of feeding a baby and accepted as part of everyday life.
3. Creating settings and environments which reflect a positive and inclusive ethos towards breastfeeding (e.g. schools, workplaces, public places/transport).
4. Controlling the advertising and managing the availability of less optimal infant feeding methods (e.g. follow-on formula milk).

This is a brilliant start. It says all the right things. But what it now needs is *investment*. Because without investment, what use is a strategy? We *know* what the barriers to breastfeeding are (if you don't you need to go back to the start of this book) and we *know* what we think will help remove them and enable women. Now let's invest in putting those ideas into practice. The best outcomes for breastfeeding are associated with *more* support, from both health professionals and peer supporters, preferably delivered face-to-face.[6] This standard of care cannot be best delivered entirely through voluntary or local provision from pockets of local funds. A clear, ring-fenced funding strategy for breastfeeding is needed that properly enables high-quality support to be delivered. Using tools such as the WBTi indices and the Becoming Breastfeeding Friendly exercise can help governments understand where they most need to target funds. It's also important that this investment is consistent and long term; it can take time for interventions to embed and work their way through to changes in behaviour and health outcomes.[7]

However, despite awareness (or at least lip service to) the importance of infant feeding for longer-term health and development, in relatively rich countries such as the UK, which are juggling numerous immediate health and social care issues, breastfeeding is often not given the priority or investment it deserves. Despite evidence of the protective impact of breastfeeding in high-income regions,[8] breastfeeding is often considered an issue for low- and middle-income regions with a disconnect between how a baby is fed and longer-term health implications.[9] Often too much investment focuses on firefighting the health emergencies of non-communicable diseases rather than tackling their origins, particularly those that arise in infancy and from infant feeding.[10] It seems so obvious to us here, but somehow we need to persuade governments to open their eyes and see how much the health of our nation could be improved by investing right at the start.

Another important part of policy around increasing breastfeeding rates and support is making sure that recommendations are not just centred around maternity care. Too often reference to breastfeeding is only seen in policies about supporting infant feeding. There will be reference to how important infant feeding is for health and development, but when you then go and look at similar policies around preventing health or developmental issues, breastfeeding is nowhere to be seen. For example, despite awareness that infant feeding plays an important role in later weight and eating behaviour, reference to breastfeeding was completely missing from the UK government's Childhood Obesity Strategy.[11] Bizarrely the policy emphasised how many children are already overweight or obese by the time they enter school and then failed to focus on aspects such as infant feeding that affect weight before school entry. Notably, Wales does refer to early experiences including infant feeding (and introducing solid foods) in its '10 steps to a healthy weight' plan.[12]

Alongside funding and investment, the government and public health organisations need to truly get behind breastfeeding by not only producing policies that promote it, but also vocalising their belief in and support of the policies and the importance of breastfeeding. Clear political leadership is needed to turn policies into action. This really does make a difference. For example, countries such as Brazil, which have seen significant improvements in breastfeeding uptake and continuation over the few last decades, have centred visible government leadership and support for breastfeeding in their strategies.[13] Direction (and investment) must come from strong leadership in directing a nuanced, woman-centred approach to breastfeeding support across a country.

Clear leadership also gives support, legitimacy and power for those working on the ground. A breastfeeding supporter working in the community will have far greater opportunity for their messages to be heard if they can refer to 'high up' voices who are on their side. We have some amazing politicians fighting for support for breastfeeding in parliament (to name and thank just a few: Alison Thewliss, SNP; Alex Davies-Jones, Welsh Labour; Cat Smith, Labour; Dave Doogan, SNP; Mhairi Black, SNP... and any other MP that has ever attended the All Party Parliamentary Group on Infant Feeding and Inequalities or stood up for breastfeeding in any other way).

A big part of that vocal leadership is to insist that legislation is in place that protects breastfeeding and families. Women cannot be expected to battle additional challenges outside of their control that can make breastfeeding too complex. We must as a country strengthen our regulations around the breastmilk substitute industry and predatory marketing towards families. We must ensure women are protected to breastfeed on return to work and have sufficient well-paid maternity leave to ensure that they have the option to do that when they want. We must fight to ensure women are not discriminated against for becoming mothers. Protective legislation (and consequences) must be fully enacted to really make a difference.

Saying that, there is actually much we can learn about promoting and supporting breastfeeding from the breastmilk substitute industry. Despite how awful many of their tactics are, there is something almost to be admired in the way companies work to reach women. Ad campaigns are based on significant research into understanding what messaging works and who for. Messages, slogans and designs are consistent with everyone in the organisation getting behind the brand. Significant investment is given, knowing there will be a return.[14] Compare these carefully planned and resourced campaigns to the breastfeeding promotions led by government. They don't come close.

In summary? We need to hold the government to account. Politicians have the power to really make a difference here. We have to continue working to persuade them that it is necessary.

For further inspiration see the appendices for our joint position statement on supporting breastfeeding (2019) and our open letter on the current crisis in breastfeeding in the UK – UK mothers are being let down (2016).

But what can *I* do?

These are all pretty high-level ideas based on encouraging a public health approach to creating the environment we need to support breastfeeding in the UK. But what can we all do to make a difference in our everyday lives when we might not be engaging with politicians and health departments?

Recognise that it is women being failed, not women failing

The first rule of moving this forward is to recognise who is to blame and keep repeating that. If you feel let down, turn that into passion to change things. Turn anger into motivation. Guilt into determination. If you look around you and feel demotivated because there are just so many women to help, know that we can get there. If you've been rejected for yet another grant, meeting request or publication, get back up. We've work to do.

Be an advocate of advocates

Three amazing authors I have read recently – Michelle Obama, Brené Brown and Caitlin Moran all talk about the importance of supporting other women, building them up and never tearing them down. Whether we like it or not, breastfeeding is a predominantly female issue. Most of the voices leading this game are women's. And we know that women, on the whole, are less likely to be given time to speak and less likely to be listened to. They're already fighting an uphill battle before they even mention that they're here to advocate for breastfeeding. We need to lift these voices up and present a united front. Our strength is in our passion and numbers. You may not be, or want to be, within 1,000 miles of giving a talk to MPs or policymakers. You may not be leading an organisation. But your voice and support can make all the difference to those who are – and ultimately breastfeeding women. Support them. Bolster them. Be part of the change.

Linked to that, we must keep repeating that breastfeeding is not a women's issue. Until we get society to realise that this affects us all and that we should have men's voices at the table advocating for more investment and support, we'll be fighting a losing battle. And not the type of male involvement 'because they've got a wife or sister' and have suddenly realised this is important. But because they've realised it's not a women's issue but a people and society issue. Start with those hanging around your house. Steadily work outwards. We can change this.

Sign stuff, support stuff and write to people about stuff

One thing you can do as an individual is to get behind petitions and movements that are working to raise awareness and investment in breastfeeding. Your signature, your time or other skills, or perhaps your donation, could make all the difference. These include:

- Support the breastfeeding charities in the UK through membership, buying stuff and just a nice donation if you can. They can't do more without more. Details at the front of the book.
- Write to your local MP and ask them to attend meetings of the All Party Parliamentary Group on Infant Feeding and Inequalities chaired by Alison Thewliss MP.
- Support the work of the charity Baby Milk Action, which fights tirelessly to stop industry from breaking the WHO Code. If you see a violation of the Code you can report it to them via their website www.babymilkaction.org/monitoring-uk
- Support the work of the Human Milk Foundation which is working to help more families feed their baby with human milk. humanmilkfoundation.org
- Sign the Baby Friendly UK Call to Action, calling on governments to take steps to enable women to breastfeed for longer. www.unicef. org.uk/babyfriendly/about/call-to-action
- Sign the Better Breastfeeding campaign to end cuts to breastfeeding support. bit.ly/2TazA3d
- Support the work of the UK World Breastfeeding Trends Initiative in collating data on key indicators of breastfeeding support for the country and campaigns for investment and change. ukbreastfeeding. org/about

Support the breastfeeding women that you know (and meet)

How many women are ending up in a bad place because they simply aren't supported? Well, you can help. Small things can mean a huge amount to others.

- Support families who have had a new baby. Rather than taking tiny baby clothes, give your time to help them recover. Or give them a good breastfeeding book as a present. May I suggest Emma

Pickett's *You've got it in you*, La Leche League's *The Womanly Art of Breastfeeding* and last but not least my own *The Positive Breastfeeding Book*.

- If you're in a role in the workplace where you are responsible for line managing any new parents, know your breastfeeding policy and what works best. If you don't have a breastfeeding policy, write one! Do everything you can to enable a woman who has returned to work to feel confident and comfortable taking breaks to express. Find her a room, a fridge and time to express if needed… and tell her what a brilliant job she is doing.

Educate

We have a major societal misunderstanding about breastfeeding, and therefore lack of acceptance and support of breastfeeding and breastfeeding women. We change that one conversation at a time. There may be an awful lot of conversations to have, but a journey of a thousand miles starts with a single comment on social media. Or something like that.

- Challenge anything negative or unhelpful you see e.g. people on social media sharing misinformation, criticising breastfeeding or simply not understanding. I don't mean get into a bunfight with them, but simple, factual statements around breastfeeding being protected by law or why it matters can help. You may not change the opinion of the individual being an idiot, but you will help share positive information and facts for those watching. At the same time, keep on sharing positive pieces.
- Share copies of the Breastfeeding Network Drugs in Breastmilk leaflets with GP surgeries, children's centres and anywhere else you think might benefit. Raise awareness of good books about supporting breastfeeding. Some people like to give copies of books such as Dr Wendy Jones's *Breastfeeding and Medication* or the book we edited together, *Breastfeeding for the Medical Profession,* to GP surgeries.
- If you're a breastfeeding mother, breastfeed! Well, err yes. But I mean breastfeed everywhere and anywhere. The more we see it, the more we accept it. If you're no longer breastfeeding, a smile and nod at a breastfeeding mother can work wonders. But don't look creepy. Maybe offer to get her a glass of water if she looks stuck under a baby without anything in reach.
- Normalise normal baby behaviour. Talk about how often your baby

wakes up. Or feeds. Or doesn't want to be put down. In a way that makes it sound normal. I won't make any suggestions of what to do with books that tell you that your baby can be programmed to be a robot. But let's normalise normal babies.

Give back

- Consider using your experience of breastfeeding to train as a peer supporter, breastfeeding counsellor or IBCLC. Each course has different requirements but there is something for everyone who wants to increase their knowledge and skills. Check out the main breastfeeding organisations for more details. If you are a medic you might like to check out the work of the GP Infant Feeding Network (GPIFN) – A National Network of Primary Care Professionals and Supportive Colleagues Advocating for Improvements in Infant Feeding Practice. gpifn.org.uk
- If you or someone you support is interested in donating their milk, they can find details of their closest milk bank at www.ukamb.org/milk-banks. At present, the Hearts Milk Bank (heartsmilkbank.org), just north of London, is the only milk bank that will recruit mothers with babies older than six months, but this may change in the near future.

Ultimately, we need to work together to make sure that our next generation of mothers don't have the negative experiences that the mothers of today have had. We need to create a society that is breastfeeding friendly, welcoming and supportive. And we need to do it now, before that next generation of mothers is damaged by the version of mothering and breastfeeding that society today presents them with. If we manage this, then we will reduce the number of women who are left with feelings of guilt and regret, simply because they won't have had to stop. Those who are unable to breastfeed will feel supported rather than outcast. We won't need to worry about upsetting anyone, because there won't be a reason to be upset.

I hope the list of action points that I introduced at the start now makes sense. We need a change in society and the way we perceive, support and encourage breastfeeding. We can't just run around, shouting louder that breast is best, and wondering why we don't get results. We need more trained professionals with more time to support all women to breastfeed. We need to ensure supportive hospital practices through birth and the early days. We need to teach everyone to understand what breastfeeding is like and how they can support it. It is our collective responsibility to support breastfeeding as a society and to shout down self-styled experts and industry with their false solutions. We need to support mothers as they transition to motherhood, to help them find their own paths through the responsibilities of raising children. Ultimately, it is up to us – all of us – to protect breastfeeding. I want to leave you with the quote I cited at the beginning of the book.

'The success or failure of breastfeeding should not be seen solely as the responsibility of the woman. Her ability to breastfeed is very much shaped by the support and the environment in which she lives. There is a broader responsibility of governments and society to support women through policies and programmes in the community.' Dr Nigel Rollins, WHO, 2016

APPENDIX 1: JOINT STATEMENT ON PROTECTING BREASTFEEDING (2019)

Statement issued by: Breastfeeding Network, National Childbirth Trust, Association of Breastfeeding Mothers, UK Association of Milk Banks, Lactation Consultants of Great Britain, La Leche League GB, HENRY, Local Infant Feeding Information Board, World Breastfeeding Trends Initiative, Better Breastfeeding, Baby Feeding Law Group UK, Best Beginnings, Swansea University, Nursing Matters, GP Infant Feeding Network: www.breastfeedingnetwork.org.uk/joint-statement-on-protecting-breastfeeding

We want the new government to invest in the health of women and children by supporting and protecting breastfeeding.

The new government needs to **prioritise the first 1001 days of a child's life**, from conception to age two, to enable children to survive and thrive. How an infant is fed and nurtured strongly influences **a child's future life chances and emotional health.** Importantly, if a woman breastfeeds there are substantial **health benefits** for her – having impacts on **her future long after breastfeeding has stopped.**

This window of opportunity cannot be missed for the future health outcomes of mothers and the next generation. In addition to well documented health outcomes, supporting breastfeeding will also contribute to a **stronger economy**– potential annual savings to the NHS are estimated at about £40 million per year from just a moderate increase in breastfeeding rates.

Support for breastfeeding is also **an environmental imperative** and recognition of the contribution breastfeeding can make to avoiding environmental degradation should be a matter of increasing global and political attention.

In the UK, the majority of women start to breastfeed but breastfeeding rates drop rapidly – **our continuation rates are some of the lowest in the world** and are even lower amongst women living in deprived areas, where increasing rates could make a real difference to health inequalities. Support for all women, parents and families with breastfeeding falls short of what is wanted and needed.

Women tell us they encounter difficulties with the **public perceptions of breastfeeding out of the home.** Families tell us they are still regularly exposed to **conflicting messaging and marketing for formula milks** that drowns out advice from healthcare professionals. Women tell us they receive **little to no help with infant feeding** and that their health visitors, midwives and doctors often have little training or knowledge about breastfeeding and limited time to support them. Recent **cuts in health visitor numbers and breastfeeding peer support services** mean many women may be left without the support they need however they choose to feed their infants.

Despite robust evidence showing that investment in breastfeeding support and protection makes sense, politically breastfeeding has been viewed by governments as a lifestyle choice and so left to parents to work out for themselves. For too many women, trying to breastfeed without support, or stopping before they want to, is deeply upsetting and the situation is made worse by **fragmented care, and poor and often conflicting advice** from those they are seeking to support them. To ensure an increase in breastfeeding rates, to help reverse obesity rates and to reduce widening health inequalities will require significant investment in breastfeeding.

We call on all political parties to commit to the following actions, if elected:-

- To appoint a **permanent, multi-sectoral infant and young child feeding strategy group** and develop, fund and implement a **national strategy to improve infant and young child feeding practices.**
- To include actions to **promote, protect and support breastfeeding in all policy areas** where breastfeeding has an impact.
- To implement the **Unicef UK Baby Friendly Initiative** across community and paediatric services, building on the recommendation for maternity services in the **NHS Long Term Plan.**
- To protect babies from harmful commercial interests by bringing the full **International Code of Marketing of Breastmilk Substitutes** into UK law and enforcing this law.
- To **commission, and sustainably fund,** universal **breastfeeding support programmes** delivered by specialist/lead midwives and health visitors or suitably qualified breastfeeding specialists, such as IBCLC lactation consultants and breastfeeding counsellors, alongside trained peer supporters with accredited qualifications.
- To maintain and expand universal, accessible, affordable and confidential breastfeeding support through the **National Breastfeeding Helpline** and sustaining the **Drugs in Breastmilk Service.**
- To deliver **universal health visiting services and the Healthy Child Programme** by **linking in with local specialist and support services.**
- To establish/re-establish universal **Children's Centres** with a focus on areas of deprivation, offering **breastfeeding peer support.**
- To make it a statutory right of working mothers and those in education **to work flexibly** as required and to access a **private space** and **paid breaks** to breastfeed and/or express breastmilk and manage its safe storage.
- To commit to **resourcing for charitable** organisations who play a **key role within the health agenda** working at a national and local level to support families and communities with infant feeding.
- To support the commitment to undertake an **Infant Feeding Survey** which builds on the data previously collected in the Infant Feeding Survey 2010 (now discontinued). To implement **the recommendations of the Becoming Breastfeeding Friendly (BBF) study.**

APPENDIX 2: OPEN LETTER ON THE CURRENT CRISIS IN BREASTFEEDING IN THE UK – UK MOTHERS ARE BEING LET DOWN (2016)

Last week it was reported in *The Lancet* that breastfeeding rates at 12 months in the UK are the lowest in the world. What was not mentioned was that rates of starting breastfeeding have been increasing since the 1990s and are relatively high (81 per cent in the last national survey, in 2010). This is thanks to better communication about the importance of breastfeeding as well as the work of health service staff through the UNICEF Baby Friendly Initiative.

However, rates plummet in the first weeks and months after birth, and most mothers say they stopped breastfeeding before they wanted to. Every mother's decision about how to feed her baby needs to be made freely and respected. The breastfeeding crisis in the UK is in fact a crisis of lack of support for those mothers who choose to breastfeed. The result is that many mothers decide, reluctantly, that they must use infant formula.

Lancet report co-author Dr Nigel Rollins of the World Health Organisation (WHO), said: "The success or failure of breastfeeding should not be seen solely as the responsibility of the woman. Her ability to breastfeed is very much shaped by the support and the environment in which she lives. There is a broader responsibility of governments and society to support women through policies and programmes in the community."

While the progress made in breastfeeding initiation is to be celebrated, the report that we have the lowest breastfeeding rates in the world at one year cannot be ignored. Yet, this news comes at a time when support services for breastfeeding mothers are being cut across the country. Each week, we hear of yet another breastfeeding drop-in or peer-support programme that has closed or is under threat of closure, and the number of infant feeding specialist staff posts has been drastically cut in recent years.

In England, the public health budget has been cut by £200 million. It is little wonder then that Local Authorities – newly charged with responsibility for public health services – are looking for savings wherever they can, and closing down the very services that help mothers to continue breastfeeding.

The Lancet series on breastfeeding – the most comprehensive review of all the evidence on breastfeeding to date – confirms what we have known for many years. The authors state: "Our systematic reviews emphasise how important breastfeeding is for all women and children, irrespective of where they live and of whether they are rich or poor. Appropriate breastfeeding practices prevent child morbidity due to diarrhoea, respiratory infections, and otitis media [ear infections]. Where infectious diseases are common causes of death, breastfeeding provides major protection, but even in high-income populations it lowers mortality from causes such as necrotising enterocolitis and sudden infant death syndrome. Available evidence shows that breastfeeding enhances human capital by increasing intelligence. It also helps nursing women by preventing breast cancer. Additionally, our review suggests likely effects on overweight and diabetes in breastfed children, and on ovarian cancer and diabetes in mothers."

It is no surprise then that most mothers want to breastfeed. If they encounter problems, but don't get support to continue, this can be devastating and increases their risk for postnatal depression. That is why skilled support, from those who are properly trained, is essential. Breastfeeding is an individual choice for mothers but, when looked at a population level, it is also an important determinant of public health. The government is rightly concerned about reducing childhood obesity; breastfeeding is the first step on the road to healthy eating for life.

The economic and environmental consequences of improving breastfeeding rates and thus public health are significant. UNICEF UK reported in 2012 that moderate increases in breastfeeding rates could save the NHS millions. But the true cost to the wider economy of our low breastfeeding rates is far greater. The Lancet series calculates that the overall savings would actually be in the order of billions, not millions of pounds. If this were not enough, in the UK poorer mothers are far less likely to breastfeed than richer mothers, which increases health and social inequality.

So, what is undermining so many mothers' intention to breastfeed? It is a lack of support and protection for breastfeeding. When there is promotion but no support, mothers can understandably feel frustrated, resentful and even angry, as reflected in a recent Save the Children report. It highlighted how the lack of protection from misleading marketing by the formula manufacturers undermines mothers' confidence. A commentary in The Lancet series suggests that a coordinated international strategy is needed to protect women from such pressure.

That's the bad news. But the good news is that what needs to be done, to turn things around and improve breastfeeding rates in the UK, is well known. The Lancet series reinforces other recent large-scale evidence reviews, such as a special issue of Acta Pediatrica in December, which found that interventions to improve breastfeeding rates are most effective when delivered in combination. Such approaches include support from peers and health professionals, the Baby Friendly Initiative, and robust restrictions on formula advertising. A shift in public attitudes is needed to prevent women feeling vulnerable when breastfeeding in public, and employment protection is needed for women who return to work while still breastfeeding.

Moreover, these measures are relatively inexpensive and would soon pay for themselves. As Keith Hansen of the World Bank said last year "In bottom-line economic terms, breastfeeding may be the single best investment a country can make."

The actions are clear – they have been spelled out in the WHO's Global Strategy for Infant and Young Child Feeding, while the UK NICE guidelines set out that all maternity hospitals and community settings should become Baby Friendly accredited and that all mothers should be offered skilled breastfeeding support.

We, the undersigned – health visitors, midwives, paediatricians, GPs, lactation consultants, breastfeeding counsellors, peer supporters, university researchers and those who work for professional organisations and charities that support families – therefore call on the governments of the UK to end this crisis by acting now to:

- Establish and sustain a multi-sectoral National Breastfeeding Committee, with co-ordination across the four countries of the UK and an expert coordinator in each, building on existing work in Scotland and Northern Ireland. The committee would develop and monitor the implementation of a National Breastfeeding Strategy that is regularly refreshed (just as is done with the National Cancer Strategy)
- Ensure that Baby Friendly accreditation becomes a minimum requirement for all maternity and community settings, as recommended by NICE and following the examples set by Scotland and Northern Ireland
- Ensure that all mothers, regardless of where they live, receive skilled evidence-based breastfeeding support, as recommended by NICE, by making this provision a mandatory responsibility of Local Authorities
- Enable Local Authorities to carry out this responsibility by safeguarding the public health budget for universal health visiting services and breastfeeding support
- Protect all families from aggressive marketing by formula manufacturers by fully enacting in UK law the International Code of Marketing of Breastmilk Substitutes and subsequent, relevant World Health Assembly resolutions
- Require employers to provide breaks to breastfeeding mothers to allow them to breastfeed or express milk at work.

9 February 2016

Signed:
Dr Cheryll Adams – Executive Director, Institute of Health Visiting
Obi Amadi – Lead Professional Officer, Community Practitioners' and
   Health Visitors' Association Professor
Neena Modi – President, Royal College of Paediatrics and Child Health
Professor Maureen Baker CBE – Chair of Council, Royal College of General
   Practitioners
Professor Nick Spencer – President, International Society for Social
   Pediatrics and Child Health Regional Coordinators – National Infant
   Feeding Network
Zoe Faulkner IBCLC – Coordinator, Lactation Consultants of Great Britain
Jacqui Tomkins – Chair, Independent Midwives UK
Dr Cathy Ashwin – Principal Editor, Midwives Information & Resource
   Service (MIDIRS)
Katherine Hales – Midwife and National Coordinator, ARM
Rosemary Dodds – Senior Policy Adviser, NCT
Shereen Fisher – Chief Executive, The Breastfeeding Network
Emma Pickett IBCLC – Chair, Association of Breastfeeding Mothers
Eden Anderson – Chair, La Leche League GB
Professor Mary Renfrew – Director, Mother and Infant Research Unit,
   University of Dundee
Dr Amy Brown – Associate Professor, Public Health And Policy Studies,

Swansea University

Dr Alison McFadden – Senior Research Fellow, Mother and Infant Research Unit, University of Dundee

Professor Fiona Dykes – Director, Maternal and Infant Nutrition and Nurture Unit, University of Central Lancashire

Dr Nigel Sherriff and Carol Williams, Centre for Health Research, University of Brighton

Shel Banks – Chair, The Local Infant Feeding Information Board

Debbie Barnett – Co-Chair, United Kingdom Association for Milk Banking

Alison Baum – Chief Executive, Best Beginnings

Dr Helen Crawley – Director, First Steps Nutrition Trust

Patti Rundall OBE – Policy Director, Baby Milk Action/IBFAN-UK

Mike Brady – Secretariat, Baby Feeding Law Group

Helen Gray IBCLC and Clare Meynell IBCLC – Coordinators, World Breastfeeding Trends Initiative UK

Dr Colin Michie – Paediatrician, Ealing Hospital, London North West Healthcare NHS Trust

Beverley Lawrence Beech – Honorary Chair, Association for Improvements in the Maternity Services

Robin Ireland – Chief Executive, Health Equalities Group

Helen Calvert – Founder, Hospital Breastfeeding Campaign

Sally Etheridge IBCLC and Aayesha Bhattay – Directors, Leicester Mammas CIC

Mindy Noble – Coordinator, Hampshire Breastfeeding Counselling

Rachel O'Leary IBCLC – Chair, Cambridge Breastfeeding Alliance

Milli Hill – Founder, The Positive Birth Movement

Maddie McMahon – Committee member, Doula UK

Sophie Brigstocke – Director, Nurturing Birth

ACKNOWLEDGEMENTS

Thank you to all the usual suspects particularly my family and friends for supporting me through everything and putting up with my confused 'what number book is this now?' questions.

Thank you again as always to everyone at Pinter & Martin for believing in this topic and book. And to my colleagues, fellow academics and researchers who contributed to this book, both directly in their expert evidence and through the research that you all do in this field. One day we won't need to research this area as there will be nothing to research. Until then, keep keeping on, until we retire to our bookshop/gin bar/allotment by the sea.

REFERENCES

Chapter 1: The issue

1. Victora, C. G., Bahl, R., Barros, A. J., França, G. V., Horton, S., Krasevec, J., ... & Group, T. L. B. S. (2016). Breastfeeding in the 21st century: epidemiology, mechanisms, and lifelong effect. *The Lancet*, *387*(10017), 475-490.
2. McAndrew, F., Thompson, J., Fellows, L., Large, A., Speed, M., & Renfrew, M. J. (2012). Infant feeding survey 2010. Leeds: health and social care information Centre, 2(1).
3. Joint statement on the cancellation of the UK Infant Feeding Survey www.breastfeedingnetwork.org.uk/wp-content/pdfs/pressreleases/2015-IFS.pdf
4. Scottish maternal and infant nutrition survey 2017: summary of key findings www.gov.scot/publications/scottish-maternal-infant-nutrition-survey-2017-summary-key-findings/
5. www.theguardian.com/us-news/2020/jan/27/maternity-leave-us-policy-worst-worlds-richest-countries
6. Hörnell A, Aarts C, Kylberg E, Hofvander Y, Gebre-Medhin M. Breastfeeding patterns in exclusively breastfed infants: a longitudinal prospective study in Uppsala, Sweden. Acta Paediatrica. 1999 Feb 1;88(2):203-11.
7. www.plunket.org.nz/plunket/news-and-research/research-from-plunket/breastfeeding-data/
8. Brown, A., Raynor, P., & Lee, M. (2011). Young mothers who choose to breast feed: the importance of being part of a supportive breast-feeding community. *Midwifery*, *27*(1), 53-59
9. Ladewig, E. L., Hayes, C., Browne, J., Layte, R., & Reulbach, U. (2014). The influence of ethnicity on breastfeeding rates in Ireland: a cross-sectional study. *J Epidemiol Community Health*, *68*(4), 356-362.
10. Li, R., Darling, N., Maurice, E., Barker, L. and Grummer-Strawn, L.M., 2005. Breastfeeding rates in the United States by characteristics of the child, mother, or family: the 2002 National Immunization Survey. *Pediatrics*, *115*(1), pp.e31-e37.
11. Gross, T.T., Powell, R., Anderson, A.K., Hall, J., Davis, M. and Hilyard, K., 2015. WIC peer counselors' perceptions of breastfeeding in African American women with lower incomes. *Journal of Human Lactation*, *31*(1), pp.99-110
12. Thomas, E. V. (2018). "Why even bother; they are not going to do it?" The structural roots of racism and discrimination in lactation care. *Qualitative health research*, *28*(7), 1050-1064.
13. Griswold, M. K., Crawford, S. L., Perry, D. J., Person, S. D., Rosenberg, L., Cozier, Y. C., & Palmer, J. R. (2018). Experiences of racism and breastfeeding initiation and duration among first-time mothers of the Black Women's Health Study. *Journal of racial and ethnic health disparities*, *5*(6), 1180-1191.
14. Beal, A. C., Kuhlthau, K., & Perrin, J. M. (2016). Breastfeeding advice given to African American and white women by physicians and WIC counselors. *Public Health Reports*.
15. Robinson, K., Fial, A., & Hanson, L. (2019). Racism, bias, and discrimination as modifiable barriers to breastfeeding for African American women: a scoping review of the literature. *Journal of midwifery & women's health*, *64*(6), 734-742.
16. Williams, D. R., & Rucker, T. D. (2000). Understanding and addressing racial disparities in health care. *Health care financing review*, *21*(4), 75.
17. Silva, M., Loureiro, A., & Cardoso, G. (2016). Social determinants of mental health: a review of the evidence. *The European Journal of Psychiatry*, *30*(4), 259-292.
18. Alexander, A., Dowling, D. and Furman, L., 2010. What do pregnant low-income women say about breastfeeding?. *Breastfeeding Medicine*, *5*(1), pp.17-23.
19. Gibson-Davis, C.M. and Brooks-Gunn, J., 2006. Couples' immigration status and ethnicity as determinants of breastfeeding. *American Journal of Public Health*, *96*(4), pp.641-646.
20. Griffiths, L.J., Tate, A.R. and Dezateux, C., 2005. The contribution of parental and community ethnicity to breastfeeding practices: evidence from the Millennium Cohort Study. *International Journal of Epidemiology*, *34*(6), pp.1378-1386*The Lancet*,

387(10017), pp.475-490

21. Wandel, M., Terragni, L., Nguyen, C., Lyngstad, J., Amundsen, M. and de Paoli, M., 2016. Breastfeeding among Somali mothers living in Norway: Attitudes, practices and challenges. *Women and Birth, 29*(6), pp.487-493.

Chapter 2: Why does breastfeeding matter anyway?

1. www.epic.iarc.fr
2. Ladomenou F, Moschandreas J, Kafatos A, Tselentis Y, Galanakis E. Protective effect of exclusive breastfeeding against infections during infancy: a prospective study. *Archives of disease in childhood.* 2010 Dec 1;95(12):1004-8.
3. Sankar MJ, Sinha B, Chowdhury R, Bhandari N, Taneja S, Martines J, Bahl R. Optimal breastfeeding practices and infant and child mortality: a systematic review and meta-analysis. *Acta Paediatrica.* 2015 Dec 1;104(S467):3-13.
4. Brown A, Lee M. Breastfeeding during the first year promotes satiety responsiveness in children aged 18–24 months. *Pediatric obesity.* 2012 Oct;7(5):382-90.
5. Colen CG, Ramey DM. Is breast truly best? Estimating the effects of breastfeeding on long-term child health and wellbeing in the United States using sibling comparisons. *Social Science & Medicine.* 2014 May 1;109:55-65.
6. Raissian KM, Su JH. The best of intentions: Prenatal breastfeeding intentions and infant health. *SSM-Population Health.* 2018 Aug 31;5:86-100.
7. Flaherman VJ, Cabana MD, McCulloch CE, Paul IM. Effect of early limited formula on breastfeeding duration in the first year of life: a randomized clinical trial. *JAMA pediatrics.* 2019 Aug 1;173(8):729-35.
8. Victora C, Barros A. Effect of breastfeeding on infant and child mortality due to infectious diseases in less developed countries. *The Lancet.* 2000 Feb 5;355(9202):451-5
9. Victora CG, Bahl R, Barros AJ, França GV, Horton S, Krasevec J, Murch S, Sankar MJ, Walker N, Rollins NC, Group TL. Breastfeeding in the 21st century: epidemiology, mechanisms, and lifelong effect. *The Lancet.* 2016 Feb 5;387(10017):475-90.
10. Bowatte G, Tham R, Allen KJ, Tan DJ, Lau MX, Dai X, Lodge CJ. Breastfeeding and childhood acute otitis media: a systematic review and meta-analysis. *Acta Paediatrica.* 2015 Dec 1;104(S467):85-95.
11. Becker S, Rutstein S, Labbok MH. Estimation of births averted due to breast-feeding and increases in levels of contraception needed to substitute for breast-feeding. *Journal of Biosocial Science.* 2003 Oct 1;35(04):559-74.
12. Ip S, Chung M, Raman G, Trikalinos TA, Lau J. A summary of the Agency for Healthcare Research and Quality's evidence report on breastfeeding in developed countries. *Breastfeeding Medicine.* 2009 Oct 1;4(S1):S-17.
13. Kramer MS, Chalmers B, Hodnett ED, Sevkovskaya Z, Dzikovich I, Shapiro S, Collet JP, Vanilovich I, Mezen I, Ducruet T, Shishko G. Promotion of Breastfeeding Intervention Trial (PROBIT): a randomized trial in the Republic of Belarus. *JAMA.* 2001 Jan 24;285(4):413-20.
14. Koch A, Mølbak K, Homøe P, Sørensen P, Hjuler T, Olesen ME, Pejl J, Pedersen FK, Olsen OR, Melbye M. Risk factors for acute respiratory tract infections in young Greenlandic children. *American Journal of Epidemiology.* 2003 Aug 15;158(4):374-84.
15. Howie PW, Forsyth JS, Ogston SA, Clark A, Florey CD. Protective effect of breast feeding against infection. *BMJ.* 1990 Jan 6;300(6716):11-6.
16. Pisacane A, Graziano L, Zona G, Granata G, Dolezalova H, Cafiero M, Coppola A, Scarpellino B, Ummarino M, Mazzarella G. Breast feeding and acute lower respiratory infection. *Acta Paediatrica.* 1994 Jul 1;83(7):714-8.
17. Bachrach VR, Schwarz E, Bachrach LR. Breastfeeding and the risk of hospitalization for respiratory disease in infancy: a meta-analysis. *Archives of pediatrics & adolescent medicine.* 2003 Mar 1;157(3):237-43.
18. Fisk CM, Crozier SR, Inskip HM, Godfrey KM, Cooper C, Roberts GC, Robinson SM. Breastfeeding and reported morbidity during infancy: findings from the Southampton Women's Survey. *Maternal & Child Nutrition.* 2011 Jan 1;7(1):61-70.
19. Scariati PD, Grummer-Strawn LM, Fein SB. A longitudinal analysis of infant morbidity and the extent of breastfeeding in the United States. *Pediatrics.* 1997 Jun

1;99(6):e5
20. Kramer MS, Kakuma R. Optimal duration of exclusive breastfeeding (Review). Cochrane database of systematic reviews. 2002;1:11-2.
21. Dewey KG, Heinig MJ, Nommsen-Rivers LA. Differences in morbidity between breast-fed and formula-fed infants. *The Journal of Pediatrics.* 1995 May 31;126(5):696-702.
22. Chivers P, Hands B, Parker H, Bulsara M, Beilin LJ, Kendall GE, Oddy WH. Body mass index, adiposity rebound and early feeding in a longitudinal cohort (Raine Study). *International Journal of Obesity.* 2010 Jul 1;34(7):1169-76.
23. Gubbels JS, Thijs C, Stafleu A, Van Buuren S, Kremers SP. Association of breast-feeding and feeding on demand with child weight status up to 4 years. *International Journal of Pediatric Obesity.* 2011 Jun 1;6(sup3):e515-522.
24. Huh SY, Rifas-Shiman SL, Taveras EM, Oken E, Gillman MW. Timing of solid food introduction and risk of obesity in preschool-aged children. *Pediatrics.* 2011 Mar 1;127(3):e544-51.
25. Zhu Y, Hernandez LM, Dong Y, Himes JH, Hirschfeld S, Forman MR. Longer breastfeeding duration reduces the positive relationships among gestational weight gain, birth weight and childhood anthropometrics. *Journal of Epidemiology and Community Health.* 2015 Jul 1;69(7):632-8.
26. Scholtens S, Gehring U, Brunekreef B, Smit HA, de Jongste JC, Kerkhof M, Gerritsen J, Wijga AH. Breastfeeding, weight gain in infancy, and overweight at seven years of age: the prevention and incidence of asthma and mite allergy birth cohort study. *American Journal of Epidemiology.* 2007 Apr 15;165(8):919-26.
27. Monasta L, Batty GD, Cattaneo A, Lutje V, Ronfani L, Van Lenthe FJ, Brug J. Early-life determinants of overweight and obesity: a review of systematic reviews. *Obesity Reviews.* 2010 Oct 1;11(10):695-708.
28. Hörnell A, Lagström H, Lande B, Thorsdottir I. Breastfeeding, introduction of other foods and effects on health: a systematic literature review for the 5th Nordic Nutrition Recommendations. *Food & Nutrition Research.* 2013 Apr 12;57.
29. Chobanian AV, Bakris GL, Black HR, Cushman WC, Green LA, Izzo Jr JL, Jones DW, Materson BJ, Oparil S, Wright Jr JT, Roccella EJ. The seventh report of the joint national committee on prevention, detection, evaluation, and treatment of high blood pressure: the JNC 7 report. *JAMA.* 2003 May 21;289(19):2560-71.
30. Cook NR, Cohen J, Hebert PR, Taylor JO, Hennekens CH. Implications of small reductions in diastolic blood pressure for primary prevention. *Archives of Internal Medicine.* 1995 Apr 10;155(7):701-9.
31. Owen CG, Whincup PH, Kaye SJ, Martin RM, Smith GD, Cook DG, Bergstrom E, Black S, Wadsworth ME, Fall CH, Freudenheim JL. Does initial breastfeeding lead to lower blood cholesterol in adult life? A quantitative review of the evidence. *The American Journal of Clinical Nutrition.* 2008 Aug 1;88(2):305-14.
32. Larsen FS, Hanifin JM. Epidemiology of atopic dermatitis. *Immunology and Allergy Clinics of North America.* 2002 Feb 28;22(1):1-24.
33. Oddy WH, De Klerk NH, Sly PD, Holt PG. The effects of respiratory infections, atopy, and breastfeeding on childhood asthma. *European Respiratory Journal.* 2002 May 1;19(5):899-905.
34. Bergmann RL, Diepgen TL, Kuss O, Bergmann KE, Kujat J, Dudenhausen JW, Wahn U. Breastfeeding duration is a risk factor for atopic eczema. *Clinical & Experimental Allergy.* 2002 Feb 1;32(2):205-9.
35. Jedrychowski W, Perera F, Jankowski J, Butscher M, Mroz E, Flak E, Kaim I, Lisowska-Miszczyk I, Skarupa A, Sowa A. Effect of exclusive breastfeeding on the development of children's cognitive function in the Krakow prospective birth cohort study. *European Journal of Pediatrics.* 2012 Jan 1;171(1):151-8.
36. Oken E, Østerdal ML, Gillman MW, Knudsen VK, Halldorsson TI, Strøm M, Bellinger DC, Hadders-Algra M, Michaelsen KF, Olsen SF. Associations of maternal fish intake during pregnancy and breastfeeding duration with attainment of developmental milestones in early childhood: a study from the Danish National Birth Cohort. *The American Journal of Clinical Nutrition.* 2008 Sep 1;88(3):789-96.
37. Whitehouse AJ, Robinson M, Li J, Oddy WH. Duration of breast feeding and

language ability in middle childhood. *Paediatric and Perinatal Epidemiology.* 2011 Jan 1;25(1):44-52.

38. Isaacs EB, Fischl BR, Quinn BT, Chong WK, Gadian DG, Lucas A. Impact of breastmilk on intelligence quotient, brain size, and white matter development. *Pediatric Research.* 2010 Apr 1;67(4):357-62.

39. Khedr EM, Farghaly WM, Amry S, Osman AA. Neural maturation of breastfed and formula-fed infants. *Acta Paediatrica.* 2004 Jun 1;93(6):734-8.

40. Horta BL, Loret de Mola C, Victora CG. Long-term consequences of breastfeeding on cholesterol, obesity, systolic blood pressure and type 2 diabetes: a systematic review and meta-analysis. *Acta Paediatrica.* 2015 Dec 1;104(S467):30-7.

41. Akobeng AK, Ramanan AV, Buchan I, Heller RF. Effect of breast feeding on risk of coeliac disease: a systematic review and meta-analysis of observational studies. *Archives of Disease in Childhood.* 2006 Jan 1;91(1):39-43.

42. Kwan ML, Buffler PA, Abrams B, Kiley VA. Breastfeeding and the risk of childhood leukemia: a meta-analysis. *Public Health Reports.* 2004 Nov;119(6):521.

43. Küçükçongar A, Oğuz A, Pınarlı FG, Karadeniz C, Okur A, Kaya Z, Çelik B. Breastfeeding and childhood cancer: is breastfeeding preventative to childhood cancer? *Pediatric hematology and oncology.* 2015 Aug 18;32(6):374-81.

44. Bahl R. Optimal feeding of low-birth-weight infants. Technical review, World Health Organization.

45. Abrams SA, Schanler RJ, Lee ML, Rechtman DJ. Greater mortality and morbidity in extremely preterm infants fed a diet containing cow milk protein products. *Breastfeeding Medicine.* 2014 Jul 1;9(6):281-5.

46. Donovan SM. Role of human milk components in gastrointestinal development: current knowledge and future needs. *The Journal of Pediatrics.* 2006 Nov 30;149(5):S49-61.

47. Narayanan I, Bala S, Prakash K, Verma RK, Gujral VV. Partial supplementation with expressed breast-milk for prevention of infection in low-birth-weight infants. *The Lancet.* 1980 Sep 13;316(8194):561-3.

48. Lucas A, Morley R, Cole TJ. Randomised trial of early diet in preterm babies and later intelligence quotient. *BMJ.* 1998 Nov 28;317(7171):1481-7.

49. Lewandowski AJ, Lamata P, Francis JM, Piechnik SK, Ferreira VM, Boardman H, Neubauer S, Singhal A, Leeson P, Lucas A. Breastmilk Consumption in Preterm Neonates and Cardiac Shape in Adulthood. *Pediatrics.* 2016 Jun 14.

50. Ballard, O., & Morrow, A. L. (2013). Human milk composition: nutrients and bioactive factors. *Pediatric Clinics,* 60(1), 49-74.

51. Simmer K, Patole SK, Rao SC. Longchain polyunsaturated fatty acid supplementation in infants born at term. *Cochrane database of systematic reviews.* 2011(12).

52. Fleith M, Clandinin MT. Dietary PUFA for preterm and term infants: review of clinical studies. *Critical Reviews in Food Science and Nutrition* 2005;45:205-29.

53. Horta BL, Loret de Mola C, Victora CG. Long-term consequences of breastfeeding on cholesterol, obesity, systolic blood pressure and type 2 diabetes: a systematic review and meta-analysis. *Acta paediatrica.* 2015 Dec;104:30-7.

54. Colao A, Di Somma C, Cascella T, Pivonello R, Vitale G, Grasso LF, Lombardi G, Savastano S. Relationships between serum IGF1 levels, blood pressure, and glucose tolerance: an observational, exploratory study in 404 subjects. *European Journal of Endocrinology.* 2008 Oct 1;159(4):389-97.

55. Devlin AM, Innis SM, Shukin R, Rioux MF. Early diet influences hepatic hydroxymethyl glutaryl coenzyme A reductase and 7α-hydroxylase mRNA but not low-density lipoprotein receptor mRNA during development. *Metabolism.* 1998 Jan 31;47(1):20-6.

56. Savino F, Liguori SA. Update on breast milk hormones: leptin, ghrelin and adiponectin. *Clinical Nutrition.* 2008 Feb 1;27(1):42-7.

57. Heijtz RD, Wang S, Anuar F, Qian Y, Björkholm B, Samuelsson A, Hibberd ML, Forssberg H, Pettersson S. Normal gut microbiota modulates brain development and behavior. *Proceedings of the National Academy of Sciences.* 2011 Feb 15;108(7):3047-52.

58. Pannaraj PS, Li F, Cerini C, Bender JM, Yang S, Rollie A, Adisetiyo H, Zabih S, Lincez PJ, Bittinger K, Bailey A. Association between breast milk bacterial communities and

establishment and development of the infant gut microbiome. *JAMA pediatrics.* 2017 Jul 1;171(7):647-54.

59. Rubio R, Collado MC, Laitinen K, Salminen S, Isolauri E, Mira A. The human milk microbiome changes over lactation and is shaped by maternal weight and mode of delivery. *The American Journal of Clinical Nutrition.* 2012 Sep 1;96(3):544-51.
60. Bode, L. (2009). Human milk oligosaccharides: prebiotics and beyond. *Nutrition reviews,* 67(suppl_2), S183-S191.
61. Engler AC, Hadash A, Shehadeh N, Pillar G. Breastfeeding may improve nocturnal sleep and reduce infantile colic: potential role of breastmilk melatonin. *European Journal of Pediatrics.* 2012 Apr 1;171(4):729-32.
62. Fomon SJ, Owen GM, Thomas LN. Milk or formula volume ingested by infants fed ad libitum. *American Journal of Diseases of Children.* 1964 Dec 1;108(6):601-4.
63. 57.Wright P, Fawcett J, Crow R. The development of differences in the feeding behaviour of bottle and breast fed human infants from birth to two months. *Behavioural Processes.* 1980 Apr 30;5(1):1-20.
64. Lavelli M, Poli M. Early mother-infant interaction during breast-and bottle-feeding. *Infant behavior and Development.* 1998 Dec 31;21(4):667-83.
65. Brown A, Lee M. Breastfeeding is associated with a maternal feeding style low in control from birth. *PloS One.* 2013 Jan 30;8(1):e54229.
66. Dewey KG, Heinig MJ, Nommsen LA, Lonnerdal B. Maternal versus infant factors related to breastmilk intake and residual milk volume: the DARLING study. *Pediatrics.* 1991 Jun 1;87(6):829-37.
67. Wood, C. T., Skinner, A. C., Yin, H. S., Rothman, R. L., Sanders, L. M., Delamater, A. M., & Perrin, E. M. (2016). Bottle size and weight gain in formula-fed infants. *Pediatrics,* 138(1).
68. Li R, Fein SB, Grummer-Strawn LM. Do infants fed from bottles lack self-regulation of milk intake compared with directly breastfed infants? *Pediatrics.* 2010 Jun 1;125(6):e1386-93.
69. Heinig MJ, Nommsen LA, Peerson JM, Lonnerdal B, Dewey KG. Intake and growth of breast-fed and formula-fed infants in relation to the timing of introduction of complementary foods: the DARLING study. *Acta Paediatrica.* 1993 Jan 1;82(s385):999-1006.
70. Collaborative Group on Hormonal Factors in Breast Cancer. Breast cancer and breastfeeding: collaborative reanalysis of individual data from 47 epidemiological studies in 30 countries, including 50 302 women with breast cancer and 96 973 women without the disease. The Lancet. 2002 Jul 20;360(9328):187-95.
71. Chowdhury R, Sinha B, Sankar MJ, Taneja S, Bhandari N, Rollins N, Bahl R, Martines J. Breastfeeding and maternal health outcomes: a systematic review and meta-analysis. *Acta Paediatrica.* 2015 Dec 1;104(S467):96-113.
72. Bartick, M. C., Schwarz, E. B., Green, B. D., Jegier, B. J., Reinhold, A. G., Colaizy, T. T., ... & Stuebe, A. M. (2017). Suboptimal breastfeeding in the United States: Maternal and pediatric health outcomes and costs. *Maternal & child nutrition,* 13(1), e12366.
73. Basree, M. M., Shinde, N., Koivisto, C., Cuitino, M., Kladney, R., Zhang, J., ... & Acero-Bedoya, S. (2019). Abrupt involution induces inflammation, estrogenic signaling, and hyperplasia linking lack of breastfeeding with increased risk of breast cancer. *Breast Cancer Research,* 21(1), 80.
74. Danforth KN, Tworoger SS, Hecht JL, Rosner BA, Colditz GA, Hankinson SE. Breastfeeding and risk of ovarian cancer in two prospective cohorts. *Cancer causes & control.* 2007 Jun 1;18(5):517-23.
75. Cramer DW, Titus-Ernstoff L, McKolanis JR, Welch WR, Vitonis AF, Berkowitz RS, Finn OJ. Conditions associated with antibodies against the tumor-associated antigen MUC1 and their relationship to risk for ovarian cancer. *Cancer Epidemiology Biomarkers & Prevention.* 2005 May 1;14(5):1125-31.
76. Cramer, D. W., Williams, K., Vitonis, A. F., Yamamoto, H. S., Stuebe, A., Welch, W. R., ... & Fichorova, R. N. (2013). Puerperal mastitis: a reproductive event of importance affecting anti-mucin antibody levels and ovarian cancer risk. *Cancer Causes & Control,* 24(11), 1911-1923.
77. Hunn, J., & Rodriguez, G. C. (2012). Ovarian cancer: etiology, risk factors, and

epidemiology. Clinical obstetrics and gynecology, 55(1), 3-23.

78. Aune D, Norat T, Romundstad P, Vatten LJ. Breastfeeding and the maternal risk of type 2 diabetes: A systematic review and dose–response meta-analysis of cohort studies. *Nutrition, Metabolism and Cardiovascular Diseases.* 2014 Feb 28;24(2):107-15.

79. Bartick, M. C., Schwarz, E. B., Green, B. D., Jegier, B. J., Reinhold, A. G., Colaizy, T. T., ... & Stuebe, A. M. (2017). Suboptimal breastfeeding in the United States: Maternal and pediatric health outcomes and costs. *Maternal & child nutrition,* 13(1), e12366.

80. Stuebe AM, Rich-Edwards JW. The reset hypothesis: Lactation and maternal metabolism. *American Journal of Perinatology.* 2009;26(1):81–8

81. Schwarz EB, Ray RM, Stuebe AM, Allison MA, Ness RB, Freiberg MS, Cauley JA. Duration of lactation and risk factors for maternal cardiovascular disease. *Obstetrics and Gynecology.* 2009 May;113(5):974.

82. Choi, S. R., Kim, Y. M., Cho, M. S., Kim, S. H., & Shim, Y. S. (2017). Association between duration of breast feeding and metabolic syndrome: The Korean National Health and Nutrition Examination Surveys. *Journal of Women's Health,* 26(4), 361-367.

83. Stuebe AM, Michels KB, Willett WC, Manson JE, Rexrode K, Rich-Edwards JW. Duration of lactation and incidence of myocardial infarction in middle to late adulthood. *Am J Obstet Gynecol* 2009; 200: 138.e131–138.e138.

84. Chowdhury, R., Sinha, B., Sankar, M. J., Taneja, S., Bhandari, N., Rollins, N., ... & Martines, J. (2015). Breastfeeding and maternal health outcomes: a systematic review and meta-analysis. *Acta paediatrica,* 104, 96-113.

85. Baker JL, Gamborg M, Heitmann BL, et al. Breastfeeding reduces postpartum weight retention. *American Journal of Clinical Nutrition.* 2008;88(6):1543–51.

86. Butte NF, Garza C, Stuff JE, Smith EO, Nichols BL. Effect of maternal diet and body composition on lactational performance. *Am J Clin Nutr.* 1984;39:296–306

87. Oken E, Fields DA, Lovelady CA, Redman LM. TOS scientific position statement: breastfeeding and obesity. *Obesity.* 2017 Nov 1;25(11):1864-6.

88. Kim, S. W., Lee, J. H., Shon, H. S., Jeon, E., & Kim, T. Y. (2020). Association of breastfeeding with thyroid function and autoimmunity in postmenopausal women. *Endocrine,* 1-9.

89. Karlson, E. W., Mandl, L. A., Hankinson, S. E., & Grodstein, F. (2004). Do breast-feeding and other reproductive factors influence future risk of rheumatoid arthritis?: Results from the Nurses' Health Study. *Arthritis & Rheumatism,* 50(11), 3458-3467.

90. Langer-Gould, A., Smith, J. B., Hellwig, K., Gonzales, E., Haraszti, S., Koebnick, C., & Xiang, A. (2017). Breastfeeding, ovulatory years, and risk of multiple sclerosis. *Neurology,* 89(6), 563-569.

91. Pope, C. J., Mazmanian, D., Bédard, M., & Sharma, V. (2016). Breastfeeding and postpartum depression: Assessing the influence of breastfeeding intention and other risk factors. *Journal of Affective Disorders,* 200, 45-50.

92. Engler A et al (2012). Breastfeeding may improve nocturnal sleep and reduce infantile colic: potential role of breastmilk melatonin. *European journal of pediatrics,* 171(4), 729-732.

93. Blyton, D et al. (2002). Lactation is associated with an increase in slow-wave sleep in women. *Journal of sleep research,* 11(4), 297-303.

94. Cong Z et al. The Effect of Feeding Method on Sleep Duration, Maternal Well. being, and Pospartum Depression. *Clinical Lactation.* 2011;2(2):22-6.

95. Kendall-Tackett K. A new paradigm for depression in new mothers: the central role of inflammation and how breastfeeding and anti-inflammatory treatments protect maternal mental health. *International breastfeeding journal.* 2007 Mar;2(1):6.

96. Groër MW et al: Immunity, inflammation and infection in post-partum breast and formula feeders. *Am J Reprod Immunol.* 2005, 54: 222-231

97. Brown A. What Do Women Lose if They Are Prevented From Meeting Their Breastfeeding Goals? *Clinical Lactation.* 2018 Nov 1;9(4):200-7.

98. Brown, A et al (2016). Understanding the relationship between breastfeeding and postnatal depression: the role of pain and physical difficulties. *Journal of advanced nursing,* 72(2), 273-282.

99. IsHak WW et al. Pain and depression: A systematic review. *Harvard review of psychiatry.* 2018 Nov 1;26(6):352-63.

100. Ahmed AH et al. Relationship between sleep quality, depression symptoms, and blood glucose in pregnant women. *Western journal of nursing research.* 2018 Nov 8:0193945918809714.
101. Brown, A. *Why breastfeeding grief and trauma matter.* Pinter & Martin ltd.
102. Labbok, M. (2008). Exploration of guilt among mothers who do not breastfeed: the physician's role. *Journal of Human Lactation,* 24(1), 80-84.
103. Pokhrel S, Quigley MA, Fox-Rushby J, McCormick F, Williams A, Trueman P, Dodds R, Renfrew MJ. Potential economic impacts from improving breastfeeding rates in the UK. *Archives of Disease in Childhood.* 2015 Apr;100(4):334–400.
104. Bartick MC, Stuebe AM, Schwarz EB, Luongo C, Reinhold AG, Foster EM. Cost analysis of maternal disease associated with suboptimal breastfeeding. *Obstetrics & Gynecology.* 2013 Jul 1;122(1):111-9.
105. Bartick M, Reinhold A. The burden of suboptimal breastfeeding in the United States: a pediatric cost analysis. *Pediatrics.* 2010 May 1;125(5):e1048-56
106. Siregar, A. Y., Pitriyan, P., & Walters, D. (2018). The annual cost of not breastfeeding in Indonesia: the economic burden of treating diarrhea and respiratory disease among children (< 24mo) due to not breastfeeding according to recommendation. *International breastfeeding journal,* 13(1), 10.
107. Mahon, J., Claxton, L., & Wood, H. (2016). Modelling the cost-effectiveness of human milk and breastfeeding in preterm infants in the United Kingdom. *Health economics review,* 6(1), 54.
108. Walters, D. D., Phan, L. T., & Mathisen, R. (2019). The cost of not breastfeeding: global results from a new tool. *Health policy and planning,* 34(6), 407-417.
109. Joffe, N., Webster, F., & Shenker, N. (2019). Support for breastfeeding is an environmental imperative. *BMJ*
110. Cassella C. No one is talking about the environmental impacts of the baby formula industry. *Science Alert.* 2018; 10 January 2019. Available from: https://www.sciencealert.com/no-one-is-talking-about-the-environmental-impacts-of-the-baby-formula-industry.
111. Karlsson JO, Garnett T, Rollins NC, Röös E. The carbon footprint of breastmilk substitutes in comparison with breastfeeding. *J Clean Prod.* 2019;222:436–45.
112. Marshall JL et al. Being a 'good mother': managing breastfeeding and merging identities. *Social Science & Medicine.* 2007 Nov 1;65(10):2147-59.
113. Flacking R et al. Trustful bonds: a key to "becoming a mother" and to reciprocal breastfeeding. Stories of mothers of very preterm infants at a neonatal unit. *Social science & medicine.* 2006 Jan 1;62(1):70-80

Chapter 3: Let's look at the biology

1. www.llli.org/how-often-does-breastfeeding-really-fail/
2. Neville, M. C., Morton, J., & Umemura, S. (2001). Lactogenesis: the transition from pregnancy to lactation. *Pediatric Clinics of North America,* 48(1), 35-52
3. Neville, M. C., Morton, J., & Umemura, S. (2001). Lactogenesis: the transition from pregnancy to lactation. *Pediatric Clinics of North America,* 48(1), 35-52
4. Arbour, M. W., & Kessler, J. L. (2013). Mammary hypoplasia: not every breast can produce sufficient milk. *Journal of midwifery & women's health,* 58(4), 457-461.
5. Huggins, K., Petok, E. S., & Mireles, O. (2000). Markers of Lactation Insufficiency. *Curr Issues Clin Lact,* 119, 1053.
6. Souto, G. C., Giugliani, E. R., Giugliani, C., & Schneider, M. A. (2003). The impact of breast reduction surgery on breastfeeding performance. *Journal of Human Lactation,* 19(1), 43-49.
7. Schiff, M., Algert, C. S., Ampt, A., Sywak, M. S., & Roberts, C. L. (2014). The impact of cosmetic breast implants on breastfeeding: a systematic review and meta-analysis. *International breastfeeding journal,* 9(1), 17.
8. NT. Sclerodermalike esophageal disease in children breast-fed by mothers with silicone breast implants. *JAMA.* 1994 Jan 19;271(3):213-6.
9. Speller, E., & Brodribb, W. (2012). Breastfeeding and thyroid disease: a literature review. *Breastfeeding Review,* 20(2), 41.

10. Stuebe, A. M., Meltzer-Brody, S., Pearson, B., Pedersen, C., & Grewen, K. (2015). Maternal neuroendocrine serum levels in exclusively breastfeeding mothers. *Breastfeeding Medicine*, 10(4), 197-202.
11. Delshad, H., & Azizi, F. (2020). Iodine nutrition in pregnant and breastfeeding women: Sufficiency, deficiency, and supplementation. *Hormones*, 19(2), 179-186.
12. Herskin, C. W., Stage, E., Barfred, C., Emmersen, P., Ladefoged Nichum, V., Damm, P., & Mathiesen, E. R. (2016). Low prevalence of long-term breastfeeding among women with type 2 diabetes. *The Journal of Maternal-Fetal & Neonatal Medicine*, 29(15), 2512-2517.
13. Nommsen-Rivers LA. A case control study of diabetes during pregnancy and low milk supply. *Breastfeeding Medicine*. 2016 Mar 1;11(2):80-5.
14. Chapman, D. J. & Perez-Escamilla, R. (1999) Identification of risk factors for delayed onset of lactation. *J. Am. Diet. Assoc.*99:450–454.
15. Rasmussen KM, Kjolhede CL: Prepregnant overweight and obesity diminish the prolactin response to suckling in the first week postpartum. *Pediatrics* 113:e465–e471, 2004
16. Matias, S. L., Dewey, K. G., Quesenberry Jr, C. P., & Gunderson, E. P. (2014). Maternal prepregnancy obesity and insulin treatment during pregnancy are independently associated with delayed lactogenesis in women with recent gestational diabetes mellitus. *The American journal of clinical nutrition*, 99(1), 115-121.
17. Taylor, J. S., Kacmar, J. E., Nothnagle, M., & Lawrence, R. A. (2005). A systematic review of the literature associating breastfeeding with type 2 diabetes and gestational diabetes. *Journal of the american college of nutrition*, 24(5), 320-326.
18. Harrison, C. L., Teede, H. J., Joham, A. E., & Moran, L. J. (2016). Breastfeeding and obesity in PCOS. *Expert review of endocrinology & metabolism*, 11(6), 449-454.
19. Vanky, E., Isaksen, H., Haase Moen, M., & Carlsen, S. M. (2008). Breastfeeding in polycystic ovary syndrome. *Acta obstetricia et gynecologica Scandinavica*, 87(5), 531-535.
20. McGuire, E., & Rowan, M. K. (2015). PCOS, breast hypoplasia and low milk supply: A case study. *Breastfeeding Review*, 23(3), 29.
21. Chandran L, Gelfer P. Breastfeeding: the essential principles. *Pediatrics in Review*. 2006 Nov 1;27(11):409.
22. Lawrence RM, Lawrence RA. Given the benefits of breastfeeding, what contraindications exist? *Pediatric Clinics of North America*. 2001 Feb 1;48(1):235-51.
23. Latham, M. C., & Greiner, T. (1998). Breastfeeding versus formula feeding in HIV infection. *The Lancet*, 352(9129), 737.
24. https://www.who.int/elena/titles/hiv_infant_feeding/en/
25. https://www.cdc.gov/breastfeeding/breastfeeding-special-circumstances/maternal-or-infant-illnesses/influenza.html
26. Lubbe, W., Botha, E., Niela-Vilen, H., & Reimers, P. (2020). Breastfeeding during the COVID-19 pandemic–a literature review for clinical practice. *International breastfeeding journal*, 15(1), 1-9.
27. Jones, W. (2018). Breastfeeding and Medication. Routledge.
28. Mitchell, J., Jones, W., Winkley, E., & Kinsella, S. M. (2020). Guideline on anaesthesia and sedation in breastfeeding women 2020: Guideline from the Association of Anaesthetists. *Anaesthesia*.
29. Kendall-Tackett, K., & Hale, T. W. (2010). The use of antidepressants in pregnant and breastfeeding women: a review of recent studies. *Journal of Human Lactation*, 26(2), 187-195.
30. Mitchell, J. L. (1999). Use of cough and cold preparations during breastfeeding. *Journal of Human Lactation*, 15(4), 347-349.
31. Jones, W. (2015). Cocaine use and the breastfeeding mother. *The practising midwife*, 18(1), 19-22.
32. Anderson, P. O. (2017). Cannabis and breastfeeding. *Breastfeeding Medicine*, 12(10), 580-581
33. https://www.breastfeedingnetwork.org.uk/smoking/
34. Haastrup, M. B., Pottegård, A., & Damkier, P. (2014). Alcohol and breastfeeding. *Basic & clinical pharmacology & toxicology*, 114(2), 168-173.

35. McCreedy, A., Bird, S., Brown, L. J., Shaw-Stewart, J., & Chen, Y. F. (2018). Effects of maternal caffeine consumption on the breastfed child: a systematic review. Swiss medical weekly, 148(3940).
36. Sellen DW. Weaning, complementary feeding, and maternal decision making in a rural east African pastoral population. Journal of Human Lactation. 2001 Aug 1;17(3):233-44.

Chapter 4: Have things always been this way?

1. Salmon, M., 1994. The cultural significance of breastfeeding and infant care in early modern England and America. *Journal of Social History*, pp.247-269.
2. Pal, M.N.: The Ayurvedic tradition of child care: pediatric wisdom of ancient India. Ind. J. Hist., 9: 22-31 (1973)
3. Laroia, N. and Sharma, D., 2006. The religious and cultural bases for breastfeeding practices among the Hindus. *Breastfeeding Medicine*, 1(2), pp.94-98.
4. Shaikh, U. and Ahmed, O., 2006. Islam and infant feeding. *Breastfeeding Medicine*, 1(3), pp.164-167.
5. Ertem, I.O., Kaynak, G., Kaynak, C., Ulukol, B. and Gulnar, S.B., 2001. Attitudes and practices of breastfeeding mothers regarding fasting in Ramadan. *Child: care, health and development*, 27(6), pp.545-554.
6. Stevens, E.E., Patrick, T.E. and Pickler, R., 2009. A history of infant feeding. *The Journal of perinatal education*, 18(2), pp.32-39.
7. Thorley, V. (2008). Sharing breastmilk: wet nursing, cross-feeding, and milk donations. *Breastfeeding Review*, 16(1), 25.
8. West, E., & Knight, R. J. (2017). Mothers' Milk: Slavery, Wet-Nursing, and Black and White Women in the Antebellum South. *Journal of Southern History*, 83(1), 37-68.
9. Fildes, V. A. (1988). *Wet nursing: a history from antiquity to the present*. B. Blackwell.
10. Minchin, M. (2018). 14 Infant Feeding in History: an Outline. *Breastfeeding and Breastmilk-From Biochemistry to Impact: A Multidisciplinary Introduction*, 219.
11. Fildes, V. (1986). *Breasts, bottles and babies-a history of infant feeding*. Edinburgh University Press.
12. Cassidy, T. (2007). *Birth: A history*. Random House.
13. Sackett, W. W. (1962). *Bringing up babies: a family doctor's practical approach to child care*. Harper & Row.
14. Crowther, S. M., Reynolds, L. A., & Tansey, E. M. (2009). *The resurgence of breastfeeding, 1975–2000* (Vol. 35, No. 35). Wellcome Trust Centre for the History of Medicine at UCL.

Chapter 5: Our birth experiences can interfere with getting breastfeeding off to a good start

1. Wen J, Yu G, Kong Y, Liu F, Wei H. An exploration of the breastfeeding behaviors of women after cesarean section: A qualitative study. *International Journal of Nursing Sciences*. 2020 Jul 20.
2. Nissen E, Lilja G, Widström AM, Uvnás-Moberg K. Elevation of oxytocin levels early post partum in women. *Acta Obstetricia et Gynecologica Scandinavica*. 1995 Jul 1;74(7):530-3.
3. Jonas J, L M, Nissen E, Ejdebäck M, Ransjö-Arvidson A, Uvnäs-Moberg K. Effects of intrapartum oxytocin administration and epidural analgesia on the concentration of plasma oxytocin and prolactin, in response to suckling during the second day postpartum. *Breastfeeding Medicine*. 2009;4(2):71–82. pmid:19210132
4. Yuksel B, Ital I, Balaban O, Kocak E, Seven A, Kucur SK, Erbakirci M, Keskin N. Immediate breastfeeding and skin-to-skin contact during cesarean section decreases maternal oxidative stress, a prospective randomized case-controlled study. *The Journal of Maternal-Fetal & Neonatal Medicine*. 2016 Aug 17;29(16):2691-6.
5. Guala A, Boscardini L, Visentin R, Angellotti P, Grugni L, Barbaglia M, Chapin E, Castelli E, Finale E. Skin-to-skin contact in cesarean birth and duration of breastfeeding: A cohort study. *The Scientific World Journal*. 2017 Jan 1;2017
6. Velandia M. Parent-infant skin-to-skin contact studies: Parent-infant interaction

and oxytocin levels during skin-to-skin contact after Cesarean section and mother-infant skin-to-skin contact as treatment for breastfeeding problems. Doctoral thesis. Karolinska Institute, Dept of Women's and Children's Health; 2012, Stockholm Sweden.

7. Bystrova K. Skin-to-skin contact and suckling in early postpartum: Effects on temperature, breastfeeding and mother-infant interaction. Institutionen för kvinnors och barns hälsa/Department of Women's and Children's Health; 2008 Jan 28.

8. Jonas W, Nissen E, Ransjö-Arvidson AB, Matthiesen AS, Uvnäs-Moberg K. Influence of oxytocin or epidural analgesia on personality profile in breastfeeding women: a comparative study. *Archives of Women's Mental Health.* 2008 Dec 1;11(5-6):335-45.

9. Cetisli NE, Arkan G, Top ED. Maternal attachment and breastfeeding behaviors according to type of delivery in the immediate postpartum period. *Revista da Associação Médica Brasileira.* 2018 Feb;64(2):164-9.

10. Sakalidis VS, Williams TM, Hepworth AR, Garbin CP, Hartmann PE, Paech MJ, Al-Tamimi Y, Geddes DT. A comparison of early sucking dynamics during breastfeeding after cesarean section and vaginal birth. *Breastfeeding Medicine.* 2013 Feb 1;8(1):79-85

11. Zhang F, Cheng J, Yan S, Wu H, Bai T. Early Feeding Behaviors and Breastfeeding Outcomes After Cesarean Section. *Breastfeeding Medicine.* 2019 Jun 1;14(5):325-33.

12. Abel, R. A., Ronca, A. E. & Alberts, J. R. (1998). Perinatal stimulation facilitates suckling onset in newborn rats. *Developmental Psychobiology* 32, 91–9.

13. Brown A, Jordan S. Impact of birth complications on breastfeeding duration: an internet survey. *Journal of advanced nursing.* 2013 Apr;69(4):828-39.

14. Wall V, Glass R. Mandibular asymmetry and breastfeeding problems: experience from 11 cases. *Journal of Human Lactation.* 2006 Aug 1;22(3):328-34.

15. Chen DC, Nommsen-Rivers L, Dewey KG, Lönnerdal B. Stress during labor and delivery and early lactation performance. *The American Journal of Clinical Nutrition.* 1998 Aug 1;68(2):335-44.

16. Taylor A, Fisk NM, Glover V. Mode of delivery and subsequent stress response. *The Lancet.* 2000 Jan 8;355(9198):120.

17. Fleet, J. A., Jones, M., & Belan, I. (2017). The influence of intrapartum opioid use on breastfeeding experience at 6 weeks post partum: a secondary analysis. *Midwifery, 50,* 106-109.

18. Ransjö-Arvidson AB, Matthiesen AS, Lilja G, Nissen E, Widström AM, Uvnäs-Moberg K. Maternal analgesia during labor disturbs newborn behavior: effects on breastfeeding, temperature, and crying. *Birth.* 2001 Mar 1;28(1):5-12.

19. Fleet J-A, Jones M, Belan I. Taking the alternative route: women's experience of intranasal fentanyl, subcutaneous fentanyl or intramuscular pethidine for labour analgesia. *Midwifery* 2017;53:15–19.

20. Moran VH, Thomson G, Cook J, Storey H, Beeson L, MacArthur C, Wilson M. Qualitative exploration of women's experiences of intramuscular pethidine or remifentanil patient-controlled analgesia for labour pain. *BMJ open.* 2019 Dec 1;9(12).

21. Fleet JA, Jones M, Belan I. The influence of intrapartum opioid use on breastfeeding experience at 6 weeks post partum: a secondary analysis. *Midwifery.* 2017 Jul 1;50:106-9.

22. Wilson MJ, MacArthur C, Hewitt CA, Handley K, Gao F, Beeson L, Daniels J, Group RT. Intravenous remifentanil patient-controlled analgesia versus intramuscular pethidine for pain relief in labour (RESPITE): an open-label, multicentre, randomised controlled trial. *The lancet.* 2018 Aug 25;392(10148):662-72.

23. Wilson MJ, MacArthur C, Hewitt CA, Handley K, Gao F, Beeson L, Daniels J, Group RT. Intravenous remifentanil patient-controlled analgesia versus intramuscular pethidine for pain relief in labour (RESPITE): an open-label, multicentre, randomised controlled trial. *The lancet.* 2018 Aug 25;392(10148):662-72.

24. Nguyen, US, Rothman, KJ, Demissie, S, Jackson, DJ, Lang, JM, Ecker, JL. Epidural analgesia and risks of cesarean and operative vaginal deliveries in nulliparous and multiparous women. Matern Child Health J. 2010;14(5):705-712.

25. Jonas W, Nissen E, Ransjö-Arvidson AB, Matthiesen AS, Uvnäs-Moberg K. Influence of oxytocin or epidural analgesia on personality profile in breastfeeding women: a comparative study. *Archives of Women's Mental Health.* 2008 Dec 1;11(5-6):335-45.

26. Levy F, Kendrick KM, Keverne EB, Piketty V, Poindron P. Intracerebral oxytocin is

important for the onset of maternal behavior in inexperienced ewes delivered under peridural anesthesia. *Behavioral Neuroscience.* 1992 Apr;106(2):427.
27. Goodfellow CF, Hull MG, Swaab DF, Dogterom J, Buijs RM. Oxytocin deficiency at delivery with epidural analgesia. *BJOG: An International Journal of Obstetrics & Gynaecology.* 1983 Mar 1;90(3):214-9.
28. Jonas , Nissen E, Ransjö-Arvidson A, Matthiesen A, Uvnäs-Moberg K. Influence of oxytocin or epidural analgesia on personality profile in breastfeeding women: a comparative study. *Archives of women's mental health.* 2008;11(5–6):335–45. pmid:18726143
29. Murray AD, Dolby RM, Nation RL, Thomas DB. Effects of epidural anesthesia on newborns and their mothers. *Child Development.* 1981 Mar 1:71-82
30. Jordan, S, Emery, S, Watkins, A, Evans, JD, Storey, M, Morgan, G. Associations of drugs routinely given in labour with breastfeeding at 48 hours: analysis of the Cardiff Births Survey. *Bjog.* 2009;116(12):1622-1632
31. Chang, ZM, Heaman, MI. Epidural analgesia during labor and delivery: effects on the initiation and continuation of effective breastfeeding. *J Hum Lact.* 2005;21(3):305-314, quiz 315-319, 326.
32. Beilin, Y, Bodian, CA, Weiser, J. Effect of labor epidural analgesia with and without fentanyl on infant breast-feeding: a prospective, randomized, double-blind study. *Anesthesiology.* 2005;103(6):1211-1217.
33. Jonas W, Nissen E, Ransjö-Arvidson AB, Matthiesen AS, Uvnäs-Moberg K. Influence of oxytocin or epidural analgesia on personality profile in breastfeeding women: a comparative study. *Arch Womens Ment Health*
34. England MJ, Tjallinks A, Hofmeyr J, Harber J. Suppression of lactation. A comparison of bromocriptine and prostaglandin E2. *J Reprod Med*1988;**33**:630–2.
35. Jordan S, Emery S, Watkins A, Evans JD, Storey M, Morgan G. Associations of drugs routinely given in labour with breastfeeding at 48 hours: analysis of the Cardiff Births Survey. *BJOG: An International Journal of Obstetrics & Gynaecology.* 2009 Nov;116(12):1622-32.
36. Gonzalez Mesa E. Hard data about the side effects of synthetic oxytocin. In: Presentation at the mid-pacific conference on birth and primal health research. Honolulu October 26–28; 2012.
37. Odent MR. Synthetic oxytocin and breastfeeding: reasons for testing an hypothesis. *Medical hypotheses.* 2013 Nov 1;81(5):889-91.
38. Thompson JF, Heal LJ, Roberts CL, Ellwood DA. Women's breastfeeding experiences following a significant primary postpartum haemorrhage: a multicentre cohort study. *International breastfeeding journal.* 2010 May 1;5(1):5.
39. Horie S, Nomura K, Takenoshita S, Nakagawa J, Kido M, Sugimoto M. A relationship between a level of hemoglobin after delivery and exclusive breastfeeding initiation at a baby friendly hospital in Japan. *Environmental health and preventive medicine.* 2017 Dec 1;22(1):40.
40. Henry L, Britz SP. Loss of Blood= Loss of Breastmilk? The Effect of Postpartum Hemorrhage on Breastfeeding Success. *Journal of Obstetric, Gynecologic & Neonatal Nursing.* 2013 Jun 1;42:S100.
41. De Groot AN, van Dongen PW, Vree TB, Hekster YA, van Roosmalen J. Ergot alkaloids. Current status and review of clinical pharmacology and therapeutic use compared with other oxytocics in obstetrics and gynaecology. *Drugs* 1998;**56**:523–35.
42. Willis CE, Livingstone V. Infant insufficient milk syndrome associated with maternal postpartum hemorrhage. *Journal of Human Lactation.* 1995 Jun;11(2):123-6.
43. Boskabadi H, Maamouri G, Ebrahimi M, Ghayour-Mobarhan M, Esmaeily H, Sahebkar A, Ferns GA. Neonatal hypernatremia and dehydration in infants receiving inadequate breastfeeding. *Asia Pacific journal of clinical nutrition.* 2010 Sep;19(3):301.
44. Fahy KM. Third stage of labour care for women at low risk of postpartum haemorrhage. *Journal of midwifery & women's health.* 2009 Sep 1;54(5):380-6.
45. Brown A, Jordan S. Active management of the third stage of labor may reduce breastfeeding duration due to pain and physical complications. *Breastfeeding Medicine.* 2014 Dec 1;9(10):494-502.
46. Begley CM, Gyte GM, Devane D, McGuire W, Weeks A, Biesty LM. Active versus

expectant management for women in the third stage of labour. *Cochrane database of systematic reviews*. 2019(2).

47. Anderson AM. Disruption of lactogenesis by retained placental fragments. *Journal of Human Lactation*. 2001 May;17(2):142-4.

48. Barrera, C.M., Kawwass, J.F., Boulet, S.L., Nelson, J.M. and Perrine, C.G. Fertility treatment use and breastfeeding outcomes. *American journal of obstetrics and gynecology* 2019; *220*(3), pp.261-e1.

49. Fisher, J., Hammarberg, K., Wynter, K., McBain, J., Gibson, F., Boivin, J. and McMahon, C., 2013. Assisted conception, maternal age and breastfeeding: an Australian cohort study. *Acta Paediatrica*, *102*(10), pp.970-976.

50. Kawwass, J.F., Drph, S.L.B. and Perrine, C.G. Fertility treatment use and breastfeeding outcomes. AJOG 2019; 261e.

51. Cromi, A., Serati, M., Candeloro, I., Uccella, S., Scandroglio, S., Agosti, M. and Ghezzi, F., 2015. Assisted reproductive technology and breastfeeding outcomes: a case-control study. *Fertility and Sterility*, 103(1), pp.89-94.

52. Barnes M, Roiko A, Reed R, Williams C, Willcocks K. Experiences of birth and breastfeeding following assisted conception. *Breast-feed Rev* 2013;21:9–15.

53. Brown, A. What do women lose if they are prevented from meeting their breastfeeding goals? *Clinical Lactation*. 2018. 9(4), 200-207.

54. Dewey KG. Maternal and fetal stress are associated with impaired lactogenesis in humans. *The Journal of Nutrition*. 2001 Nov 1;131(11):3012S-5S

55. Grajeda R, Pérez-Escamilla R. Stress during labor and delivery is associated with delayed onset of lactation among urban Guatemalan women. *The Journal of Nutrition*. 2002 Oct 1;132(10):3055-60.

56. Türkmen H, Yalniz Dilcen H, Akin B. The Effect of Labor Comfort on Traumatic Childbirth Perception, Post-Traumatic Stress Disorder, and Breastfeeding. *Breastfeeding Medicine*. 2020 Sep 3.

57. Molloy, E., Biggerstaff, D. L., & Sidebotham, P. (2020). A phenomenological exploration of parenting after birth trauma: Mothers perceptions of the first year. *Women and Birth*.

58. Hinic K. Predictors of breastfeeding confidence in the early postpartum period. Journal of Obstetric, Gynecologic & Neonatal Nursing. 2016 Sep 1;45(5):649-60.

59. Ayers S, Wright DB, Thornton A. Development of a measure of postpartum PTSD: the city birth trauma scale. *Frontiers in psychiatry*. 2018 Sep 18;9:409.

60. Brown A, Rance J, Bennett P. Understanding the relationship between breastfeeding and postnatal depression: the role of pain and physical difficulties. *Journal of advanced nursing*. 2016 Feb;72(2):273-82.

61. Hodgkinson EL, Smith DM, Wittkowski A. Women's experiences of their pregnancy and postpartum body image: a systematic review and meta-synthesis. *BMC pregnancy and childbirth*. 2014 Dec 1;14(1):330.

62. NHS England. National maternity review. better births; improving outcomes of maternity services in England. London: NHS England. 2016.

Chapter 6: Our early postnatal environments are not always conducive to supporting breastfeeding

1. www.who.int/activities/promoting-baby-friendly-hospitals/ten-steps-to-successful-breastfeeding

2. www.unicef.org.uk/babyfriendly/wp-content/uploads/sites/2/2014/02/Guide-to-the-Unicef-UK-Baby-Friendly-Initiative-Standards.pdf

3. Pérez-Escamilla R, Martinez JL, Segura-Pérez S. Impact of the Baby-friendly Hospital Initiative on breastfeeding and child health outcomes: a systematic review. *Maternal & Child Nutrition*. 2016 Jan 1.

4. Kramer MS, Fombonne E, Igumnov S, Vanilovich I, Matush L, Mironova E, Bogdanovich N, Tremblay RE, Chalmers B, Zhang X, Platt RW. Effects of prolonged and exclusive breastfeeding on child behavior and maternal adjustment: evidence from a large, randomized trial. *Pediatrics*. 2008 Mar 1;121(3):e435-40.

5. Wright A, Rice S, Wells S. Changing hospital practices to increase the duration of breastfeeding. *Pediatrics*. 1996 May 1;97(5):669-75

6. Munn, A. C., Newman, S. D., Mueller, M., Phillips, S. M., & Taylor, S. N. (2016). The impact in the United States of the baby-friendly hospital initiative on early infant health and breastfeeding outcomes. *Breastfeeding Medicine, 11*(5), 222-230.

7. Wouk, K., Tully, K. P., & Labbok, M. H. (2017). Systematic review of evidence for baby-friendly hospital initiative step 3: prenatal breastfeeding education. *Journal of Human Lactation, 33*(1), 50-82.

8. Balogun, O. O., Dagvadorj, A., Yourkavitch, J., da Silva Lopes, K., Suto, M., Takemoto, Y., ... & Ota, E. (2017). Health facility staff training for improving breastfeeding outcome: A systematic review for step 2 of the Baby-Friendly Hospital initiative. *Breastfeeding Medicine, 12*(9), 537-546.

9. Robert, E., Michaud-Létourneau, I., Dramaix-Wilmet, M., Swennen, B., & Devlieger, R. (2019). A comparison of exclusive breastfeeding in Belgian maternity facilities with and without Baby-friendly Hospital status. *Maternal & child nutrition, 15*(4), e12845.

10. Marinelli, A., Del Prete, V., Finale, E., Guala, A., Pelullo, C. P., & Attena, F. (2019). Breastfeeding with and without the WHO/UNICEF baby-friendly hospital initiative: A cross-sectional survey. *Medicine, 98*(44).

11. de Carvalho, M. L., Boccolini, C. S., de Oliveira, M. I. C., & do Carmo Leal, M. (2016). The baby-friendly hospital initiative and breastfeeding at birth in Brazil: a cross sectional study. *Reproductive health, 13*(3), 119.

12. Nobari, T. Z., Jiang, L., Wang, M. C., & Whaley, S. E. (2017). Baby-Friendly Hospital Initiative and breastfeeding among WIC-participating infants in Los Angeles county. *Journal of Human Lactation, 33*(4), 677-683.

13. Charpak N, Ruiz-Peláez JG, Charpak Y. A randomized, controlled trial of kangaroo mother care: results of follow-up at 1 year of corrected age. *Pediatrics.* 2001 Nov 1;108(5):1072-9.

14. Christensson K, Cabrera T, Christensson E, Uvnäs–Moberg K, Winberg J. Separation distress call in the human neonate in the absence of maternal body contact. *Acta Paediatrica.* 1995 May 1;84(5):468-73.

15. Moore ER, Anderson GC, Bergman N. Early skin-to-skin contact for mothers and their healthy newborn infants (Review). *Cochrane database of systematic reviews.* 2007;3:1-63.

16. Anderzen-Carlsson A, Lamy ZC, Eriksson M. Parental experiences of providing skin-to-skin care to their newborn infant—Part 1: A qualitative systematic review. International Journal of Qualitative Studies on Health and Well-being. 2014;9.

17. Moore ER, Anderson GC, Bergman N, Dowswell T. Early skin-to-skin contact for mothers and their healthy newborn infants. *Cochrane database of systematic reviews.* 2012 May;5(3).

18. Srivastava S, Gupta A, Bhatnagar A, Dutta S. Effect of very early skin to skin contact on success at breastfeeding and preventing early hypothermia in neonates. Indian *Journal of Public Health.* 2014 Jan 1;58(1):22.

19. Gregson S, Meadows J, Teakle P, Blacker J. Skin-to-skin contact after elective caesarean section: Investigating the effect on breastfeeding rates. *British Journal of Midwifery.* 2016 Jan 1;24(1).

20. Phillips R. The sacred hour: uninterrupted skin-to-skin contact immediately after birth. *Newborn and Infant Nursing Reviews.* 2013 Jun 30;13(2):67-72.

21. Khan J, Vesel L, Bahl R, Martines JC. Timing of breastfeeding initiation and exclusivity of breastfeeding during the first month of life: effects on neonatal mortality and morbidity—a systematic review and meta-analysis. *Maternal and Child Health Journal.* 2015 Mar 1;19(3):468-79.

22. Perrine CG, Scanlon KS, Li R, Odom E, Grummer-Strawn LM. Baby-friendly hospital practices and meeting exclusive breastfeeding intention. *Pediatrics.* 2012 Jul 1;130(1):54-60.

23. www.rcm.org.uk/media/2289/infant-feeding.pdf

24. DiGirolamo AM, Grummer-Strawn LM, Fein SB. Effect of maternity-care practices on breastfeeding. *Pediatrics.* 2008 Oct 1;122(Supplement 2):S43-9.

25. Righard L, Alade MO. Effect of delivery room routines on success of first breast-feed. *The Lancet.* 1990 Nov 3;336(8723):1105-7.

26. Rojas MA, Kaplan M, Quevedo M, Sherwonit E, Foster LB, Ehrenkranz RA, Mayes L.

Somatic growth of preterm infants during skin-to-skin care versus traditional holding: A randomized, controlled trial. *Journal of Developmental & Behavioral Pediatrics.* 2003 Jun 1;24(3):163-8.

27. Hillier K. Babies and bacteria: phage typing, bacteriologists, and the birth of infection control. *Bulletin of the History of Medicine.* 2006;80(4):733-61.

28. Jaafar SH, Lee KS, Ho JJ. Separate care for new mother and infant versus rooming-in for increasing the duration of breastfeeding. *Cochrane database of systematic reviews.* 2012 Jan 1;9.

29. Bystrova K, Ivanova V, Edhborg M, Matthiesen AS, Ransjö-Arvidson AB, Mukhamedrakhimov R, Uvnäs-Moberg K, Widström AM. Early contact versus separation: effects on mother–infant interaction one year later. *Birth.* 2009 Jun 1;36(2):97-109

30. Chantry CJ, Dewey KG, Peerson JM, Wagner EA, Nommsen-Rivers LA. In-hospital formula use increases early breastfeeding cessation among first-time mothers intending to exclusively breastfeed. The Journal of Pediatrics. 2014 Jun 30;164(6):1339-45

31. Howard CR, Howard FM, Lanphear B, et al. Randomized clinical trial of pacifier use and bottle-feeding or cupfeeding and their effect on breastfeeding. *Pediatrics* 2003; 111: 511-518

32. Brown A, Jordan S. Impact of birth complications on breastfeeding duration: an internet survey. *Journal of advanced nursing.* 2013 Apr;69(4):828-39.

33. Tender JA, Janakiram J, Arce E, Mason R, Jordan T, Marsh J, Kin S, He J, Moon RY. Reasons for in-hospital formula supplementation of breastfed infants from low-income families. *Journal of Human Lactation.* 2009 Feb;25(1):11-7.

34. Centers for Disease Control and Prevention (CDC. Vital signs: hospital practices to support breastfeeding - United States, 2007 and 2009. MMWR. *Morbidity and Mortality Weekly Report.* 2011 Aug 5;60(30):1020.

35. Parry JE, Ip DK, Chau PY, Wu KM, Tarrant M. Predictors and consequences of in-hospital formula supplementation for healthy breastfeeding newborns. Journal of *Human Lactation.* 2013 Nov 1;29(4):527-36.

36. Gagnon AJ, Leduc G, Waghorn K, Yang H, Platt RW. In-hospital formula supplementation of healthy breastfeeding newborns. *Journal of Human Lactation.* 2005 Nov;21(4):397-405.

37. Forster DA, Johns HM, McLachlan HL, Moorhead AM, McEgan KM, Amir LH. Feeding infants directly at the breast during the postpartum hospital stay is associated with increased breastfeeding at 6 months postpartum: a prospective cohort study. *BMJ Open.* 2015 May 1;5(5):e007512.

38. Flaherman VJ, Cabana MD, McCulloch CE, Paul IM. Effect of early limited formula on breastfeeding duration in the first year of life: a randomized clinical trial. *JAMA pediatrics.* 2019 Aug 1;173(8):729-35.

39. Flaherman VJ, Aby J, Burgos AE, Lee KA, Cabana MD, Newman TB. Effect of early limited formula on duration and exclusivity of breastfeeding in at-risk infants: an RCT. *Pediatrics.* 2013 Jun 1;131(6):1059-65.

40. Bodley V, Powers D. Long-term nipple shield use—A positive perspective. *Journal of Human Lactation.* 1996 Dec 1;12(4):301-4.

41. Pincombe J, Baghurst P, Antoniou G, Peat B, Henderson A, Reddin E. Baby Friendly Hospital Initiative practices and breast feeding duration in a cohort of first-time mothers in Adelaide, Australia. *Midwifery.* 2008 Mar 31;24(1):55-61.

42. Amatayakul K, Vutyavanich T, Tanthayaphinant O, Tovanabutra S, Yutabootr Y, Drewett RF. Serum prolactin and cortisol levels after suckling for varying periods of time and the effect of a nipple shield. *Acta Obstetricia et Gynecologica Scandinavica.* 1987 Jan 1;66(1):47-51.

43. Auerbach KG. The effect of nipple shields on maternal milk volume. *Journal of Obstetric, Gynecologic, & Neonatal Nursing.* 1990 Sep 1;19(5):419-30.

44. Woolridge MW, Baum JD, Drewett RF. Effect of a traditional and of a new nipple shield on sucking patterns and milk flow. *Early Human Development.* 1980 Dec 1;4(4):357-64.

45. Clum D, Primomo J. Use of a silicone nipple shield with premature infants. *Journal of Human Lactation.* 1996 Dec 1;12(4):287-90.

46. Meier PP, Brown LP, Hurst NM, Spatz DL, Engstrom JL, Borucki LC, Krouse AM. Nipple shields for preterm infants: effect on milk transfer and duration of breastfeeding. *Journal of Human Lactation*. 2000 May 1;16(2):106-14.
47. Hassan MI. Exclusive Breast feeding & non-nutritive sucking (pacifier) affect the nutritional status of infants. In 3rd International Conference on Nutrition and Food Sciences-ICNFS 2014 Jun (pp. 18-20).
48. Jenik AG, Vain NE, Gorestein AN, Jacobi NE. Pacifier and Breastfeeding Trial Group. Does the recommendation to use a pacifier influence the prevalence of breastfeeding?. *The Journal of Pediatrics*. 2009 Sep 30;155(3):350-4.
49. Fukumoto E, Fukumoto S, Kawasaki K, Furugen R, Kitamura M, Kawashita Y, Hayashida H, Fukuda H, Iijima Y, Saito T. Cessation age of breast-feeding and pacifier use is associated with persistent finger-sucking. *Pediatric Dentistry*. 2013 Nov 15;35(7):506-9
50. www.unicef.org.uk/babyfriendly/baby-friendly-resources/bottle-feeding-resources/guide-to-bottle-feeding/
51. Bass, J., Gartley, Y., & Kleinman, R. Unintended Consequences of Current Breastfeeding Initiatives. *JAMA*, doi:1001/jamapediatrics.2016.1529
52. Herlenius, E., & Kuhn, P. (2013). Sudden unexpected postnatal collapse of newborn infants: a review of cases, definitions, risks, and preventive measures. *Translational stroke research*, 4(2), 236-247.
53. Helsley, L., McDonald, J. V., & Stewart, V. T. (2010). Addressing In-Hospital. *The Joint Commission Journal on Quality and Patient Safety*, 36(7), 327-333.
54. Ball, H. L., Ward-Platt, M. P., Heslop, E., Leech, S. J., & Brown, K. A. (2006). Randomised trial of infant sleep location on the postnatal ward. *Archives of Disease in Childhood*, 91(12), 1005-1010.
55. Driscoll CA, Pereira N, Lichenstein R. In-hospital neonatal falls: an unintended consequence of efforts to improve breastfeeding. *Pediatrics*. 2019 Jan 1;143(1):e20182488.
56. Vohr BR, Poindexter BB, Dusick AM, McKinley LT, Higgins RD, Langer JC, Poole WK. Persistent beneficial effects of breastmilk ingested in the neonatal intensive care unit on outcomes of extremely low birth weight infants at 30 months of age. *Pediatrics*. 2007 Oct 1;120(4):e953-9.
57. Nyqvist KH, Sjödén PO, Ewald U. The development of preterm infants' breastfeeding behavior. *Early Human Development*. 1999 Jul 31;55(3):247-64.
58. Baxter J, Cooklin AR, Smith J. Which mothers wean their babies prematurely from full breastfeeding? An Australian cohort study. *Acta Paediatrica*. 2009 Aug 1;98(8):1274-7.
59. Conde-Agudelo A, Diaz-Rosello JL, Belizan JM. Kangaroo mother care to reduce morbidity and mortality in low birthweight infants. Review. *The Cochrane Library*. 2000(4):3.
60. Shin H, White-Traut R. The conceptual structure of transition to motherhood in the neonatal intensive care unit. *Journal of Advanced Nursing*. 2007 Apr 1;58(1):90-94
61. Flacking R, Ewald U, Starrin B. "I wanted to do a good job": experiences of 'becoming a mother' and breastfeeding in mothers of very preterm infants after discharge from a neonatal unit. *Social Science & Medicine*. 2007 Jun 30;64(12):2405-16.
62. Dewey, K. G. (2001). Maternal and fetal stress are associated with impaired lactogenesis in humans. *The Journal of nutrition*, 131(11), 3012S-3015S.
63. Flacking, R., Ewald, U., Nyqvist, K. H., & Starrin, B. (2006). Trustful bonds: a key to "becoming a mother" and to reciprocal breastfeeding. Stories of mothers of very preterm infants at a neonatal unit. *Social science & medicine*, 62(1), 70-80.

Chapter 7: A lack of investment in skilled support means that too many women experience pain and difficulty

1. McClellan HL, Hepworth AR, Garbin CP, Rowan MK, Deacon J, Hartmann PE, Geddes DT. Nipple pain during breastfeeding with or without visible trauma. *Journal of Human Lactation*. 2012 Nov 1;28(4):511-21.
2. Amir LH, Dennerstein L, Garland SM, Fisher J, Farish SJ. Psychological aspects of nipple pain in lactating women. *Journal of Psychosomatic Obstetrics & Gynecology*. 1996 Jan 1;17(1):53-8.

3. Riordan J, Gill-Hopple K, Angeron J. Indicators of effective breastfeeding and estimates of breast milk intake. *Journal of Human Lactation*. 2005 Nov 1;21(4):406-12.

4. Page T, Lockwood C, Guest K. Management of nipple pain and/or trauma associated with breast-feeding. *JBI Reports*. 2003 Sep 1;1(4):127-47.

5. Buck ML, Amir LH, Cullinane M, Donath SM. Nipple pain, damage, and vasospasm in the first 8 weeks postpartum. *Breastfeeding Medicine*. 2014 Mar 1;9(2):56-62.

6. McClellan HL, Hepworth AR, Garbin CP, Rowan MK, Deacon J, Hartmann PE, Geddes DT. Nipple pain during breastfeeding with or without visible trauma. *Journal of Human Lactation*. 2012 Nov 1;28(4):511-21.

7. De Vries L. Breastfeeding frequency, milk volume, and duration in mother-infant dyads with persistent nipple pain. *Breastfeeding Review*. 2013 Mar 1;21(1):40-2.

8. Li R, Fein SB, Chen J, Grummer-Strawn LM. Why mothers stop breastfeeding: mothers' self-reported reasons for stopping during the first year. *Pediatrics*. 2008 Oct 1;122(Supplement 2):S69-76.

9. Brown A, Rance J, Bennett P. Understanding the relationship between breastfeeding and postnatal depression: the role of pain and physical difficulties. *Journal of Advanced Nursing*. 2016 Feb 1;72(2):273-82.

10. Woolridge MW. The 'anatomy' of infant sucking. Midwifery. 1986 Dec 31;2(4):164-71.

11. Sakalidis VS, Williams TM, Garbin CP, Hepworth AR, Hartmann PE, Paech MJ, Geddes DT. Ultrasound imaging of infant sucking dynamics during the establishment of lactation. *Journal of Human Lactation*. 2013 May 1;29(2):205-13.

12. Kent JC, Ashton E, Hardwick CM, Rowan MK, Chia ES, Fairclough KA, Menon LL, Scott C, Mather-McCaw G, Navarro K, Geddes DT. Nipple pain in breastfeeding mothers: incidence, causes and treatments. *International Journal of Environmental Research and Public Health*. 2015 Sep 29;12(10):12247-63.

13. McClellan HL, Kent JC, Hepworth AR, Hartmann PE, Geddes DT. Persistent nipple pain in breastfeeding mothers associated with abnormal infant tongue movement. *International Journal of Environmental Research and Public Health*. 2015 Sep 2;12(9):10833-45

14. Darmangeat V. The frequency and resolution of nipple pain when latch is improved in a private practice. *Clinical Lactation*. 2011 Sep 1;2(3):22-4

15. Cadwell K, Turner-Maffei C, Blair A, Brimdyr K, Maja McInerney Z. Pain reduction and treatment of sore nipples in nursing mothers. *The Journal of Perinatal Education*. 2004;13(1):29-35

16. Thompson R, Kruske S, Barclay L, Linden K, Gao Y, Kildea S. Potential predictors of nipple trauma from an in-home breastfeeding programme: A cross-sectional study. *Women and Birth*. 2016 Feb 16.

17. Amir LH, Dennerstein L, Garland SM, Fisher J, Farish SJ. Psychological aspects of nipple pain in lactating women. *Journal of Psychosomatic Obstetrics & Gynecology*. 1996 Jan 1;17(1):53-8.

18. Spencer JP. Management of mastitis in breastfeeding women. *Am Fam Physician*. 2008 Sep 15;78(6):727-31.

19. Jacobs LA, Dickinson JE, Hart PD, Doherty DA, Faulkner SJ. Normal nipple position in term infants measured on breastfeeding ultrasound. *Journal of Human Lactation*. 2007 Feb 1;23(1):52-9.

20. Gunther M. Sore nipples causes and prevention. *The Lancet*. 1945 Nov 10;246(6376):590-3

21. Mizuno K, Fujimaki K, Sawada M. Sucking behavior at breast during the early newborn period affects later breast-feeding rate and duration of breast-feeding. *Pediatrics International*. 2004 Feb;46(1):15-20.

22. Gunther M. Sore nipples causes and prevention. *The Lancet*. 1945 Nov 10;246(6376):590-3

23. McClellan HL, Geddes DT, Kent JC, Garbin CP, Mitoulas LR, Hartmann PE. Infants of mothers with persistent nipple pain exert strong sucking vacuums. *Acta Paediatrica*. 2008 Sep 1;97(9):1205-9.

24. Qi Y, Zhang Y, Fein S, Wang C, Loyo-Berríos N. Maternal and breast pump factors associated with breast pump problems and injuries. *Journal of Human Lactation*. 2013 Oct 28:0890334413507499.

25. Snyder JB. Bubble palate and failure to thrive: A case report. *Journal of Human Lactation.* 1997 Jun 1;13(2):139-43.
26. Mills, N., Pransky, S. M., Geddes, D. T., & Mirjalili, S. A. (2019). What is a tongue tie? Defining the anatomy of the in-situ lingual frenulum. *Clinical Anatomy,* 32(6), 749-761.
27. Burrows S, Lanlehin R. Is frenotomy effective in improving breastfeeding in newborn babies with tongue-tie? A literature review. *British Journal of Midwifery.* 2015 Nov 2;23(11):790-7.
28. Ghaheri, Cole, Fausel, Chuop & Mace 2017
29. Geddes DT, Kent JC, Mitoulas LR, Hartmann PE. Tongue movement and intra-oral vacuum in breastfeeding infants. *Early Human Development.* 2008 Jul 31;84(7):471-7.
30. Amitai Y, Shental H, Atkins-Manelis L, Koren G, Zamir CS. Pre-conceptional folic acid supplementation: a possible cause for the increasing rates of ankyloglossia. *Medical hypotheses.* 2020 Jan 1;134:109508.
31. Sari LN, Auerkari EI. Molecular Genetics and Epigenetics of Ankyloglossia. In 11th International Dentistry Scientific Meeting (IDSM 2017) 2018 May. Atlantis Press.
32. Dai J, Xu C, Wang G, Liang Y, Wan T, Zhang Y, Xu X, Yu L, Che Z, Han Q, Wu D. Novel TBX22 mutations in Chinese nonsyndromic cleft lip/palate families. *Journal of genetics.* 2018 Jun;97(2):411-7.
33. Lenormand A, Khonsari R, Corre P, Perrin JP, Boscher C, Nizon M, Pichon O, David A, Le Caignec C, Bertin H, Isidor B. Familial autosomal dominant severe ankyloglossia with tooth abnormalities. *American Journal of Medical Genetics Part A.* 2018 Jul;176(7):1614-7.
34. Greenberg JA, Bell SJ. Multivitamin Supplementation during pregnancy: emphasis on folic acid and L-methylfolate. *Reviews in Obstetrics and Gynecology.* 2011;4(3-4):126.
35. Messner AH, Walsh J, Rosenfeld RM, Schwartz SR, Ishman SL, Baldassari C, Brietzke SE, Darrow DH, Goldstein N, Levi J, Meyer AK. Clinical consensus statement: Ankyloglossia in children. *Otolaryngology–Head and Neck Surgery.* 2020 May;162(5):597-611.
36. Edmunds JE, Fulbrook P, Miles S. Understanding the experiences of mothers who are breastfeeding an infant with tongue-tie: a phenomenological study. *Journal of Human Lactation.* 2013 May;29(2):190-5.
37. Wong K, Patel P, Cohen MB, Levi JR. Breastfeeding infants with ankyloglossia: insight into mothers' experiences. *Breastfeeding Medicine.* 2017 Mar 1;12(2):86-90.
38. Finigan V, Long T. The effectiveness of frenulotomy on infant-feeding outcomes: a systematic literature review. *Midirs Midwifery Digest.* 2013 Apr;23(4).
39. McGoldrick R, Solari D, Hogan M, Corrigan I, Cutting A, Shadbolt B, Todd DA. Tongue-tie in the newborn: Follow-up in the first 6 months. *Breastfeeding Review.* 2016 Nov;24(3):33.
40. Berry J, Griffiths M, Westcott C. A double-blind, randomized, controlled trial of tongue-tie division and its immediate effect on breastfeeding. *Breastfeeding Medicine.* 2012 Jun 1;7(3):189-93.
41. Geddes DT, Langton DB, Gollow I, Jacobs LA, Hartmann PE, Simmer K. Frenulotomy for breastfeeding infants with ankyloglossia: effect on milk removal and sucking mechanism as imaged by ultrasound. *Pediatrics.* 2008 Jul 1;122(1):e188-94.
42. Emond A, Ingram J, Johnson D, Blair P, Whitelaw A, Copeland M, Sutcliffe A. Randomised controlled trial of early frenotomy in breastfed infants with mild–moderate tongue-tie. *Archives of Disease in Childhood-Fetal and Neonatal Edition.* 2014 May 1;99(3):F189-95.
43. Constantine AH, Williams C, Sutcliffe AG. A systematic review of frenotomy for ankyloglossia (tongue tie) in breast fed infants. *Archives of Disease in Childhood.* 2011 Apr 1;96(Suppl 1):A62-3.
44. Bin-Nun A, Kasirer YM, Mimouni FB. A dramatic increase in tongue tie-related articles: a 67 years systematic review. *Breastfeeding Medicine.* 2017 Sep 1;12(7):410-4.
45. Burns E, Fenwick J, Sheehan A, Schmied V. Mining for liquid gold: midwifery language and practices associated with early breastfeeding support. *Maternal & Child Nutrition.* 2013 Jan 1;9(1):57-73.
46. McFadden A, Gavine A, Renfrew MJ, Wade A, Buchanan P, Taylor JL, Veitch

E, Rennie AM, Crowther SA, Neiman S, MacGillivray S. Support for healthy breastfeeding mothers with healthy term babies. *Cochrane Database of Systematic Reviews*. 2017(2).

47. Dykes F. A critical ethnographic study of encounters between midwives and breastfeeding women in postnatal wards in England. *Midwifery*. 2005 Sep 30;21(3):241-52.

48. Hoddinott P, Pill R. A qualitative study of women's views about how health professionals communicate about infant feeding. *Health Expectations*. 2000 Dec 1;3(4):224-33.

49. Graffy J, Taylor J. What information, advice, and support do women want with breastfeeding? *Birth*. 2005 Sep 1;32(3):179-86.

50. Swerts M, Westhof E, Bogaerts A, Lemiengre J. Supporting breast-feeding women from the perspective of the midwife: A systematic review of the literature. *Midwifery*. 2016 Jun 30;37:32-40.

51. Ingram J, Johnson D, Greenwood R. Breastfeeding in Bristol: teaching good positioning, and support from fathers and families. *Midwifery*. 2002 Jun 30;18(2):87-101.

52. Palmer G. *The Politics of Breastfeeding: When Breasts are Bad for Business*. 2009 Second edition. London: Pinter & Martin

53. McLelland G, Hall H, Gilmour C, Cant R. Support needs of breast-feeding women: Views of Australian midwives and health nurses. *Midwifery*. 2015 Jan 31;31(1):e1-6.

54. Nelson AM. Maternal-newborn nurses' experiences of inconsistent professional breastfeeding support. *Journal of Advanced Nursing*. 2007 Oct 1;60(1):29-38.

55. Lee E, Furedi F. Mothers' experience of, and attitudes to, using infant formula in the early months. School of Social Policy, Sociology and Social Research, University of Kent, UK. Retrieved December. 2005;8:2011.

56. Lee E. Health, morality, and infant feeding: British mothers' experiences of formula milk use in the early weeks. *Sociology of Health & Illness*. 2007 Nov 1;29(7):1075-90.

57. Brown A, Raynor P, Lee M. Healthcare professionals' and mothers' perceptions of factors that influence decisions to breastfeed or formula feed infants: a comparative study. *Journal of Advanced Nursing*. 2011 Sep 1;67(9):1993-2003.

58. Thomson G, Ebisch-Burton K, Flacking R. Shame if you do–shame if you don't: women's experiences of infant feeding. *Maternal & Child Nutrition*. 2015 Jan 1;11(1):33-46.

59. Smale M, Renfrew MJ, Marshall JL, Spiby H. Turning policy into practice: more difficult than it seems. The case of breastfeeding education. *Maternal & child nutrition*. 2006 Apr 1;2(2):103-13.

60. Marshall JL, Green JM, Spiby H. Parents' views on how health professionals should work with them now to get the best for their child in the future. *Health Expectations*. 2014 Aug 1;17(4):477-87.

61. Gustafsson I, Nyström M, Palmér L. Midwives' lived experience of caring for new mothers with initial breastfeeding difficulties: A phenomenological study. *Sexual & Reproductive Healthcare*. 2017 Jun 1;12:9-15.1

62. Cloherty M, Alexander J, Holloway I. Supplementing breast-fed babies in the UK to protect their mothers from tiredness or distress. *Midwifery*. 2004 Jun 30;20(2):194-204.

63. Kronborg H, Væth M, Olsen J, Iversen L, Harder I. Effect of early postnatal breastfeeding support: a cluster-randomized community based trial. *Acta Paediatrica*. 2007 Jul 1;96(7):1064-70.

64. Ekström A, Matthiesen AS, Widström AM, Nissen E. Breastfeeding attitudes among counselling health professionals Development of an instrument to describe breastfeeding attitudes. *Scandinavian Journal of Public Health*. 2005 Oct 1;33(5):353-9.

65. Amir LH. Medicines for breastfeeding women: risky business. Breastfeeding: Methods,Benefits to the Infant and Mother and Difficulties. *International Breastfeeding Journal*. 2010:129-41.

66. Rutter PM, Jones W. Enquiry analysis and user opinion of the Drugs in Breastmilk Helpline: a prospective study. *International breastfeeding journal*. 2012 May;7(1):6.

67. McDonald K, Amir LH, Davey MA. Maternal bodies and medicines: a commentary on risk and decision-making of pregnant and breastfeeding women and health professionals. *BMC public health*. 2011 Dec;11(5):S5.

68. Brown, A., Finch, G., Trickey, H., Hopkins, R. (2019) 'A lifeline when no one else wants to give you an answer: an evaluation of the Breastfeeding Network drugs in breastmilk service'. Breastfeeding Network: Scotland

69. Holtzman O, Usherwood T. Australian general practitioners' knowledge, attitudes and practices towards breastfeeding. *PloS one*. 2018 Feb 28;13(2):e0191854.

70. Biggs KV, Fidler KJ, Shenker NS, Brown H. Are the doctors of the future ready to support breastfeeding? A cross-sectional study in the UK. *International breastfeeding journal*. 2020 Dec;15:1-8.

71. Moukarzel S, Mamas C, Farhat A, Abi Abboud A, Daly AJ. A qualitative examination of barriers against effective medical education and practices related to breastfeeding promotion and support in Lebanon. *Medical education online*. 2020 Jan 1;25(1):1723950.

72. Viaro VD, Linhares FMP, Marinus MWLC, Guedes TG, Vanderley LSL. Limitsand possibilities for teaching and learning about breastfeeding. *Rev BrasEnferm*. 2019;72(1):3–8.

73. Chao SM, Goldfinger J, Gozalians SA, Sun SY, Thaker P. Evaluating the impact of provider breastfeeding encouragement timing: Evidence from a large population-based study. *Journal of Epidemiological Research*. 2016 Feb 16;2(2):p56.

74. Hannula L, Kaunonen M, Tarkka MT. A systematic review of professional support interventions for breastfeeding. Journal of clinical nursing. 2008 May 1;17(9):1132-43.

75. Hoddinott P, Pill R, Chalmers M. Health professionals, implementation and outcomes: reflections on a complex intervention to improve breastfeeding rates in primary care. *Family Practice*. 2007 Feb 1;24(1):84-91.

76. Sjarif DR, Yuliarti K, Wahyuni LK, Wiguna T, Prawitasari T, Devaera Y, et al. Effectiveness of a comprehensive integrated module using interactive lectures and workshops in understanding and knowledge retention about infant feeding practice in fifth year medical students: a quasi-experimental study. *BMC Med Educ*. 2016;16:210.

77. Sadovnikova A, Chuisano SA, Ma K, Grabowski A, Stanley KP, Mitchell KB, et al. Development and evaluation of a high-fidelity lactation simulation model for health professional breastfeeding education. *Int Breastfeed J*. 2020;15:8.

78. Becker GE, Quinlan G, Ward F, O'Sullivan EJ. Dietitians supporting breastfeeding: a survey of education, skills, knowledge and attitudes. *Irish Journal of Medical Science* (1971-). 2020 Sep 29:1-2.

79. National Nutrition Surveillance Centre (2010) Assessment of training needs of health care professionals who provide foetal, maternal and infant nutrition advice. National Nutrition Surveillance Centre as part of the HSE Framework for action on obesity, University College Dublin. www.ucd.ie/nnsc/t4media/Assessment%20of%20training%20needs%20of%20health%20care%20professionals%20who%20provide%20foetal,%20maternal%20and%20infant%20nutrition%20advice.pdf

80. Pugh LC, Milligan RA, Frick KD, Spatz D, Bronner Y. Breastfeeding duration, costs, and benefits of a support program for low-income breastfeeding women. *Birth*. 2002 Jun 1;29(2):95-100.

81. Labarere J, Gelbert-Baudino N, Ayral AS, Duc C, Berchotteau M, Bouchon N, Schelstraete C, Vittoz JP, Francois P, Pons JC. Efficacy of breastfeeding support provided by trained clinicians during an early, routine, preventive visit: a prospective, randomized, open trial of 226 mother-infant pairs. *Pediatrics*. 2005 Feb 1;115(2):e139-46.

82. Ingram J. Multiprofessional training for breastfeeding management in primary care in the UK. *International Breastfeeding Journal*. 2006 Apr 28;1(1):1.

83. Haase B, Brennan E, Wagner CL. Effectiveness of the IBCLC: Have we Made an Impact on the Care of Breastfeeding Families Over the Past Decade? *Journal of Human Lactation*. 2019 Aug;35(3):441-52.

84. Gray KD, Hannon EA, Erickson E, Stewart AB, Wood CT, Fisher K, Shaikh SK, Tanaka D. Influence of Early Lactation Assistance on Inpatient Exclusive Breastfeeding Rates. *Journal of Human Lactation*. 2020 Sep 14:0890334420957967.

85. Sanchez A, Farahi N, Flower K, Page C. Improved Breastfeeding Outcomes Following an On-site Support Intervention in an Academic Family Medicine Center. *Family medicine*. 2019;51(10):836-40.

86. Bunik M, Gao D, Moore L. An investigation of the field trip model as a method for teaching breastfeeding to pediatric residents. *Journal of Human Lactation.* 2006 May 1;22(2):195-202.

87. McKeever P, Stevens B, Miller KL, MacDonell JW, Gibbins S, Guerriere D, Dunn MS, Coyte PC. Home versus hospital breastfeeding support for newborns: a randomized controlled trial. *Birth.* 2002 Dec 1;29(4):258-65.

88. Fallon AB, Hegney D, O'Brien M, Brodribb W, Crepinsek M, Doolan J. An evaluation of a telephone-based postnatal support intervention for infant feeding in a regional Australian city. *Birth.* 2005 Dec 1;32(4):291-8.

89. Stevens B, Guerriere D, McKeever P, Croxford R, Miller KL, Watson-MacDonell J, Gibbins S, Dunn M, Ohlsson A, Ray K, Coyte P. Economics of home vs. hospital breastfeeding support for newborns. *Journal of advanced nursing.* 2006 Jan 1;53(2):233-43.

90. Lee YH, Chang GL, Chang HY. Effects of education and support groups organized by IBCLCs in early postpartum on breastfeeding. *Midwifery.* 2019 Aug 1;75:5-11.

91. Patel S, Patel S. The effectiveness of lactation consultants and lactation counselors on breastfeeding outcomes. *Journal of Human Lactation.* 2016 Aug;32(3):530-41.

Chapter 8: A lack of understanding of normal breastfed baby behaviour leads to people thinking something is wrong

1. Kent JC, Prime DK, Garbin CP. Principles for maintaining or increasing breastmilk production. *Journal of Obstetric, Gynecologic & Neonatal Nursing.* 2012 Jan 1;41(1):114-21.

2. Dewey KG, Lönnerdal B. Infant self-regulation of breastmilk intake. *Acta Paediatrica.* 1986 Nov 1;75(6):893-8.

3. Woolridge MW, Greasley V, Silpisornkosol S. The initiation of lactation: the effect of early versus delayed contact for suckling on milk intake in the first week post-partum. A study in Chiang Mai, Northern Thailand. *Early Human Development.* 1985 Dec 31;12(3):269-78.

4. Illingworth RS. Self-demand feeding. *BMJ.* 1952 Dec 20;2(4798):1355.

5. De Carvalho M, Klaus MH, Merkatz RB. Frequency of breast-feeding and serum bilirubin concentration. *American Journal of Diseases of Children.* 1982 Aug 1;136(8):737-8.

6. Hörnell A, Aarts C, Kylberg E, Hofvander Y, Gebre-Medhin M. Breastfeeding patterns in exclusively breastfed infants: a longitudinal prospective study in Uppsala, Sweden. *Acta Paediatrica.* 1999 Feb 1;88(2):203-11.

7. Tay CC, Glasier AF, McNeilly AS. Twenty-four hour patterns of prolactin secretion during lactation and the relationship to suckling and the resumption of fertility in breast-feeding women. *Human Reproduction.* 1996 May 1;11(5):950-5.

8. De Carvalho M, Klaus MH, Merkatz RB. Frequency of breast-feeding and serum bilirubin concentration. *American Journal of Diseases of Children.* 1982 Aug 1;136(8):737-8.)

9. Aarts C, Hörnell A, Kylberg E, Hofvander Y, Gebre-Medhin M. Breastfeeding patterns in relation to thumb sucking and pacifier use. *Pediatrics.* 1999 Oct 1;104(4):e50-.

10. Kent JC, Ashton E, Hardwick CM, Rowan MK, Chia ES, Fairclough KA, Menon LL, Scott C, Mather-McCaw G, Navarro K, Geddes DT. Nipple pain in breastfeeding mothers: incidence, causes and treatments. *International Journal of Environmental Research and Public Health.* 2015 Sep 29;12(10):12247-63.

11. Konner M, Worthman C. Nursing frequency, gonadal function, and birth spacing among !Kung hunter-gatherers. *Science.* 1980 Feb 15;207(4432):788-91.

12. Ghosh, R., Mascie-Taylor, C. N., & Rosetta, L. (2006). Longitudinal study of the frequency and duration of breastfeeding in rural Bangladeshi women. *American Journal of Human Biology: The Official Journal of the Human Biology Association, 18*(5), 630-638.

13. Zeitlin, M. F., & Ahmed, N. U. (1995). Nutritional correlates of frequency and length of breastfeeds in rural Bangladesh. *Early Human Development, 41*(2), 97-110

14. Hörnell A, Hofvander Y, Kylberg E. Solids and formula: association with pattern and

duration of breastfeeding. *Pediatrics.* 2001 Mar 1;107(3):e38.

15. Hörnell A, Aarts C, Kylberg E, Hofvander Y, Gebre-Medhin M. Breastfeeding patterns in exclusively breastfed infants: a longitudinal prospective study in Uppsala, Sweden. *Acta Paediatrica.* 1999 Feb 1;88(2):203-11.

16. Kent JC, Mitoulas LR, Cregan MD, Ramsay DT, Doherty DA, Hartmann PE. Volume and frequency of breastfeedings and fat content of breastmilk throughout the day. *Pediatrics.* 2006 Mar 1;117(3):e387-95.

17. Noonan M. Breastfeeding: Is my baby getting enough milk? *British Journal of Midwifery.* 2011 Feb;19(2):82-9.

18. Lozoff B, Brittenham G. Infant care: cache or carry. *The Journal of Pediatrics.* 1979 Sep 30;95(3):478-83.

19. Agras WS, Kraemer HC, Berkowitz RI, Korner AF, Hammer LD. Does a vigorous feeding style influence early development of adiposity? *The Journal of Pediatrics.* 1987 May 31;110(5):799-804.

20. Casiday RE, Wright CM, Panter-Brick C, Parkinson KN. Do early infant feeding patterns relate to breast-feeding continuation and weight gain? Data from a longitudinal cohort study. *European Journal of Clinical Nutrition.* 2004 Sep 1;58(9):1290-6.

21. Li R, Fein SB, Grummer-Strawn LM. Do infants fed from bottles lack self-regulation of milk intake compared with directly breastfed infants? *Pediatrics.* 2010 Jun 1;125(6):e1386-93.

22. Brown A, Lee M. Breastfeeding during the first year promotes satiety responsiveness in children aged 18–24 months. *Pediatric Obesity.* 2012 Oct 1;7(5):382-90.

23. Barr RG, Elias MF. Nursing interval and maternal responsivity: effect on early infant crying. Pediatrics. 1988 Apr 1;81(4):529-36.

24. Casiday RE, Wright CM, Panter-Brick C, Parkinson KN. Do early infant feeding patterns relate to breast-feeding continuation and weight gain? Data from a longitudinal cohort study. *European Journal of Clinical Nutrition.* 2004 Sep 1;58(9):1290-6.

25. Gartner LM, Morton J, Lawrence RA, Naylor AJ, O'Hare D, Schanler RJ, Eidelman AI. Breastfeeding and the use of human milk. *Pediatrics.* 2005 Feb;115(2):496-506.

26. Shealy KR, Scanlon KS, Labiner-Wolfe J, Fein SB, Grummer-Strawn LM. Characteristics of breastfeeding practices among US mothers. *Pediatrics.* 2008 Oct 1;122(Supplement 2):S50-5. Paul, Dittrichova & Papousek, 1996

27. Richards MP, Bernal JF. Social interaction in the first days of life. *The Origins of Human Relations,* Academic Press, New York. 1971:3-13.

28. Van Den Driessche M, Peeters K, Marien P, Ghoos Y, Devlieger H, Veereman-Wauters G. Gastric emptying in formula-fed and breast-fed infants measured with the 13C-octanoic acid breath test. *Journal of Pediatric Gastroenterology and Nutrition.* 1999 Jul;29(1):46-51.

29. Zangen S, Di Lorenzo C, Zangen T, Mertz H, Schwankovsky L, Hyman PE. Rapid maturation of gastric relaxation in newborn infants. *Pediatric Research.* 2001 Nov 1;50(5):629-32.

30. Sievers E, Oldigs HD, Santer RE, Schaub JU. Feeding patterns in breast-fed and formula-fed infants. Annals of Nutrition and Metabolism. 2002 Dec 11;46(6):243-8.

31. Dollberg S, Lahav S, Mimouni FB. A comparison of intakes of breast-fed and bottle-fed infants during the first two days of life. *Journal of the American College of Nutrition.* 2001 Jun 1;20(3):209-11.

32. Riordan J, Gill-Hopple K, Angeron J. Indicators of effective breastfeeding and estimates of breastmilk intake. *Journal of Human Lactation.* 2005 Nov 1;21(4):406-12.

33. Brown A, Raynor P, Lee M. Maternal control of child-feeding during breast and formula feeding in the first 6 months post-partum. *Journal of Human Nutrition and Dietetics.* 2011 Apr 1;24(2):177-86.

34. Fomon SJ, Owen GM, Thomas LN. Milk or formula volume ingested by infants fed ad libitum. *American Journal of Diseases of Children.* 1964 Dec 1;108(6):601-4.

35. Anders TF. Night-waking in infants during the first year of life. *Pediatrics.* 1979 Jun 1;63(6):860-4.

36. Price AM, Wake M, Ukoumunne OC, Hiscock H. Outcomes at six years of age for

children with infant sleep problems: longitudinal community-based study. *Sleep Medicine*. 2012 Sep 30;13(8):991-8.

37. Barry H, Paxson, LM. Infancy and early childhood: cross-cultural codes 2, *Ethnology*. 1971 10: 466-508

38. Morelli GA, Rogoff B, Oppenheim D, Goldsmith D. Cultural variations in infants' sleeping arrangements: questions of independence, *Developmental Psychology*. 1992 28(4): 604 -613

39. Blair PS, Fleming PJ, Smith IJ, Ward Platt M. Young J, Nadin P, Berry P J, Golding J, CESDI SUDI Research Group. Babies sleeping with parents: case-control study of factors influencing the risk of the sudden infant death syndrome. *BMJ*, 1999 319: 1457 -1461

40. Hoppenbrouwers T, Jensen D, Hodgman J, Harper R, Sterman M. Body movements during quiet sleep (QS) in subsequent siblings of SIDS. *Clinical Research* 1982 Jan 1 Vol. 30, No. 1, 136-136

41. Keefe MR. Comparison of neonatal nighttime sleep-wake patterns in nursery versus rooming-in environments. *Nursing research*. 1987 May 1;36(3):140-4.

42. Lozoff B, Brittenham G. Infant care: cache or carry? *Journal of Pediatrics*, 1979 95(3): 478-483

43. Liamputtong Rice P, Naksook C. Child rearing and cultural beliefs and practices amongst Thai mothers in Victoria, Australia: implications for the sudden infant death syndrome. *Journal of Paediatric Child Health*, 1998 34: 320-324.

44. Abbott S. Holding on and pushing away, Ethos, 1992 20: 33-65

45. Blair PS, Ball HL, McKenna JJ, Feldman-Winter L, Marinelli KA, Bartick MC, Academy of Breastfeeding Medicine. Bedsharing and Breastfeeding: The Academy of Breastfeeding Medicine Protocol# 6, Revision 2019. *Breastfeeding Medicine*. 2020 Jan 1;15(1):5-16.

46. www.nice.org.uk/guidance/cg37/evidence/full-guideline-addendum-485782238

47. Smith LA, Geller NL, Kellams AL, Colson ER, Rybin DV, Heeren T, Corwin MJ. Infant sleep location and breastfeeding practices in the United States, 2011–2014. *Academic Pediatrics*. 2016 Feb 4.

48. Carpenter RG, Irgens LM, Blair PS, England PD, Fleming P, Huber J, Jorch G, Schreuder P. Sudden unexplained infant death in 20 regions in Europe: case control study. *The Lancet*. 2004 Jan 17;363(9404):185-91.

49. Drago DA, Dannenberg AL. Infant mechanical suffocation deaths in the United States, 1980–1997. *Pediatrics*. 1999 May 1;103(5):e59.

50. Richard C, Mosko S, McKenna J, Drummond S. Sleeping position, orientation, and proximity in bedsharing infants and mothers. *Sleep*. 1996 Nov;19(9):685-90.

51. McKenna JJ, Mosko SS. Sleep and arousal, synchrony and independence, among mothers and infants sleeping apart and together (same bed): an experiment in evolutionary medicine. *Acta Paediatrica*. 1994 Jun 1;83(s397):94-102.

52. Lee NN, Chan YF, Davies DP, Lau E, Yip DC. Sudden infant death syndrome in Hong Kong: confirmation of low incidence. *BMJ*. 1989 Mar 18;298(6675):721.

53. Balarajan R, Raleigh VS, Botting B. Sudden infant death syndrome and postneonatal mortality in immigrants in England and Wales. *BMJ*. 1989 Mar 18;298(6675):716-20.

54. Grether JK, Schulman J, Croen LA. Sudden infant death syndrome among Asians in California. *The Journal of Pediatrics*. 1990 Apr 30;116(4):525-8.

55. Tuffnell CS, Petersen SA, Wailoo MP. Higher rectal temperatures in co-sleeping infants. *Archives of Disease in Childhood*. 1996 Sep 1;75(3):249-50.

56. Reite M, Short RA. Nocturnal sleep in separated monkey infants. *Archives of General Psychiatry*. 1978 Oct 1;35(10):1247-53.

57. Coe CL, Levine S. Normal responses to mother-infant separation in non-human primates. In Anxiety: New research and changing concepts 1981 (pp. 155-177). Raven Press New York.

58. Horne JA. A review of the biological effects of total sleep deprivation in man. *Biological Psychology*. 1978 Sep 30;7(1):55-102.

59. Richard CA, Mosko SS. Mother-infant bedsharing is associated with an increase in infant heart rate. *Sleep* 2004 May 1;27(3):507-11.

60. Richard CA, Mosko SS, McKenna JJ. Apnea and periodic breathing in bed-sharing and

solitary sleeping infants. *Journal of Applied Physiology*. 1998 Apr 1;84(4):1374-80.
61. Mosko S, Richard C, McKenna J, Drummond S, Mukai D. Maternal proximity and infant CO 2 environment during bedsharing and possible implications for SIDS research. *American Journal of Physical Anthropology*. 1997 Jul 1;103(3):315-28.
62. Tollenaar MS, Beijers R, Jansen J, Riksen-Walraven JM, de Weerth C. Solitary sleeping in young infants is associated with heightened cortisol reactivity to a bathing session but not to a vaccination. *Psychoneuroendocrinology*. 2012 Feb 29;37(2):167-77.
63. Lewis RJ, Janda LH. The relationship between adult sexual adjustment and childhood experiences regarding exposure to nudity, sleeping in the parental bed, and parental attitudes toward sexuality. *Archives of Sexual Behavior*. 1988 Aug 1;17(4):349-62.
64. Keller MA, Goldberg WA. Co-sleeping: Help or hindrance for young children's independence? *Infant and Child Development*. 2004 Dec 1;13(5):369-88.
65. Ball HL. Breastfeeding, bed-sharing, and infant sleep. *Birth*. 2003 Sep 1;30(3):181-8.
66. Butte NF, Jensen CL, Moon JK, Glaze DG, Frost Jr JD. Sleep organization and energy expenditure of breast-fed and formula-fed infants. *Pediatric Research*. 1992 Nov 1;32(5):514-9.
67. Doan T, Gay CL, Kennedy HP, Newman J, Lee KA. Nighttime breastfeeding behavior is associated with more nocturnal sleep among first-time mothers at one month postpartum. *Journal of Clinical Sleep Medicine*. 2014 Mar 15;10(3):313-9.
68. Galbally M, Lewis AJ, McEgan K, Scalzo K, Islam FM. Breastfeeding and infant sleep patterns: an Australian population study. *Journal of Paediatrics and Child Health*. 2013 Feb 1;49(2):E147-52.
69. Brown A, Harries V. Infant sleep and night feeding patterns during later infancy: Association with breastfeeding frequency, daytime complementary food intake, and infant weight. *Breastfeeding Medicine*. 2015 Jun 1;10(5):246-52.
70. Moore T, Ucko LE. Night waking in early infancy: Part I. *Archives of Disease in Childhood*. 1957 Aug;32(164):333.
71. Rudzik, A. E., Robinson-Smith, L., & Ball, H. L. (2018). Discrepancies in maternal reports of infant sleep vs. actigraphy by mode of feeding. *Sleep medicine*, *49*, 90-98.
72. Sellen DW. Comparison of infant feeding patterns reported for nonindustrial populations with current recommendations. *The Journal of Nutrition*. 2001 Oct 1;131(10):2707-15.
73. Brown KH, Black RE, Robertson AD, Akhtar NA, Ahmed G, Becker S. Clinical and field studies of human lactation: methodological considerations. *The American Journal of Clinical Nutrition*. 1982 Apr 1;35(4):745-56.
74. Imong SM, Jackson DA, Wongsawasdii L, Ruckphaophunt S, Tansuhaj A, Chiowanich P, Woolridge MW, Drewett RF, Baum JD, Amatayakul K. Predictors of breastmilk intake in rural northern Thailand. *Journal of Pediatric Gastroenterology and Nutrition*. 1989 Apr 1;8(3):359-70.
75. McKenna JJ, Gettler LT. There is no such thing as infant sleep, there is no such thing as breastfeeding, there is only breastsleeping. *Acta Paediatrica*. 2016 Jan 1;105(1):17-21.
76. Matheny RJ, Picciano MF. Assessment of abbreviated techniques for determination of milk volume intake of the human milk-fed infant. *Journal of Pediatric Gastroenterology and Nutrition*. 1985 Oct 1;4(5):808-12.
77. Hörnell A, Aarts C, Kylberg E, Hofvander Y, Gebre-Medhin M. Breastfeeding patterns in exclusively breastfed infants: a longitudinal prospective study in Uppsala, Sweden. *Acta Paediatrica*. 1999 Feb 1;88(2):203-11.
78. Konner M, Worthman C. Nursing frequency, gonadal function, and birth spacing among !Kung hunter-gatherers. *Science*. 1980 Feb 15;207(4432):788-91.
79. Blair PS, Ball HL. The prevalence and characteristics associated with parent–infant bed-sharing in England. *Archives of Disease in Childhood*. 2004 Dec 1;89(12):1106-10.
80. McKenna JJ, Mosko SS, Richard CA. Bedsharing promotes breastfeeding. *Pediatrics*. 1997 Aug 1;100(2):214-9.
81. Ball HL, Ward-Platt MP, Heslop E, Leech SJ, Brown KA. Randomised trial of infant sleep location on the postnatal ward. *Archives of Disease in Childhood*. 2006 Dec 1;91(12):1005-10.
82. Quillin SI, Glenn LL. Interaction between feeding method and co-sleeping on maternal-newborn sleep. *Journal of Obstetric, Gynecologic & Neonatal Nursing*. 2004

Sep 1;33(5):580-8.
83. Yamouchi Y, Yamnouchi I. The relationship between rooming-in/not rooming-in and breast-feeding variables. *Acta Pædiatrica.* 1990 Nov 1;79(11):1017-22.
84. McKenna JJ, McDade T. Why babies should never sleep alone: a review of the co-sleeping controversy in relation to SIDS, bedsharing and breast feeding. *Paediatric Respiratory Reviews.* 2005 Jun 30;6(2):134-52.
85. Morelli GA, Rogoff B, Oppenheim D, Goldsmith D. Cultural variation in infants' sleeping arrangements: Questions of independence. *Developmental Psychology.* 1992 Jul;28(4):604.
86. Hall WA, Saunders RA, Clauson M, Carty EM, Janssen PA. Effects of an intervention aimed at reducing night waking and signaling in 6- to 12-month-old infants. *Behavioral Sleep Medicine.* 2006 Nov 1;4(4):242-61.

Chapter 9: Our obsession with big babies and rapid weight gain leads to unnecessary supplementation

1. Stettler N, Stallings VA, Troxel AB, Zhao J, Schinnar R, Nelson SE, Ziegler EE, Strom BL. Weight gain in the first week of life and overweight in adulthood a cohort study of European American subjects fed infant formula. *Circulation.* 2005 Apr 19;111(15):1897-903.
2. Kools EJ, Thijs C, Kester AD, de Vries H. The motivational determinants of breast-feeding: predictors for the continuation of breast-feeding. *Preventive Medicine.* 2006 Nov 30;43(5):394-401.
3. Flaherman VJ, Beiler JS, Cabana MD, Paul IM. Relationship of newborn weight loss to milk supply concern and anxiety: the impact on breastfeeding duration. *Maternal & Child Nutrition.* 2015 Apr 1.
4. Sachs M, Dykes F, Carter B. Feeding by numbers: an ethnographic study of how breastfeeding women understand their babies' weight charts. *International Breastfeeding Journal.* 2006 Dec 22;1(1):1.
5. Wright CM. Who comes to be weighed: an exception to the inverse care law. *The Lancet.* 1997 Aug 30;350(9078):642.
6. Sharpe H, Loewenthal D. Reasons for attending GP or health authority clinics. *Health Visitor.* 1992 Oct;65(10):349-51.
7. Hamlyn B. Infant feeding 2000: A survey conducted on behalf of the Department of Health, the Scottish Executive, the National Assembly for Wales and the Department of Health, Social Services and Public Safety in Northern Ireland. TSO; 2002.
8. Sanderson D, Wright D, Acton C, Duree D. Cost analysis of child health surveillance. National Co-ordinating Centre for HTA. Great Britain; 2001.
9. De Onis M, Garza C, Victora CG, Onyango AW, Frongillo EA, Martines J. The WHO Multicentre Growth Reference Study: planning, study design, and methodology. *Food and Nutrition Bulletin.* 2004 Mar 1;25(1 suppl1):S15-26.
10. Bertini G, Breschi R, Dani C. Physiological weight loss chart helps to identify high-risk infants who need breastfeeding support. *Acta Paediatrica.* 2015 Oct 1;104(10):1024-7.
11. Wright CM, Parkinson KN. Postnatal weight loss in term infants: what is "normal" and do growth charts allow for it? *Archives of Disease in Childhood-Fetal and Neonatal Edition.* 2004 May 1;89(3):F254-7.
12. Macdonald PD, Ross SR, Grant L, Young D. Neonatal weight loss in breast and formula fed infants. *Archives of Disease in Childhood-Fetal and Neonatal Edition.* 2003 Nov 1;88(6):F472-6.
13. Yamauchi Y, Yamanouchi I. Breast-feeding frequency during the first 24 hours after birth in full-term neonates. *Pediatrics.* 1990 Aug 1;86(2):171-5.
14. Noel-Weiss J, Woodend AK, Peterson WE, Gibb W, Groll DL. An observational study of associations among maternal fluids during parturition, neonatal output, and breastfed newborn weight loss. *International Breastfeeding Journal.* 2011 Aug 15;6(1):1
15. Dahlenburg GW, Burnell RH, Braybrook R. The relation between cord serum sodium levels in newborn infants and maternal intravenous therapy during labour. BJOG: An *International Journal of Obstetrics & Gynaecology.* 1980 Jun 1;87(6):519-22.
16. Chantry CJ, Nommsen-Rivers LA, Peerson JM, Cohen RJ, Dewey KG. Excess weight

loss in first-born breastfed newborns relates to maternal intrapartum fluid balance. *Pediatrics*. 2010 Dec 10:peds-2009.

17. Manganaro R, Mamì C, Marrone T, Marseglia L, Gemelli M. Incidence of dehydration and hypernatremia in exclusively breast-fed infants. *The Journal of Pediatrics*. 2001 Nov 30;139(5):673-5.

18. Bystrova K, Matthiesen AS, Widström AM, Ransjö-Arvidson AB, Welles-Nyström B, Vorontsov I, Uvnäs-Moberg K. The effect of Russian maternity home routines on breastfeeding and neonatal weight loss with special reference to swaddling. *Early Human Development*. 2007 Jan 31;83(1):29-39.

19. Martens PJ. Increasing breastfeeding initiation and duration at a community level: an evaluation of Sagkeeng First Nation's community health nurse and peer counselor programs. *Journal of Human Lactation*. 2002 Aug 1;18(3):236-46.

20. Davanzo R, Cannioto Z, Ronfani L, Monasta L, Demarini S. Breastfeeding and neonatal weight loss in healthy term infants. *Journal of Human Lactation*. 2013 Feb 1;29(1):45-53.

21. Lamp JM, Macke JK. Relationships among intrapartum maternal fluid intake, birth type, neonatal output, and neonatal weight loss during the first 48 hours after birth. *Journal of Obstetric, Gynecologic, & Neonatal Nursing*. 2010 Mar 1;39(2):169-77.

22. Noel-Weiss J, Courant G, Woodend AK. Physiological weight loss in the breastfed neonate: a systematic review. *Open Medicine*. 2008 Oct 27;2(4):99-110.

23. Flaherman VJ, Schaefer EW, Kuzniewicz MW, Li SX, Walsh EM, Paul IM. Early weight loss nomograms for exclusively breastfed newborns. *Pediatrics*. 2015 Jan 1;135(1):e16-23.

24. Laing IA. Hypernatremic dehydration in newborn infants. *Acta Pharmacol Sin*. 2002;23(suppl):48-51.

25. Oddie S, Richmond S, Coulthard M. Hypernatraemic dehydration and breast feeding: a population study. *Archives of Disease in Childhood*. 2001 Oct 1;85(4):318-20.

26. Livingstone VH, Willis CE, Abdel-Wareth LO, Thiessen P, Lockitch G. Neonatal hypernatremic dehydration associated with breast-feeding malnutrition: a retrospective survey. *Canadian Medical Association Journal*. 2000 Mar 7;162(5):647-52.

27. Dewey KG, Nommsen-Rivers LA, Heinig MJ, Cohen RJ. Risk factors for suboptimal infant breastfeeding behavior, delayed onset of lactation, and excess neonatal weight loss. *Pediatrics*. 2003 Sep 1;112(3):607-19.

28. Chapman DJ, Perez-Escamilla R. Identification of risk factors for delayed onset of lactation. *Journal of the American Dietetic Association*. 1999 Apr 30;99(4):450-4.

29. Dewey KG, Nommsen-Rivers LA, Heinig MJ, Cohen RJ. Lactogenesis and infant weight change in the first weeks of life. In *Integrating Population Outcomes, Biological Mechanisms and Research Methods in the Study of Human Milk and Lactation* 2002 (pp. 159-166). Springer US.

30. Manganaro R, Mamì C, Marrone T, Marseglia L, Gemelli M. Incidence of dehydration and hypernatremia in exclusively breast-fed infants. *J Pediatr*. 2001;139(5):673-675.

31. Oddie SJ, Craven V, Deakin K, Westman J, Scally A. Severe neonatal hypernatraemia: a population based study. *Arch Dis Child Fetal Neonatal Ed*. 2013;98(5):F384-F387.

32. Pelleboer RA, Bontemps ST, Verkerk PH, Van Dommelen P, Pereira RR, Van Wouwe JP. A nationwide study on hospital admissions due to dehydration in exclusively breastfed infants in the Netherlands: its incidence, clinical characteristics, treatment and outcome. *Acta Paediatr*. 2009;98(5):807-811.

33. Moritz ML, Manole MD, Bogen DL, Ayus JC. Breastfeeding-associated hypernatremia: are we missing the diagnosis? *Pediatrics*. 2005 Sep 1;116(3):e343-7.

34. www.nice.org.uk/guidance/ng75

35. Rebhan B, Kohlhuber M, Schwegler U, Fromme H, Abou-Dakn M, Koletzko BV. Breastfeeding duration and exclusivity associated with infants' health and growth: data from a prospective cohort study in Bavaria, Germany. *Acta Paediatrica*. 2009 Jun 1;98(6):974-80.

36. Kramer MS. Exclusive bottle feeding of either formula or breastmilk is associated with greater infant weight gain than exclusive breastfeeding, but findings may not reflect a causal effect of bottle feeding. *Evidence Based Medicine*. 2012 Sep 21:ebmed-2012.

37. Durmuş B, van Rossem L, Duijts L, Arends LR, Raat H, Moll HA, Hofman A, Steegers

EA, Jaddoe VW. Breast-feeding and growth in children until the age of 3 years: the Generation R Study. *British Journal of Nutrition.* 2011 Jun 14;105(11):1704-11.

38. Mihrshahi S, Battistutta D, Magarey A, Daniels LA. Determinants of rapid weight gain during infancy: baseline results from the NOURISH randomised controlled trial. *BMC Pediatrics.* 2011 Nov 7;11(1):1.

39. Griffiths LJ, Smeeth L, Hawkins SS, Cole TJ, Dezateux C. Effects of infant feeding practice on weight gain from birth to 3 years. *Archives of Disease in Childhood.* 2009 Aug 1;94(8):577-82.

40. Johnson L, van Jaarsveld CH, Llewellyn CH, Cole TJ, Wardle J. Associations between infant feeding and the size, tempo and velocity of infant weight gain: SITAR analysis of the Gemini twin birth cohort. *International Journal of Obesity.* 2014 Jul 1;38(7):980-7.

41. Li R, Magadia J, Fein SB, Grummer-Strawn LM. Risk of bottle-feeding for rapid weight gain during the first year of life. *Archives of Pediatrics & Adolescent medicine.* 2012 May 1;166(5):431-6.

Chapter 10: Our obsession with routines and good babies causes unnecessary problems

1. Szyf M, Weaver IC, Champagne FA, Diorio J, Meaney MJ. Maternal programming of steroid receptor expression and phenotype through DNA methylation in the rat. *Frontiers in Neuroendocrinology.* 2005 Dec 31;26(3):139-62.

2. Haley DW, Stansbury K. Infant stress and parent responsiveness: regulation of physiology and behavior during still-face and reunion. *Child Development.* 2003 Oct 1;74(5):1534 46.

3. Loman MM, Gunnar MR. Early experience and the development of stress reactivity and regulation in children. *Neuroscience & Biobehavioral Reviews.* 2010 May 31;34(6):867-76.

4. Spock, Benjamin. *The Common Sense Book of Baby and Child Care.* New York: Duell, Sloan, and Pearce, 1946

5. Hall T. *Save Our Sleep: Helping your baby to sleep through the night, from birth to two years.* Vermillon.

6. Ford G. *The New Contented Little Baby Book: The Secret to Calm and Confident Parenting.* Vermillon.

7. Weissbluth, M. Sleep duration and infant temperament. *Brief Clinical and Laboratory Observations,* 99, 817 – 818

8. Morelli GA, Rogoff B, Oppenheim D, Goldsmith D. Cultural variation in infants' sleeping arrangements: Questions of independence. *Developmental Psychology.* 1992 Jul;28(4):604.

9. Gaertner BM, Spinrad TL, Eisenberg N. Focused attention in toddlers: Measurement, stability, and relations to negative emotion and parenting. *Infant and Child Development.* 2008 Aug 1;17(4):339-63.

10. Evans CA, Porter CL. The emergence of mother–infant co-regulation during the first year: Links to infants' developmental status and attachment. *Infant Behavior and Development.* 2009 Apr 30;32(2):147-58.

11. Engert V, Efanov SI, Dedovic K, Dagher A, Pruessner JC. Increased cortisol awakening response and afternoon/evening cortisol output in healthy young adults with low early life parental care. *Psychopharmacology.* 2011 Mar 1;214(1):261-8.

12. Schore AN. Effects of a secure attachment relationship on right brain development, affect regulation, and infant mental health. *Infant Mental Health Journal.* 2001 Jan 1;22(1-2):7-66.

13. Cheng CY, Li Q. Integrative review of research on general health status and prevalence of common physical health conditions of women after childbirth. *Women's Health Issues.* 2008 Aug 31;18(4):267-80.

14. Kurth E, Spichiger E, Cignacco E, Kennedy H, Glanzmann R, Schmid M, Staehlin K, Schindler C, Stutz E. (2010). Predictors of crying problems in the early postpartum period. *Journal of Obstetric Gynecologic and Neonatal Nursing,* 39(3), 250–262.

15. Chan S, Levy V. Postnatal depression: A qualitative study of the experiences of a group of Hong Kong Chinese women. *Journal of Clinical Nursing.* 2004 13, 120–123.

16. Brockington IF, Oates J, George S, Turner D, Vostanis P, Sullivan M, Loh C, Murdoch

C. (2001). A screening questionnaire for mother–infant bonding disorders. *Archives of Women's Mental Health*, 3, 133–140.

17. Beck CT. Maternal depression and child behaviour problems: a meta-analysis. *Journal of Advanced Nursing*. 1999 Mar 1;29(3):623-9.

18. Hiscock H, Bayer J, Gold L, Hampton A, Ukoumunne OC, Wake M. Improving infant sleep and maternal mental health: a cluster randomised trial. *Archives of disease in childhood*. 2007 Nov 1;92(11):952-8.

19. Harries V, Brown A. The association between use of infant parenting books that promote strict routines, and maternal depression, self-efficacy, and parenting confidence. *Early Child Development and Care*. 2019 Jul 3;189(8):1339-50.

20. Arnott B, Brown A. An exploration of parenting behaviours and attitudes during early infancy: Association with maternal and infant characteristics. *Infant and Child Development*. 2013 Jul;22(4):349-61.

21. Brown A, Arnott B. Breastfeeding duration and early parenting behaviour: the importance of an infant-led, responsive style. *PloS one*. 2014 Feb 12;9(2):e83893.

22. Harries, V., & Brown, A. (2019). The association between baby care books that promote strict care routines and infant feeding, night-time care, and maternal–infant interactions. *Maternal & Child Nutrition*, 15(4), e12858.

Chapter 11: Our lack of value for new mothers makes everything feel more difficult

1. Kitzinger S. *Ourselves as mothers*. Bantam books; 1992.

2. Brown S, ed. *Missing voices: The experience of motherhood*. Oxford University Press, USA; 1994.

3. Oakley A. *Social support and motherhood: the natural history of a research project*. Blackwell Publishers; 1992 Dec 1.

4. Maushart S. *The mask of motherhood: How becoming a mother changes our lives and why we never talk about it*.

5. Rossiter JC. Promoting breastfeeding: the perceptions of Vietnamese mothers in Sydney, Australia. *Journal of Advanced Nursing*. 1998 Sep 1;28(3):598-605.

6. Bergum V. The phenomenology from woman to mother. Unpublished doctoral dissertation. Alberta: University of Alberta. 1986.

7. Nelson AM. Transition to motherhood. Journal of Obstetric, Gynecologic, & Neonatal Nursing. 2003 Jul 1;32(4):465-77.

8. Cowan CP, Cowan PA. *When partners become parents: The big life change for couples*. Lawrence Erlbaum Associates Publishers; 2000.

9. Deutsch FM, Ruble DN, Fleming A, Brooks-Gunn J, Stangor C. Information-seeking and maternal self-definition during the transition to motherhood. *Journal of Personality and Social Psychology*. 1988 Sep;55(3):420

10. Rubin R. Body image and self-esteem. *Nursing Outlook*. 1968 Jun;16(6):20.

11. Mercer RT. A theoretical framework for studying factors that impact on the maternal role. *Nursing Research*. 1981 Mar 1;30(2):73-7.

12. Mercer RT. *First-time motherhood: Experiences from teens to forties*. New York: Springer Publishing Company; 1986.

13. SM, Hudson DB, Bouffard C. Marital and parenting satisfaction and infant care self-efficacy during the transition to parenthood: The effect of infant sex. *Issues in Comprehensive Pediatric Nursing*. 2003 Jan 1;26(1):45-57

14. Salmela-Aro K, Nurmi JE, Saisto T, Halmesmäki E. Goal reconstruction and depressive symptoms during the transition to motherhood: evidence from two cross-lagged longitudinal studies. *Journal of Personality and Social Psychology*. 2001 Dec;81(6):1144.

15. Nelson AM. Transition to motherhood. *Journal of Obstetric, Gynecologic, & Neonatal Nursing*. 2003 Jul 1;32(4):465-77.

16. Connelly CD, Straus MA. Mother's age and risk for physical abuse. *Child Abuse & Neglect*. 1992 Oct 31;16(5):709-18.

17. Dew J, Wilcox WB. If momma ain't happy: Explaining declines in marital satisfaction among new mothers. *Journal of Marriage and Family*. 2011 Feb;73(1):1-2.

18. Lee E, Furedi F. Mothers' experience of, and attitudes to, using infant formula in the

early months. School of Social Policy, Sociology and Social Research, University of Kent, UK. Retrieved December. 2005;8:2011

19. Smith JP, Forrester R. Who pays for the health benefits of exclusive breastfeeding? An analysis of maternal time costs. *Journal of Human Lactation.* 2013 Jul 17:0890334413495450.

20. Brown A, Rance J, Bennett P. Understanding the relationship between breastfeeding and postnatal depression: the role of pain and physical difficulties. *Journal of Advanced Nursing.* 2016 Feb 1;72(2):273-82.

21. O'Hara MW. Postpartum depression: what we know. *Journal of Clinical Psychology.* 2009 Dec 12;65(12):1258-69.

22. Gonidakis F, Rabavilas AD, Varsou E, Kreatsas G, Christodoulou GN. A 6-month study of postpartum depression and related factors in Athens Greece. *Comprehensive Psychiatry.* 2008 Jun 30;49(3):275-82.

23. Shakespeare J, Blake F, Garcia J. Breast-feeding difficulties experienced by women taking part in a qualitative interview study of postnatal depression. *Midwifery.* 2004 Sep 30;20(3):251-60.

24. Bigelow A, Power M, MacLellan-Peters J, Alex M, McDonald C. Effect of mother/infant skin-to-skin contact on postpartum depressive symptoms and maternal physiological stress. *Journal of Obstetric, Gynecologic, & Neonatal Nursing.* 2012 May 1;41(3):369-82.

25. Hart SL, Jackson SC, Boylan LM. Compromised weight gain, milk intake, and feeding behavior in breastfed newborns of depressive mothers. *Journal of Pediatric Psychology.* 2011 Sep 1;36(8):942 50.

26. Jones NA, McFall BA, Diego MA. Patterns of brain electrical activity in infants of depressed mothers who breastfeed and bottle feed: The mediating role of infant temperament. *Biological Psychology.* 2004 Oct 31;67(1):103-24.

27. Kroenke K, Wu J, Bair MJ, Krebs EE, Damush TM, Tu W. Reciprocal relationship between pain and depression: a 12-month longitudinal analysis in primary care. *The Journal of Pain.* 2011 Sep 30;12(9):964-73.

28. Watkins S, Meltzer-Brody S, Zolnoun D, Stuebe A. Early breastfeeding experiences and postpartum depression. *Obstetrics & Gynecology.* 2011 Aug 1;118(2, Part 1):214 21.

29. Maes M, Lin AH, Ombelet W, Stevens K, Kenis G, De Jongh R, Cox J, Bosmans E. Immune activation in the early puerperium is related to postpartum anxiety and depressive symptoms. *Psychoneuroendocrinology.* 2000 Feb 29;25(2):121-37.

30. Kendall-Tackett K. A new paradigm for depression in new mothers: the central role of inflammation and how breastfeeding and anti-inflammatory treatments protect maternal mental health. International Breastfeeding Journal. 2007 Mar 30;2(1):1.

31. Lau C. Effects of stress on lactation. *Pediatric Clinics of North America.* 2001 Feb 1;48(1):221-34.

32. Newton M, Newton NR. The let-down reflex in human lactation. *The Journal of pediatrics.* 1948 Dec 31;33(6):698-704.

33. Ueda T, Yokoyama Y, Irahara M, Aono T. Influence of psychological stress on suckling-induced pulsatile oxytocin release. *Obstetrics & Gynecology.* 1994 Aug 1;84(2):259-62.

34. Feher SD, Berger LR, Johnson JD, Wilde JB. Increasing breastmilk production for premature infants with a relaxation/imagery audiotape. *Pediatrics.* 1989 Jan 1;83(1):57-60

35. Dias CC, Figueiredo B. Breastfeeding and depression: A systematic review of the literature. *Journal of Affective Disorders.* 2015 Jan 15;171:142-54.

36. Kendall-Tackett K. Childbirth-related posttraumatic stress disorder: Symptoms and impact on breastfeeding. *Clinical Lactation.* 2014 May 1;5(2):51-5.

37. Fenwick J, Gamble J, Creedy D, Barclay L, Buist A, Ryding EL. Women's perceptions of emotional support following childbirth: A qualitative investigation. *Midwifery.* 2013 Mar 31;29(3):217-24.

38. Dennis CL, McQueen K. The relationship between infant-feeding outcomes and postpartum depression: a qualitative systematic review. *Pediatrics.* 2009 Apr 1;123(4):e736-51.

39. Dorheim SK, Bondevik GT, Eberhard-Gran M, Bjorvatn B. Sleep and depression in postpartum women: a population-based study. *Sleep.* 2009 Jul 1;32(7):847-55.

Chapter 12: Pressure on women to doubt their body or get their 'pre baby body' back

1. Godart NT, Flament MF, Perdereau F, Jeammet P. Comorbidity between eating disorders and anxiety disorders: a review. *International Journal of Eating Disorders.* 2002 Nov;32(3):253-70.
2. McAndrew F, Thompson J, Fellows L, Large A, Speed M, Renfrew, MJ. *Infant feeding survey 2010.* Leeds: Health and Social Care Information Centre. 2012.
3. Brouwer MA, Drummond C, Willis E. Using Goffman's theories of social interaction to reflect first-time mothers' experiences with the social norms of infant feeding. *Qualitative health research.* 2012 Oct 1;22(10):1345-54.
4. Soltanian HT, Liu MT, Cash AD, Iglesias RA. Determinants of breast appearance and aging in identical twins. *Aesthetic Surgery Journal.* 2012 Sep 1;32(7):846-60.
5. Brown A. Maternal restraint and external eating behaviour are associated with formula use or shorter breastfeeding duration. *Appetite.* 2014 76, 30-35.
6. Durham HA, Lovelady CA, Brouwer RJ, Krause KM, Østbye T. (2011). Comparison of dietary intake of overweight postpartum mothers practicing breastfeeding or formula feeding. *Journal of the American Dietetic Association,* 111(1), 67-74.
7. Lovelady CA, Garner KE, Moreno KL, Williams JP. The effect of weight loss in overweight, lactating women on the growth of their infants. *New England Journal of Medicine.* 2000 342(7), 449-453.
8. AAP. Breastfeeding and the use of human milk. *Pediatrics.* 2012 129, 827 – 841.
9. Baker JL, Gamborg M, Heitmann BL, Lissner L, Sørensen TI, Rasmussen, KM. (2008). Breastfeeding reduces postpartum weight retention. *The American Journal of Clinical Nutrition,* 88(6), 1543-1551.
10. Daly SE, Hartmann PE. Infant demand and milk supply. Part 2: The short-term control of milk synthesis in lactating women. *Journal of Human Lactation.* 1995 11(1), 27-37.
11. Micali N, Simonoff E, Stahl D, Treasure J. (2011). Maternal eating disorders and infant feeding difficulties: maternal and child mediators in a longitudinal general population study. *Journal of Child Psychology and Psychiatry,* 52(7), 800-807.
12. Krešić G, Dujmović M, Mandić ML, Delaš I. Relationship between Mediterranean diet and breastmilk fatty acid profile: a study in breastfeeding women in Croatia. *Dairy Science & Technology.* 2013 May 1;93(3):287-301.
13. Xiang M, Harbige LS, Zetterström R. Long-chain polyunsaturated fatty acids in Chinese and Swedish mothers: diet, breastmilk and infant growth. *Acta Paediatrica.* 2005 Nov;94(11):1543-9.
14. Setterquist H. Fish Oil Supplementation during Pregnancy and Lactation. *Nutrition.* 2020 Jul 23.
15. Quin C, Vollman DM, Ghosh S, Haskey N, Estaki M, Pither J, Barnett JA, Jay MN, Birnie BW, Gibson DL. Fish oil supplementation reduces maternal defensive inflammation and predicts a gut bacteriome with reduced immune priming capacity in infants. *The ISME Journal.* 2020 May 12:1-5.
16. Berger PK, Plows JF, Jones RB, Alderete TL, Rios C, Pickering TA, Fields DA, Bode L, Peterson BS, Goran MI. Associations of maternal fructose and sugar-sweetened beverage and juice intake during lactation with infant neurodevelopmental outcomes at 24 months. *The American Journal of Clinical Nutrition.* 2020 Oct 6.
17. well.blogs.nytimes.com/2015/08/09/coca-cola-funds-scientists-who-shift-blame-for-obesity-away-from-bad-diets/
18. Garcia AL, McLean K, Wright CM. Types of fruits and vegetables used in commercial baby foods and their contribution to sugar content. *Maternal & Child Nutrition.* 2016 Oct;12(4):838-47.
19. Marangoni F, Cetin I, Verduci E, Canzone G, Giovannini M, Scollo P, Corsello G, Poli A. Maternal diet and nutrient requirements in pregnancy and breastfeeding. An Italian consensus document. *Nutrients.* 2016 Oct;8(10):629.
20. Fields DA, George B, Williams M, Whitaker K, Allison DB, Teague A, Demerath EW. Associations between human breastmilk hormones and adipocytokines and infant growth and body composition in the first 6 months of life. *Pediatric obesity.* 2017 Aug;12:78-85.

21. Babakobi MD, Reshef L, Gihaz S, Belgorodsky B, Fishman A, Bujanover Y, Gophna U. Effect of Maternal Diet and Milk Lipid Composition on the Infant Gut and Maternal Milk Microbiomes. *Nutrients.* 2020 Sep;12(9):2539.
22. Jeurink PV, Knipping K, Wiens F, Barańska K, Stahl B, Garssen J, Krolak-Olejnik B. Importance of maternal diet in the training of the infant's immune system during gestation and lactation. *Critical reviews in food science and nutrition.* 2019 Apr 28;59(8):1311-9.
23. Evans J, Le Grange D. Body size and parenting in eating disorders: a comparative study of the attitudes of mothers toward their children. *International Journal of Eating Disorder.* 1995;18:39–48.
24. Brown A, Rance J, Bennett P. Postnatal depression and breastfeeding: the role of specific physical difficulties and pain. *Journal of Advanced Nursing* (in press)
25. Sachs M, Dykes F, Carter B. Feeding by numbers: an ethnographic study of how breastfeeding women understand their babies' weight charts. *International Breastfeeding Journal.* 2006 1(1), 29.
26. Brown A.. Maternal trait personality and breastfeeding duration: the importance of confidence and social support. *Journal of Advanced Nursing.* 2014 70(3), 587-598.
27. O'Brien M, Buikstra E, Hegney D.The influence of psychological factors on breastfeeding duration. *Journal of Advanced Nursing.* 2008 63(4), 397-408.
28. Boone L, Soenens B, Braet C. Perfectionism, body dissatisfaction, and bulimic symptoms: The intervening role of perceived pressure to be thin and thin ideal internalization. *Journal of Social and Clinical Psychology.* 2011 30(10), 1043-1068.
29. Fredrickson BL, Roberts TA. Objectification theory. *Psychology of Women Quarterly.* 1997 Jun 1;21(2):173-206.
30. Roberts TA, Waters PL. Self-Objectification and That "Not So Fresh Feeling" Feminist Therapeutic Interventions for Healthy Female Embodiment. *Women & Therapy.* 2004 Mar 3;27(3-4):5-21.
31. Acker M. Breast is best… but not everywhere: ambivalent sexism and attitudes toward private and public breastfeeding. *Sex Roles.* 2009 Oct 1;61(7-8):476-90.

Chapter 13: Family and friends: when it's not you, it's them

1. Darwent KL, McInnes RJ, Swanson V. The Infant Feeding Genogram: a tool for exploring family infant feeding history and identifying support needs. *BMC pregnancy and childbirth.* 2016 Dec 1;16(1):315.
2. Thomson G, Ingram J, Clarke JL, Johnson D, Trickey H, Dombrowski SU, Hoddinott P, Darwent K, Jolly K. Exploring the use and experience of an infant feeding genogram to facilitate an assets-based approach to support infant feeding. *BMC Pregnancy and Childbirth.* 2020 Dec;20(1):1-2.
3. Ekström A, Widström AM, Nissen E. Breastfeeding support from partners and grandmothers: perceptions of Swedish women. *Birth.* 2003 Dec 1;30(4):261-6.
4. Grassley J, Eschiti V. Grandmother breastfeeding support: what do mothers need and want? *Birth.* 2008 Dec 1;35(4):329-35.
5. Hoddinott P, Pill R. Qualitative study of decisions about infant feeding among women in east end of London. *BMJ.* 1999 Jan 2;318(7175):30-4.
6. Grassley JS, Nelms TP. Understanding maternal breastfeeding confidence: A Gadamerian hermeneutic analysis of women's stories. *Health Care for Women International.* 2008 Sep 3;29(8-9):841-62.
7. Amir LH, Donath S. A systematic review of maternal obesity and breastfeeding intention, initiation and duration. *BMC Pregnancy and Childbirth.* 2007 Jul 4;7(1):1.
8. Grassley JS, Eschiti VS. Two Generations Learning Together: Facilitating Grandmothers' Support of Breastfeeding. *International Journal of Childbirth Education.* 2007 Sep 1;22(3).
9. Bentley M, Gavin L, Black MM, Teti L. Infant feeding practices of low-income, African-American, adolescent mothers: an ecological, multigenerational perspective. *Social Science & Medicine.* 1999 Oct 31;49(8):1085-100.
10. Bica OC, Giugliani ER. Influence of counseling sessions on the prevalence of breastfeeding in the first year of life: a randomized clinical trial with adolescent

mothers and grandmothers. *Birth.* 2014 Mar 1;41(1):39-45.

11. Pontes CM, Osório MM, Alexandrino AC. Building a place for the father as an ally for breast feeding. *Midwifery.* 2009 Apr 30;25(2):195-202.

12. Stapleton LR, Schetter CD, Westling E, Rini C, Glynn LM, Hobel CJ, Sandman CA. Perceived partner support in pregnancy predicts lower maternal and infant distress. *Journal of Family Psychology.* 2012 Jun;26(3):453.

13. Robertson E, Grace S, Wallington T, Stewart DE. Antenatal risk factors for postpartum depression: a synthesis of recent literature. *General Hospital Psychiatry.* 2004 Aug 31;26(4):289-95.

14. Mitchell-Box K, Braun KL. Fathers' thoughts on breastfeeding and implications for a theory-based intervention. *Journal of Obstetric, Gynecologic, & Neonatal Nursing.* 2012 Nov 1;41(6):E41-50.

15. Brown A, Lee M. An exploration of the attitudes and experiences of mothers in the United Kingdom who chose to breastfeed exclusively for 6 months postpartum. *Breastfeeding Medicine.* 2011 Aug 1;6(4):197-204.

16. Hauck Y, Hall WA, Jones C. Prevalence, self-efficacy and perceptions of conflicting advice and self-management: effects of a breastfeeding journal. *Journal of Advanced Nursing.* 2007 Feb 1;57(3):306-17.

17. Brown A, Davies R. Fathers' experiences of supporting breastfeeding: challenges for breastfeeding promotion and education. *Maternal & Child Nutrition.* 2014 Oct 1;10(4):510-26.

18. Avery AB, Magnus JH. Expectant fathers' and mothers' perceptions of breastfeeding and formula feeding: a focus group study in three US cities. *Journal of Human Lactation.* 2011 May 1;27(2):147-54.

19. Harner HM, McCarter-Spaulding D. Teenage mothers and breastfeeding: does paternal age make a difference? *Journal of Human Lactation.* 2004 Nov 1;20(4):404-8.

20. Finnbogadóttir H, Svalenius EC, Persson EK. Expectant first-time fathers' experiences of pregnancy. *Midwifery.* 2003 Jun 30;19(2):96-105.

21. Sherriff N, Hall V. Engaging and supporting fathers to promote breastfeeding: a new role for Health Visitors? *Scandinavian Journal of Caring Sciences.* 2011 Sep 1;25(3):467-75.

22. Tohotoa J, Maycock B, Hauck YL, Howat P, Burns S, Binns CW. Dads make a difference: an exploratory study of paternal support for breastfeeding in Perth, Western Australia. *International Breastfeeding Journal.* 2009 Nov 29;4(1):1.

23. Sherriff N, Panton C, Hall V. A new model of father support to promote breastfeeding. *Community Practice.* 2014 May 1;87(5):20-4.

24. Brown A, Davies R. Fathers' experiences of supporting breastfeeding: challenges for breastfeeding promotion and education. *Maternal & Child Nutrition.* 2014 Oct 1;10(4):510-26.

25. Coltrane S, Miller EC, DeHaan T, Stewart L. Fathers and the flexibility stigma. *Journal of Social Issues.* 2013 Jun 1;69(2):279-302.

26. Datta J, Graham B, Wellings K. The role of fathers in breastfeeding: Decision-making and support. *British Journal of Midwifery.* 2012 Mar 1;20(3).

27. Rempel LA, Rempel JK. The breastfeeding team: the role of involved fathers in the breastfeeding family. *Journal of Human Lactation.* 2011 May 1;27(2):115-21.

28. Maycock B, Binns CW, Dhaliwal S, Tohotoa J, Hauck Y, Burns S, Howat P. Education and support for fathers improves breastfeeding rates a randomized controlled trial. *Journal of Human Lactation.* 2013 Nov 1;29(4):484-90.

29. Pisacane A, Continisio GI, Aldinucci M, D'Amora S, Continisio P. A controlled trial of the father's role in breastfeeding promotion. *Pediatrics.* 2005 Oct 1;116(4):e494-8.

30. Susin LR, Giugliani ER. Inclusion of fathers in an intervention to promote breastfeeding: impact on breastfeeding rates. *Journal of Human Lactation.* 2008 Sep 10..

31. Schmied V, Myors K, Wills J, Cooke M. Preparing expectant couples for new-parent experiences: a comparison of two models of antenatal education. *The Journal of Perinatal Education.* 2002 Jul 1;11(3):20-7.

32. Henderson L, McMillan B, Green JM, Renfrew MJ. Men and infant feeding: Perceptions of embarrassment, sexuality, and social conduct in white low-income

British men. *Birth*. 2011 Mar 1;38(1):61-70.

33. Turan JM, Nalbant H, Bulut A, Sahip Y. Including expectant fathers in antenatal education programmes in Istanbul, Turkey. *Reproductive Health Matters*. 2001 Nov 30;9(18):114-25.

34. Buist A, Morse CA, Durkin S. Men's adjustment to fatherhood: implications for obstetric health care. *Journal of Obstetric*, Gynecologic, & Neonatal Nursing. 2003 Mar 1;32(2):172-80.

35. Longworth HL, Kingdon CK. Fathers in the birth room: what are they expecting and experiencing? A phenomenological study. *Midwifery*. 2011 Oct 31;27(5):588-94.

36. May C, Fletcher R. Preparing fathers for the transition to parenthood: Recommendations for the content of antenatal education. *Midwifery*. 2013 May 31;29(5):474-8.

37. Emmott EH, Mace R. Practical support from fathers and grandmothers is associated with lower levels of breastfeeding in the UK Millennium Cohort Study. *PloS One*. 2015 Jul 20;10(7):e0133547.

38. Hammond C. Exploring same sex couples' experiences of maternity care. *British Journal of Midwifery*. 2014 Jul 2;22(7):495-500.

39. Wells MB, Lang SN. Supporting same-sex mothers in the Nordic child health field: A systematic literature review and meta-synthesis of the most gender equal countries. *Journal of clinical nursing*. 2016 Dec;25(23-24):3469-83.

40. abm.me.uk/breastfeeding-information/tips-for-supporting-lgbtq-families/

41. Juntereal NA, Spatz DL. Same-sex mothers and lactation. *MCN: The American Journal of Maternal/Child Nursing*. 2019 May 1;44(3):164-9.

Chapter 14: We *still* have ridiculous attitudes to breastfeeding in public spaces

1. www.channel4.com/programmes/dispatches
2. www.unicef.org.uk/babyfriendly/still-talking-about-a-womans-right-to-breastfeed-in-public/
3. Brown A, Shenker N. Experiences of breastfeeding during COVID-19: Lessons for future practical and emotional support. *Maternal & child nutrition*. 2020 Sep 23:e13088.
4. www.gov.uk/government/publications/equality-strategy
5. www.legislation.gov.uk/asp/2005/1/contents
6. yougov.co.uk/news/2014/12/08/public-breastfeeding-scotlands-drink-drive-limit-p
7. CDC (2013) HealthStyles Survey — Public Beliefs and Attitudes About Breastfeeding: 2013 www.cdc.gov/breastfeeding/data/healthstyles_survey/survey_2013.htm
8. Lansinoh global breastfeeding survey www.lansinoh.com/uploads/files/articles/US_Survey_Press_Release_-_FINAL.pdf
9. Li R, Hsia J, Fridinger F, Hussain A, Benton-Davis S, Grummer-Strawn L. (2004). Public beliefs about breastfeeding policies in various settings. *Journal of the American Dietetic Association*, 104, 1162–1168
10. Meng X, Daly,A, Pollard C, Binns C. (2013). Community Attitudes toward Breastfeeding in Public Places among Western Australia Adults, 1995-2009 *Journal of Human Lactation*, 29 (2), 183-189 DOI: 10.1177/0890334413478835
11. Scott JA, Kwok YY, Synnott K, Bogue J, Amarri S, Norin E. Edwards CA. (2014). A Comparison of Maternal Attitudes to Breastfeeding in Public and the Association with Breastfeeding Duration in Four European Countries: Results of a Cohort Study. *Birth*.
12. McIntyre E, Hiller JE, Turnbull D. (2001). Community attitudes to infant feeding. *Breastfeeding Review*, 9(3), 27–33.
13. cdn.yougov.com/cumulus_uploads/document/flpxe9qagv/YG-Archive-breastfeeding-results-310713.pdf
14. Spurles PK, Babineau J. (2011). A qualitative study of attitudes toward public breastfeeding among young Canadian men and women. *Journal of Human Lactation*, 27(2), 131-137.
15. Vaaler ML, Castrucci BC, Parks SE, Clark J, Stagg J, Erickson T. (2011). Men's attitudes toward breastfeeding: findings from the 2007 Texas Behavioral Risk Factor Surveillance System. *Maternal and Child Health Journal*, 15(2), 148-157.

16. Kavanagh KF, Lou Z, Nicklas JC, Habibi MF, Murphy LT. (2012). Breastfeeding knowledge, attitudes, prior exposure, and intent among undergraduate students. *Journal of Human Lactation*, 28(4), 556-564.
17. Acker M. (2009) Breast is best… but not everywhere: ambivalent sexism and attitudes towards private and public breastfeeding. *Sex Roles*, 61, 476 – 490.
18. Spear HJ. Baccalaureate nursing students' breast-feeding knowledge: A descriptive survey. *Nurse Education Today* 2006;26:332–337
19. today.yougov.com/topics/politics/articles-reports/2014/09/17/poll-results-punishment
20. yougov.co.uk/topics/politics/articles-reports/2013/08/19/no-breastfeeding-swimming-pool
21. www.dailymail.co.uk/femail/article-2172493/Why-This-Mornings-penis-enlargement-feature-brought-tear-eyes-right-reasons.html
22. Grant A. "I… don't want to see you flashing your bits around": exhibitionism, othering and good motherhood in perceptions of public breastfeeding. *Geoforum*. 2016 May 1;71:52-61.
23. NCT (2009) nctwatch.wordpress.com/2009/07/24/mother-and-baby-survey-reveals-mothers-worries-about-breastfeeding-in-public/#_msocom_1
24. Unity Law Breastfeeding Cultural Attitudes Survey 2014 www.unity-law.co.uk/news.htm?id=2166
25. Johnston-Robledo I, Wares S, Fricker J, Pasek L. (2007). Indecent exposure: Self-objectification and young women's attitudes toward breastfeeding. *Sex Roles*, 56(7-8), 429-437.
26. Thomson G, Dykes F. (2011). Women's sense of coherence related to their infant feeding experiences. *Maternal & Child Nutrition*, 7(2), 160-174.
27. metro.co.uk/2020/08/02/one-sixth-mums-say-unwanted-sexual-attention-breastfeeding-public-13071528/
28. www.dailymail.co.uk/news/article-9317469/Facebook-BLOCKS-baby-bottle-company-Tommee-Tippees-new-breastfeeding-advert-showing-nudity.html
29. McAndrew F, Thompson J, Fellows L, Large A, Speed M, Renfrew MJ. (2012). *Infant feeding survey 2010*. Leeds: Health and Social Care Information Centre.
30. Hoddinott P, Craig LC, Britten J, McInnes RM. (2012). A serial qualitative interview study of infant feeding experiences: idealism meets realism. *BMJ Open*, 2(2).
31. Daly SE, Hartmann PE. (1995). Infant demand and milk supply. Part 1: Infant demand and milk production in lactating women. *Journal of Human Lactation*, 11(1), 21-26.
32. Ortiz J, McGilligan K, Kelly P. (2004). Duration of breastmilk expression among working mothers enrolled in an employer-sponsored lactation program. *Pediatric nursing*, 30(2), 111-119.
33. Neifert M, Lawrence RA, Seacat J. Nipple confusion: toward a formal definition. *Journal of Pediatrics*. 1995;126:S125–S129

Chapter 15: A lack of protection for breastfeeding women on return to work

1. Haider SJ, Jacknowitz A, Schoeni RF. Welfare work requirements and child well-being: Evidence from the effects on breast-feeding. *Demography*. 2003 Aug 1;40(3):479-97.
2. Renfrew MJ, Pokhrel S, Quigley M, McCormick F, Fox-Rushby J, Dodds R, Duffy S, Trueman P, Williams A. Preventing disease and saving resources: the potential contribution of increasing breastfeeding rates in the UK. UNICEF; 2012.
3. Kosmala-Anderson J, Wallace LM. Breastfeeding works: the role of employers in supporting women who wish to breastfeed and work in four organizations in England. *Journal of Public Health*. 2006 Sep 1;28(3):183-91
4. Weber D, Janson A, Nolan M, Wen LM, Rissel C. Female employees' perceptions of organisational support for breastfeeding at work: findings from an Australian health service workplace. International Breastfeeding Journal. 2011 Nov 30;6(1):1.
5. Chatterji P, Frick KD. Does returning to work after childbirth affect breastfeeding practices? Review of Economics of the Household. 2005 Sep 1;3(3):315-35.
6. Mirkovic KR, Perrine CG, Scanlon KS. Paid maternity leave and breastfeeding outcomes. *Birth*. 2016 Mar 1.
7. Hausman B. The feminist politics of breastfeeding. Australian Feminist Studies. 2004

Nov 1;19(45):273-85.

8. McGovern P, Dowd B, Gjerdingen D, Moscovice I, Kochevar L, Lohman W. Time off work and the postpartum health of employed women. *Medical Care*. 1997 May 1;35(5):507-21.

9. Burns E, Triandafilidis Z. Taking the path of least resistance: a qualitative analysis of return to work or study while breastfeeding. International breastfeeding journal. 2019 Dec 1;14(1):15.

10. maternityaction.org.uk/advice/continuing-to-breastfeed-when-you-return-to-work/

11. archive.acas.org.uk/media/3924/Accommodating-breastfeeding-employees-in-the-workplace/pdf/Acas-guide-on-accommodating-breastfeeding-in-the-workplace.pdf

12. Ball TM, Wright AL. Health care costs of formula-feeding in the first year of life. Pediatrics. 1999 Apr 1;103(Supplement 1):870-6.

13. Chapman DJ, Pérez-Escamilla R. US national breastfeeding monitoring and surveillance: current status and recommendations. *Journal of Human Lactation*. 2009 Mar 13.

14. Dunn BF, Zavela KJ, Cline AD, Cost PA. Breastfeeding practices in Colorado businesses. *Journal of Human Lactation*. 2004 May 1;20(2):170-7.

15. Libbus MK, Bullock LF. Breastfeeding and employment: an assessment of employer attitudes. *J Hum Lact*. 2002 Aug;18(3): 247-51

16. Witters-Green R. Increasing breastfeeding rates in working mothers. *Families, Systems, & Health*. 2003;21(4):415.

17. Puwar N. Space invaders: Race, gender and bodies out of place. Berg; 2004..

18. Shildrick M. *Leaky bodies and boundaries: Feminism, postmodernism and (bio) ethics*. Routledge; 2015 Dec 22.

19. Martin E. *The woman in the body: A cultural analysis of reproduction*. Beacon Press; 2001.

20. Gatrell CJ. Secrets and lies: breastfeeding and professional paid work. *Social Science & Medicine*. 2007 Jul 31;65(2):393-404.

21. uwe-repository.worktribe.com/output/803514

22. Weber D, Janson A, Nolan M, Wen LM, Rissel C. Female employees' perceptions of organisational support for breastfeeding at work: findings from an Australian health service workplace. *International Breastfeeding Journal*. 2011 Nov 30;6(1):1.

23. Cohen R, Mrtek MB, Mrtek RG. Comparison of maternal absenteeism and infant illness rates among breast-feeding and formula-feeding women in two corporations. *American Journal of Health Promotion*. 1995 Nov 1;10(2):148-53.

24. Cohen R, Mrtek MB. The impact of two corporate lactation programs on the incidence and duration of breast-feeding by employed mothers. *American Journal of Health Promotion*. 1994 Jul;8(6):436-41.

25. kenyalaw.org/kl/fileadmin/pdfdownloads/bills/2017/BreastfeedingMothersBill_2017.pdf

Chapter 16: Industry influences are allowed to spread inaccurate messaging

1. www.hexaresearch.com/research-report/infant-formula-market#utm_source=referral&utm_medium=prnewswire.com&utm_campaign=prn_infantformula_18Mar_rd2

2. www.savethechildren.org.uk/content/dam/gb/reports/health/dont-push-it.pdf

3. www.dairyreporter.com/Article/2020/05/11/New-market-potential-Huge-growth-opportunities-for-infant-formula-in-China-s-lower-tier-cities

4. Piwoz EG, Huffman SL. The impact of marketing of breast-milk substitutes on WHO-recommended breastfeeding practices. *Food and nutrition bulletin*. 2015 Aug 27:0379572115602174.

5. Allain A, Kean YJ. The youngest market: baby food peddlers undermine breastfeeding. *Multinational Monitor*. 2008 Jul 1;29(1):17.

6. www.who.int/nutrition/publications/code_english.pdf

7. www.gov.uk/government/uploads/system/uploads/attachment_data/file/204314/Infant_formula_guidance_2013_-_final_6_March.pdf

8. www.who.int/publications/i/item/9789240006010

9. Kean YJ. Commentary: Stewart Forsyth's article-Non-compliance with the International Code of Marketing of Breastmilk Substitutes is not confined to the infant formula industry. *Journal of Public Health.* 2013 Jun 1;35(2):193-4.

10. Salasibew M, Kiani A, Faragher B, Garner P. Awareness and reported violations of the WHO International Code and Pakistan's national breastfeeding legislation; a descriptive cross-sectional survey. *International breastfeeding journal.* 2008 Oct 17;3(1):1.

11. Sobel HL, Iellamo A, Raya RR, Padilla AA, Olivé JM, Nyunt-U S. Is unimpeded marketing for breastmilk substitutes responsible for the decline in breastfeeding in the Philippines? An exploratory survey and focus group analysis. *Social Science & Medicine.* 2011 Nov 30;73(10):1445-8.

12. Merewood A, Grossman X, Cook J, Sadacharan R, Singleton M, Peters K, Navidi T. US hospitals violate WHO policy on the distribution of formula sample packs: results of a national survey. *Journal of Human Lactation.* 2010 Nov 1;26(4):363-7.

13. Sadacharan R, Grossman X, Matlak S, Merewood A. Hospital discharge bags and breastfeeding at 6 months: data from the Infant Feeding Practices Study II. *Journal of Human Lactation.* 2013 Dec 4:0890334413513653.

14. Fein SB, Labiner-Wolfe J, Shealy KR, Li R, Chen J, Grummer-Strawn LM. Infant feeding practices study II: study methods. *Pediatrics.* 2008 Oct 1;122(Supplement 2):S28-35.

15. www.babymilkaction.org/archives/704

16. Stang J, Hoss K, Story M. Health Statements Made in Infant Formula Advertisements in Pregnancy and Early Parenting Magazines: A Content Analysis. *ICAN: Infant, Child, & Adolescent Nutrition.* 2010;2(1):16-25.

17. Berry NJ, Gribble KD. Health and nutrition content claims on websites advertising infant formula available in Australia: A content analysis. *Maternal & child nutrition.* 2017;13(4):e12383.

18. Smith J, Blake M. Infant food marketing strategies undermine effective regulation of breast-milk substitutes: trends in print advertising in Australia, 1950–2010. *Australian and New Zealand Journal of Public Health.* 2013 Aug 1;37(4):337-44.

19. Park CW, Milberg S, Lawson R. Evaluation of brand extensions: the role of product feature similarity and brand concept consistency. *Journal of consumer research.* 1991 Sep 1;18(2):185-93.

20. Kardes F. *Consumer behavior and managerial decision making.* 2002. Prentice Hall, New Jersey

21. Berry NJ, Jones SC, Iverson D. Toddler milk advertising in Australia: Infant formula advertising in disguise? *Australasian Marketing Journal (AMJ).* 2012;20(1):24-7.

22. Cattaneo A, Pani P, Carletti C, Guidetti M, Mutti V, Guidetti C. Follow-on Formula Research Group. Advertisements of follow-on formula and their perception by pregnant women and mothers in Italy. *Archives of disease in childhood.* 2015;100(4):323-8.

23. Brown, A., Jones. S. & Evans, E. (2020) *Marketing of infant milk in the UK: what do parents see and believe?* A report for First Steps Nutrition Trust: London

24. Suleiman A. A study of marketing and its effect on infant feeding practices. *The Medical journal of Malaysia.* 2001 Sep;56(3):319-23.

25. Stang J, Hoss K, Story M. Health Statements Made in Infant Formula Advertisements in Pregnancy and Early Parenting Magazines: A Content Analysis. *ICAN: Infant, Child, & Adolescent Nutrition.* 2010;2(1):16-25.

26. Berry NJ, Gribble KD. Health and nutrition content claims on websites advertising infant formula available in Australia: A content analysis. *Maternal & child nutrition.* 2017;13(4):e12383.

27. Belamarich PF, Bochner, RE, Racine AD. A critical review of the marketing claims of infant formula products in the United States. Clinical Pediatrics. 2016;55(5):437-42.

28. Yilmaz B, Li H. Gut microbiota and iron: the crucial actors in health and disease. *Pharmaceuticals.* 2018 Dec;11(4):98.

29. www.nutraingredients.com/Article/2020/05/07/Experts-call-for-ban-on-infant-formula-marketing-claims

30. EFSA. Scientific Opinion on the substantiation of a health claim related

Immunofortis® and strengthening of the baby's immune system pursuant to Article 14 of Regulation (EC) No 1924/2006. *EFSA Journal.* 2010;8(2)

31. Munblit D, Crawley H, Hyde R, Bole RJ. Health and nutritional claims for infant formula are poorly substantiated and potentially harmful. *BMJ.* 2020;369.

32. Berry NJ. Got milk?: the influence of toddler formula advertising on attitudes and beliefs about infant feeding : University of Wollongong Thesis Collection; 2010.

33. Moossavi S, Miliku K, Sepehri S, Khafipour E, Azad MB. The Prebiotic and Probiotic Properties of Human Milk: Implications for Infant Immune Development and Pediatric Asthma. *Frontiers in Pediatrics.* 2018;6.

34. www.babymilkaction.org/archives/20974

35. Romo-Palafox MJ, Pomeranz JL, Harris JL. Infant formula and toddler milk marketing and caregiver's provision to young children. *Maternal & Child Nutrition.* 2020;16(3):e12962.

36. infantmilkinfo.org/costs/

37. www.channel4.com/press/news/channel-4-dispatches-asks-if-ps40billion-infant-formula-industry-putting-profit-babies

38. Brown A, Shenker N. Experiences of breastfeeding during COVID-19: Lessons for future practical and emotional support. *Maternal & child nutrition.* 2020 Sep 23:e13088.

39. van Tulleken C, Wright C, Brown A, McCoy D, Costello A. Marketing of breastmilk substitutes during the COVID-19 pandemic. *Lancet.* 2020 Oct 8.

40. Hastings G, Angus K, Eadie D, Hunt K. Selling second best: how infant formula marketing works. Globalization and Health. 2020 Dec;16(1):1-2.

41. www.theguardian.com/commentisfree/2007/may/30/comment. internationalaidanddevelopment

42. Gribble K, Fernandes C. Considerations regarding the use of infant formula products in infant and young child feeding in emergencies (IYCF-E) programs. *World Nutrition.* 2018 Dec 29;9(3):261-83.

43. www.unicef.org.uk/babyfriendly/wp-content/uploads/sites/2/2019/05/Provision-of-formula-milk-at-food-banks-Unicef-UK-Baby-Friendly-Initiative.pdf

44. Grummer-Strawn LM, Holliday F, Jungo KT, Rollins N. Sponsorship of national and regional professional paediatrics associations by companies that make breast-milk substitutes: evidence from a review of official websites. *BMJ open.* 2019 Aug 1;9(8):e029035.

45. Save the Children. *Breastfeeding and the IGBM code violations survey.* London: Save the Children; 2013

46. Harney A. Special report: How Big Formula bought China. *Reuters Business and Financial News.* 2013 Nov;7.

47. unicef.org.uk/Documents/Baby_Friendly/Statements/formula_sponsored_study_days.pdf

48. Godlee F. No more infant formula advertising in The BMJ 2019;364:l1279

49. www.rcpch.ac.uk/news-events/news/rcpch-statement-relationship-formula-milk-companies

50. PrescQIPP. Appropriate prescribing of specialist infant formulae (foods for special medical purposes). 2016. www.prescqipp.info/media/1346/b146-infant-feeds-21.pdf

51. NHS Digital. Prescription cost analysis— England, 2017. digital.nhs.uk/data-and-information/publications/statistical/prescription-cost-analysis/prescription-cost-analysis-england-2017

52. Venter C, Patil V, Grundy J, etal . Prevalence and cumulative incidence of food hyper-sensitivity in the first 10 years of life. Pediatr Allergy Immunol 2016;27:452-8.

53. van Tulleken C. Overdiagnosis and industry influence: how cow's milk protein allergy is extending the reach of infant formula manufacturers. *BMJ.* 2018 Dec 5;363.

54. www.firststepsnutrition.org/making-infant-milk-safely

55. www.ofcom.org.uk/__data/assets/pdf_file/0017/129050/Issue-367-of-Ofcoms-Broadcast-and-On-Demand-Bulletin.pdf

56. www.irishexaminer.com/news/arid-30927503.html

57. Koletzko B, Bhutta ZA, Cai W, Cruchet S, Guindi ME, Fuchs GJ, et al. Compositional requirements of follow-up formula for use in infancy: Recommendations of an

international expert group coordinated by the Early Nutrition Academy. *Ann Nutr Metab.* 2013;62(1):44-54.

58. www.dailymail.co.uk/news/article-8927847/Formula-milk-firms-bombarded-parents-social-media-coronavirus-lockdown.html
59. www.dailymail.co.uk/news/article-9317469/Facebook-BLOCKS-baby-bottle-company-Tommee-Tippees-new-breastfeeding-advert-showing-nudity.html
60. www.aptaclub.co.uk/baby/diet-and-nutrition/breastfeeding/alcohol-and-breastfeeding.html
61. WHO Collaborative Study Team. Effect of breastfeeding on infant and child mortality due to infectious diseases in less developed countries. *The Lancet.* 2000 Feb 5;355(9202):451-5.
62. Palmer G. *The politics of breastfeeding: When breasts are bad for business.* Pinter & Martin Publishers; 2009.
63. Donnelly A, Snowden HM, Renfrew MJ, Woolridge MW. Commercial hospital discharge packs for breastfeeding women. The Cochrane Library. 2000.
64. Feldman-Winter L, Grossman X, Palaniappan A, Kadokura E, Hunter K, Milcarek B, Merewood A. Removal of industry-sponsored formula sample packs from the hospital: does it make a difference? *Journal of Human Lactation.* 2012 Aug 1;28(3):380-8.
65. Rosenberg KD, Eastham CA, Kasehagen LJ, Sandoval AP. Marketing infant formula through hospitals: the impact of commercial hospital discharge packs on breastfeeding. *American Journal of Public Health.* 2008 Feb;98(2):290-5.
66. www.alisonthewliss.scot/bill-published-to-crack-down-on-formula-milk-promotion/
67. Carignan, C. C., Karagas, M. R., Punshon, T., Gilbert-Diamond, D., & Cottingham, K. L. (2016). Contribution of breastmilk and formula to arsenic exposure during the first year of life in a US prospective cohort. *Journal of exposure science & environmental epidemiology, 26*(5), 452-457.
68. www.theguardian.com/lifeandstyle/2020/nov/14/i-want-to-give-my-child-the-best-the-race-to-grow-human-breast-milk-in-a-lab
69. Ahmed AH, Roumani AM, Szucs K, Zhang L, King D. The effect of interactive web-based monitoring on breastfeeding exclusivity, intensity, and duration in healthy, term infants after hospital discharge. *Journal of Obstetric, Gynecologic & Neonatal Nursing.* 2016 Apr 30;45(2):143-54.
70. Giglia R, Cox K, Zhao Y, Binns CW. Exclusive breastfeeding increased by an internet intervention. *Breastfeeding Medicine.* 2015 Feb 1;10(1):20-5.

Chapter 17: How has the COVID-19 pandemic affected all of this?

1. Babies in Lockdown: listening to parents to build back better (2020). Best Beginnings, Home-Start UK, and the Parent-Infant Foundation UK.
2. Brown, A., & Shenker, N. (2021). Experiences of breastfeeding during COVID-19: Lessons for future practical and emotional support. *Maternal & child nutrition, 17*(1), e13088.
3. Vazquez-Vazquez, A., Dib, S., Rougeaux, E., Wells, J. C., & Fewtrell, M. S. (2021). The impact of the Covid-19 lockdown on the experiences and feeding practices of new mothers in the UK: Preliminary data from the COVID-19 New Mum Study. *Appetite, 156,* 104985.
4. Mollard, E., & Wittmaack, A. (2021). Experiences of Women Who Gave Birth in US Hospitals During the COVID-19 Pandemic. *Journal of Patient Experience, 8,* 2374373520981492.
5. www.unicef.org/rosa/stories/misinformation-and-formula-milk-donations-are-threatening-breastfeeding-during-covid-19
6. Chen, H., Guo, J., Wang, C., Luo, F., Yu, X., Zhang, W., ... & Zhang, Y. (2020). Clinical characteristics and intrauterine vertical transmission potential of COVID-19 infection in nine pregnant women: a retrospective review of medical records. *The lancet, 395*(10226), 809-815.
7. www.cdc.gov/breastfeeding/breastfeeding-special-circumstances/maternal-or-infant-illnesses/covid-19-and-breastfeeding.html

8. Smith, H. A. (2020). Impact of COVID-19 on neonatal health: are we causing more harm than good. *Eur J Midwifery, 4*(9).

9. Lowe, B., & Bopp, B. (2020). COVID-19 vaginal delivery–a case report. *Australian and New Zealand Journal of Obstetrics and Gynaecology, 60*(3), 465-466.

10. Goldman AS. The immune system of human milk: antimicrobial, antiinflammatory and immunomodulating properties. Pediatr Infect Dis J 1993 Aug;12(8):664-71.

11. Robertson, C. A., Lowther, S. A., Birch, T., Tan, C., Sorhage, F., Stockman, L., ... & Bresnitz, E. (2004). SARS and pregnancy: a case report. *Emerging infectious diseases, 10*(2), 345.

12. Kimberlin, D. W., & Puopolo, K. M. (2021). Breast Milk and COVID-19: What Do We Know. Clinical Infectious Diseases, 72, 131–132

13. Centers for Disease Control and Prevention. Severe outcomes among patients with coronavirus disease 2019 (COVID-19)—United States, February 12–March 16, 2020. *MMWR Morb Mortal Wkly Rep*

14. Bartick, M. (2020) COVID-19: Separating infected mothers from newborns: Weighing the risks and benefits. trends.hms.harvard.edu/2020/03/31/covid-19-separating-infected-mothers-from-newborns-weighing-the-risks-and-benefits/

15. AAP. (2020) AAP updates guidance on newborns whose mothers have suspected or confirmed COVID-19 www.aappublications.org/news/2020/05/21/covid19newborn052120

16. Tomori, C., Gribble, K., Palmquist, A. E., Ververs, M. T., & Gross, M. S. (2020). When separation is not the answer: Breastfeeding mothers and infants affected by COVID-19. *Maternal & Child Nutrition, 16*(4), e13033.

17. Renfrew, M. J., Cheyne, H., Craig, J., Duff, E., Dykes, F., Hunter, B., … Downe, S. (2020). Sustaining quality midwifery care in a pandemic and beyond. *Midwifery*, **88**, 102759.

18. Victora, C. G., Bahl, R., Barros, A. J., França, G. V., Horton, S., Krasevec, J., … Group, T. L. B. S. (2016). Breastfeeding in the 21st century: Epidemiology, mechanisms, and lifelong effect. *The Lancet, 387*(10017), 475– 490

19. Kendall-Tackett, K. (2007). A new paradigm for depression in new mothers: The central role of inflammation and how breastfeeding and anti-inflammatory treatments protect maternal mental health. *International Breastfeeding Journal, 2*(1), 1– 14.

20. Brown, A. (2018). What do women lose if they are prevented from meeting their breastfeeding goals? *Clinical Lactation, 9*(4), 200– 207.

21. Hare, H., & Womersley, K. (2021). Why were breastfeeding women in the UK denied the covid-19 vaccine?. *BMJ, 372*.

22. www.theguardian.com/world/2020/dec/20/breastfeeding-mothers-will-not-be-offered-covid-vaccine-say-regulators

23. Kroger, A. T. (2013). General recommendations on immunization. General Recommendations Work Group CDC.

24. assets.publishing.service.gov.uk/government/uploads/system/uploads/attachment_data/file/965177/COVID-19_vaccination_programme_guidance_for_healthcare_workers_26_February_2021_v3.4.pdf

25. www.bfmed.org/abm-statement-considerations-for-covid-19-vaccination-in-lactation?fbclid=IwAR1qG7rS66IyTDyDlxGIOrwQsoSqDRuXWMWnjgBXwhOJuSofk13veeT3jl8

26. www.infantrisk.com/covid-19-vaccine-pregnancy-and-breastfeeding?fbclid=IwAR030ND0pMXbF76x1zjCzj22HCrGGIUCirCFZ-ijHBFUBOeAECkVJQpMds0

27. Karavadra, B., Stockl, A., Prosser-Snelling, E., Simpson, P., & Morris, E. (2020). Women's perceptions of COVID-19 and their healthcare experiences: a qualitative thematic analysis of a national survey of pregnant women in the United Kingdom. *BMC Pregnancy and Childbirth, 20*(1), 1-8.

28. Ravaldi, C., Wilson, A., Ricca, V., Homer, C., & Vannacci, A. (2020). Pregnant women voice their concerns and birth expectations during the COVID-19 pandemic in Italy. *Women and Birth 69*, 343 - 346

29. www.nhs.uk/conditions/coronavirus-covid-19/people-at-higher-risk/pregnancy-and-coronavirus/

30. www.birthrights.org.uk/wp-content/uploads/2020/03/Final-Covid-19-

Birthrights-31.3.20.pdf
31. Mollard, E., & Wittmaack, A. (2021). Experiences of Women Who Gave Birth in US Hospitals During the COVID-19 Pandemic. *Journal of Patient Experience, 8*, 2374373520981492.
32. www.nature.com/articles/d41586-020-02618-5
33. Been, J. V., Ochoa, L. B., Bertens, L. C., Schoenmakers, S., Steegers, E. A., & Reiss, I. K. (2020). Impact of COVID-19 mitigation measures on the incidence of preterm birth: a national quasi-experimental study. *The Lancet Public Health, 5*(11), e604-e611.
34. Martenot, A., Labbassi, I., Delfils-Stern, A., Monroy, O., Langlet, C., Pichault-Klein, V., ... & Kuhn, P. (2020). Favorable outcomes among neonates not separated from their symptomatic SARS-CoV-2-infected mothers. *Pediatric research*, 1-4.
35. Bartick, M. C., Valdés, V., Giusti, A., Chapin, E. M., Bhana, N. B., Hernández-Aguilar, M. T., ... & Feldman-Winter, L. (2021). Maternal and Infant Outcomes Associated with Maternity Practices Related to COVID-19: The COVID Mothers Study. *Breastfeeding Medicine*.
36. McFadden, A., Gavine, A., Renfrew, M. J., Wade, A., Buchanan, P., Taylor, J. L., ... & MacGillivray, S. (2017). Support for healthy breastfeeding mothers with healthy term babies. *Cochrane Database of Systematic Reviews*, (2).
37. www.dailymail.co.uk/news/article-8927847/Formula-milk-firms-bombarded-parents-social-media-coronavirus-lockdown.html
38. van Tulleken, C., Wright, C., Brown, A., McCoy, D., & Costello, A. (2020). Marketing of breastmilk substitutes during the COVID-19 pandemic. *The Lancet*, 396(10259), e58.
39. Davenport, M. H., Meyer, S., Meah, V. L., Strynadka, M. C., & Khurana, R. (2020). Moms are not ok: COVID-19 and maternal mental health. *Frontiers in Global Women's Health*, 1, 1.
40. Dib, S., Rougeaux, E., Vázquez-Vázquez, A., Wells, J. C., & Fewtrell, M. (2020). The impact of the COVID-19 lockdown on maternal mental health and coping in the UK: Data from the COVID-19 New Mum Study. medRxiv.
41. Fallon, V., Davies, S. M., Silverio, S. A., Jackson, L., De Pascalis, L., & Harrold, J. A. (2021). Psychosocial experiences of postnatal women during the COVID-19 pandemic. A UK-wide study of prevalence rates and risk factors for clinically relevant depression and anxiety. *Journal of Psychiatric Research*.
42. Adisa, T. A., Aiyenitaju, O., & Adekoya, O. D. (2021). The work–family balance of British working women during the COVID-19 pandemic. *Journal of Work-Applied Management*.
43. Collins, C., Landivar, L. C., Ruppanner, L., & Scarborough, W. J. (2021). COVID-19 and the gender gap in work hours. Gender, Work & Organization, 28, 101-112.
44. babiesinlockdown.info/a-call-to-action/

Chapter 18: How can we move forward and protect mothers and babies?

1. Brown A. What do women really want? Lessons for breastfeeding promotion and education. *Breastfeeding medicine*. 2016 Apr 1;11(3):102-10.
2. Wiessinger D. Watch your language. *Journal of Human Lactation*. 1996 Mar 1;12(1):1-4.
3. McNiel ME, Labbok MH, Abrahams SW. What are the risks associated with formula feeding? A re-analysis and review. *Birth*. 2010 Mar 1;37(1):50-8.
4. Hannan A, Li R, Benton-Davis S, Grummer-Strawn L. Regional variation in public opinion about breastfeeding in the United States. *Journal of Human Lactation*. 2005 Aug 1;21(3):284-8.
5. Quigley MA, Kelly YJ, Sacker A. Breastfeeding and hospitalization for diarrheal and respiratory infection in the United Kingdom Millennium Cohort Study. *Pediatrics*. 2007 Apr 1;119(4):e837-42.
6. Sheehan A. Complex decisions: deconstructing best a grounded theory study of infant feeding decisions in the first six weeks post-birth (Doctoral dissertation

Chapter 19: How do we handle supporting *all* families?

1. Brown A. *Why breastfeeding grief and trauma matter*. Pinter & Martin. 2019.

2. Brown A. What do women lose if they are prevented from meeting their breastfeeding goals?. *Clinical Lactation*. 2018 Nov 1;9(4):200-7.

Chapter 20: So, what can we actually do about this? What can I do?

1. Brown A. Breastfeeding as a public health responsibility: a review of the evidence. *Journal of Human Nutrition and Dietetics*. 2017 Dec;30(6):759-70.
2. publichealth.yale.edu/bfci/
3. www.gov.scot/publications/becoming-breastfeeding-friendly-scotland-report/pages/14/
4. ukbreastfeeding.org/wbtiuk2016/
5. gov.wales/sites/default/files/publications/2019-06/all-wales-breastfeeding-five-year-action-plan-july-2019_0.pdf
6. McFadden, A., Gavine, A., Renfrew, M. J., Wade, A., Buchanan, P., Taylor, J. L., ... & MacGillivray, S. (2017). Support for healthy breastfeeding mothers with healthy term babies. *Cochrane Database of Systematic Reviews*, (2).
7. Pérez-Escamilla R. & Chapman D.J. (2012) Breastfeeding pro- tection, promotion, and support in the United States: a time to nudge, a time to measure. *J Hum Lact* 28 (2), 118–121.
8. Ip, S., Chung, M., Raman, G., Trikalinos, T. A., & Lau, J. (2009). A summary of the Agency for Healthcare Research and Quality's evidence report on breastfeeding in developed countries. *Breastfeeding medicine*, 4(S1), S-17.
9. Azad, M. B., Nickel, N. C., Bode, L., Brockway, M., Brown, A., Chambers, C., ... & Zuccolo, L. (2020). Breastfeeding and the origins of health: Interdisciplinary perspectives and priorities. *Maternal & child nutrition*, e13109.
10. Hanson, M. A., & Gluckman, P. D. (2015). Developmental origins of health and disease–global public health implications. *Best practice & research Clinical obstetrics & gynaecology*, 29(1), 24-31.
11. www.gov.uk/government/publications/childhood-obesity-a-plan-for-action-chapter-2
12. www.dewis.wales/ResourceDirectory/ViewResource.aspx?id=11159
13. Rollins, N. C., Bhandari, N., Hajeebhoy, N., Horton, S., Lutter, C. K., Martines, J. C., ... & Group, T. L. B. S. (2016). Why invest, and what it will take to improve breastfeeding practices? *TLancet*, 387(10017), 491-504.
14. Nguyen P.H., Kim S.S., Keithly S.C., Hajeebhoy N., Tran L.M., Ruel M.T. et al. (2014) Incorporating elements of social fran- chising in government health services improves the quality of infant and young child feeding counselling services at commune health centres in Vietnam. *Health Policy and Planning* 29 (8), 1008–1020.

INDEX